The
Power of Sound

Other Books and CDs by Joshua Leeds

BOOKS

Sonic Alchemy: Conversations with Leading Sound Practitioners

CDs

1986	*Songs of Affirmation* (with Louise L. Hay)
1987	*Gift of the Present* (with Louise L. Hay)
1989	*Rhapsody*
1991	*Safe Passage* (with Louise L. Hay)
1996	*Masterworks for Relaxation*
1997	*Eight Meditations for Optimum Health* (with Andrew Weil, M.D.)
1997	*Sound Health/Concentration*
1997	*Sound Health/Learning*
1997	*A Baroque Garden*
1998	*Sound Body, Sound Mind: Music for Healing* (with Andrew Weil, M.D.)
1998	*Sound Health/De-Stress*
1998	*Sound Health/Thinking*
1999	*Sound Health/Relax*
1999	*Sound Health/Productivity*
1999	*The Listening Program* (8-CD set)

The Power of Sound

How to Manage Your Personal Soundscape for a Vital, Productive, and Healthy Life

JOSHUA LEEDS

Healing Arts Press
Rochester, Vermont

Healing Arts Press
One Park Street
Rochester, Vermont 05767
www.InnerTraditions.com

Healing Arts Press is a division of Inner Traditions International

Note to the reader: This book is intended as an informational guide. The remedies, approaches, and techniques described herein are meant to supplement, and not to be a substitute for, professional medical care or treatment. They should not be used to treat a serious ailment without prior consultation with a qualified healthcare professional.

Library of Congress Cataloging-in-Publication Data

Leeds, Joshua.
The power of sound : how to manage your personal soundscape for a vital, productive, and healthy life / Joshua Leeds.
p. cm.
Includes bibliographical references and index.
ISBN 0-89281-768-2 (alk. paper)
1. Sound—Therapeutic use. 2. Psychoacoustics. 3. Learning. I. Title.

RZ999 .L36 2001
615.8'3—dc21

00-050573

Grateful acknowledgement is given for permission to republish pieces from the following works: Chapter 2, Conceptual Physics, Paul G. Hewitt, © 1993, Addison Wesley Longman, Inc.; Chapter 6, The Story of Dawn, Robert J. Doman, © 1980, National Academy of Child Development; "The Birth of a Sound Therapy," Alexander Doman, reprinted from The Listening Program Guidebook, © 1999, Advanced Brain Technologies, LLC (many thanks to Terry Patten for editorial assistance); "FAQ on Music Therapy," © 1999, American Music Therapy Association; Music for The Power of Sound features selections from the Sound Health Series, courtesy of Advanced Brain Technologies, LLC.

Cover concept and illustration on page 28 by
DESIGN/communications, Ross, CA (www.descomstudios.com)
Photograph of Joshua Leeds by Rick Cobb, Sausalito, CA

Printed and bound in the United States

10 9 8 7 6 5 4 3 2 1

Text design and layout by Virginia Scott-Bowman
This book was typeset in Caslon with Centaur as the display typeface

The graphic symbol 𝓖 used throughout this book is actually an early version of the G clef, also known as the violin or treble clef. Clef signs evolved from the letters they stand for. Notice the similarity of this seventeenth-century European "G" with the outline of an ear.

For Ben and Rachel

Contents

Appendices

Acknowledgments

First and foremost, profound gratitude and respect to Dr. Alfred Tomatis, the grandfather of modern psychoacoustics.

Humble recognition of the musicians/magicians who comprise The Arcangelos Chamber Ensemble.

Heartfelt appreciation to Ron Minson, M.D., and Kate O'Brien-Minson, directors of The Center for InnerChange, for the generous sharing of their Tomatis-based soundwork and valuable perspectives.

I gratefully acknowledge the contributions of many fine and dedicated Tomatis practitioners without whom the preparation of the Tomatis chapters contained within this book would not have been possible. Many thanks to Billie Thompson, Ph.D., Paul Madaule, L.Ps., Timothy Gilmore, Ph.D., and Pierre Sollier, M.F.C.C.

Special thanks to professional colleagues for invaluable peer review: Sheila Smith Allen, M.A., O.T.R., B.C.P.; H. Holmes Atwater; Mike Boles; Dorinne S. Davis, M.A., CCC-A; Alexander Doman; Rachel Leah; Ron Minson, M.D.; Laurie Monroe; Suzanne Evans Morris, Ph.D.; and Lori Riggs, M.A., CCC/SLP.

Without the expertise of the following individuals and organizations, this book would have been sorely lacking. Hats off to: Mary Jo Burtka, M.A., CCC-A, and Kathleen L. Yaremchuk, M.D., of Self Help for Hard of Hearing People, Inc., for their contributions to chapter eight; The Medical and Sports Music

Institute of America; author and composer Kay Gardner; Davis Center for Hearing, Speech & Learning; The Center for Biological Timing at the University of Virginia; The House Ear Institute; and the Noise Pollution Clearinghouse. A very special acknowledgment to Therese Schroeder-Sheker of The Chalice of Repose, Dr. Jeffrey Thompson of Brain/Mind Research, Alex Doman of Advanced Brain Technologies, Robert J. Doman Jr. of The National Academy of Child Development, and Dr. Fred Schwartz of Transitions Music.

Loving thanks to honored mentors, teachers, family, and friends: Susan Alexjander, John Bishop, Barbara Borden, Hovey Burgess, Miriam Cutler, Janine Del Arte, Vickie Dodd, Ronna Dragon, Lyric Kaela Grace, Robert Gass, Steven Gold, Jonathan Goldman, Dick Grove, Dorothy Gundling, Joe Harnell, Louise L. Hay, JaLolo, Sanda Jasper, Dennis Lambert, Deborah Leeds, Sharon Leeds, Kenny Levine, Randall McClellan, Faizi Medeiros, Terry Patten, Evie Sands, Molly Scott, Morgan Cantrell Smith, Margaret Tucker, David Tcimpedes, C. Davey Utter, Andrew Weil, Anna Wise, and Boyd Willat.

No acknowledgments would be complete without expressions of warm gratitude to the Inner Traditions/Healing Arts Press team: Ehud Sperling and Deborah Kimbell, and editors Jon Graham, Cannon Labrie, Laura Jorstad, and Jeanie Levitan. A very special "hats off" to managing editor Rowan Jacobsen, who took such a genuine interest in this project, performing way beyond the call. Thank you all for your indefatigable efforts in bringing this book to fruition.

To my friends at DESIGN/communications, whose graphic imprint graces this book and website from cover to cover: Nick French, Bill Shore, Barbara Stenson, and Cyndie Wooley. My appreciation for humoring my linear thinking and for doing what you thought was best anyway.

And finally, blessings upon Kiki La Porta—image wizard, eager research associate, literary cheerleader, heart partner, and patient friend. This project would not have been completed without your uplifting spirit and loving support.

Thank you all for gracing the pages of this book with your generous wisdom and loving heartspace.

Introduction

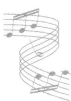 Our basic survival depends on legs for running, fingers for gathering, and sexual organs for reproducing, along with that most amazing computer that coordinates millions of messages every second of every day—the brain.

In addition, our four sensory organs, the eyes, nose, mouth, and ears, inform the brain of surrounding conditions. The seven orifices of the head sample different octaves of frequency—light, aroma, taste, and sound. With this information, the brain adjusts physiological mechanisms to function optimally. "Am I safe?" asks the reptilian brain. With the primary question of survival addressed, this ancient brain relaxes like a lazy lizard in the sun, allowing us to focus on secondary aesthetic considerations: Does this light feel good? Do I prefer these smells? Yum . . . got any more chocolate? Turn up that music!

Once the determinations of safety and personal preference are established, our attention turns to utility. This third tier of sensory perception involves conscious employment of the elements. The creation of tools distinguishes human beings from other animals. People know how to put things to work. In this context, frequencies of light, smell, taste, and sound can be perceived as utilities. Through heightened awareness and specific application, these frequencies become highly refined tools for the enhancement of human function. *How can we use these elements for a better life?* Thomas Edison asked about light. In the hands of a chef, taste becomes elevated to a fine art. Aromatherapists have built an industry on the efficacy of fragrance. The ways that sound serves us run the gamut from background ambience to a potent surgical replacement.

Although all of our sensory organs and their frequencies deserve exploration, *The Power of Sound* focuses on the domain of sound. Humans cannot manufacture light or taste directly, and our repertoire of creative odors is quite limited. We can, however, *make* sound. Not only can we perceive it, but we can also create it: Music, laughter, and words turn sound into a friendly, practical, and interactive medium.

As a child I did what comes naturally—I made a lot of noise. My early fascination with sound was channeled into music. Since then, through elementary school orchestras, teenage rock bands, classical guitar and piano in my twenties, the study of jazz in my thirties, conservatory explorations of classical composition and orchestration in my forties, I've honed that primal instinct to create and mold sound. As a composer drawn to the essence of music, I experience sound as the clay from which musical sculpture evolves. Although music comprises sound, sound is not always musical. *What is sound? What does it do* to *us? What can it do* for *us?* are questions I propose to answer.

Psychoacoustics is the study of the effect of music and sound on the nervous system. Using extensive databases of psychoacoustic research, *The Power of Sound* explains *why* we hear and feel sound, and how we can use it purposefully to enhance our lives.

To explore the many applications of sound, I will discuss the entire spectrum—heard and unheard. Their mutual substance is *vibration,* a rapid rhythmic motion back and forth, and *frequency,* the periodic speed at which an object vibrates. *Resonance* refers to the frequency at which an object most naturally vibrates. These sonic identifiers are our basic building blocks.

Consider the following: Anything that moves has a vibration. Though invisible, every aspect of our material world at the atomic level moves constantly. Wherever there is motion, there is frequency. Though inaudible at times, all frequencies make a sound. All sounds resonate and can affect one another. In the spectrum of sound—from the movement of atomic particles to the sensory phenomenon we call music—there is a chain of vibration:

- All atomic matter vibrates.
- Frequency is the speed at which matter vibrates.
- The frequency of vibration creates sound (sometimes inaudible).
- Sounds can be molded into music.

This chain explains the omnipresence of sound.

PSYCHOACOUSTICS

As I noted, psychoacoustics is the study of the perception of sound. This includes how we listen, our psychological responses, and the physiological impact of music and sound on the human nervous system. In the realm of psychoacoustics, the terms *music, sound, frequency,* and *vibration* are essentially interchangeable, because they are different approximations of the same essence. The study of psychoacoustics dissects the listening experience.

Traditionally, *psychoacoustics* is broadly defined as "pertaining to the perception of sound and the production of speech." The abundant research that has been done in the field has focused primarily on the exploration of speech and of the psychological effects of music therapy. Currently, however, there is renewed interest in sound as vibration.

An important distinction is the difference between a *psychological* and a *neurological* perception. A song or melody associated with childhood, a teenage romance, or some peak emotional experience creates a memory-based psychological reaction. There is also a *physiological* response to sounds, however. Slightly detuned tones can cause brain waves to speed up or slow down, for instance. Additionally, soundtracks that are filtered and gated—this is a sophisticated engineering process—create a random sonic event. It triggers an active listening response and thus tonifies the auditory mechanism, including the tiny muscles of the middle ear. As a result, sounds are perceived more accurately, and speech and communication skills improve. While a psychological response may occur with filtered and gated sounds, or detuned tones, the primary effect is physiological, or neurological, in nature.

Research on the neurological component of sound is currently attracting many to the field of psychoacoustics. A growing school of thought—based on the teachings of the French doctor Alfred Tomatis—values the examination of both neurological and psychological effects of resonance and frequencies on the human body.

Thanks to the groundbreaking findings of Dr. Tomatis, we have come to understand the extraordinary power of the ear. In addition to its critical functions of communication and balance, the ear's primary purpose is to recycle sound and so recharge our inner batteries. According to Tomatis, the ear's first function in utero is to govern the growth of the rest of the physical organism. After birth, sound is to the nervous system what food is to our physical bodies: Food provides nourishment at the cellular level of the organism, and sound feeds us the electrical impulses that charge the neocortex. I will discuss the theories and practices of Tomatis at length; indeed, psychoacoustics cannot be described at all without reference to the man known as the Einstein of the ear.

HEARING AND LISTENING LOSS— PLAYING WITH FIRE

My overarching theme in *The Power of Sound* is the tremendous—yet unacknowledged—influence that sound and hearing have over human functionality. But what happens if our ability to hear is diminished? In Western culture, auditory dysfunction is growing at an unprecedented rate, due mainly to noise and stress. Our delicate auditory mechanism serves as a barometer of physiological status as well as of our emotional state of mind. The result of auditory malfunction is more than a diminution of hearing.

A weakened auditory system endangers *auditory sequential processing*. This function affects short-term memory—the critical ability to link pieces of auditory information.

Auditory sequential processing is critically affected by *auditory tonal processing*. Difficulty interpreting tone may create sequential processing issues. The neurodevelopmental specialist Robert J. Doman Jr. believes that the inability to focus our listening—a symptom of auditory dysfunction—diminishes communication, language, and attention skills in adults and children. Is it a coincidence that the explosive growth in learning disabilities—a sequential processing issue—is paralleled by an accelerating rate of food allergies that cause children's ear infections?

According to Tomatis, Doman, and other pioneers, sound is a vital stimulant, a "nutrient" for the nervous system. Consequently, weakened auditory function depletes a major fuel system for the brain.

Of the many causes of hearing and listening impairment, I will discuss two primary forms. *Noise-induced hearing loss* (NIHL) contributes to approximately 35 percent of all hearing loss in America.[1] Too many protracted loud sounds damage the inner ear. NIHL is physiological damage: The delicate cilia hair cells cannot be repaired.

In addition, stress can impede the active absorption of sound. I label this phenomenon *stress-induced auditory dysfunction* (SIAD). According to Billie Thompson, a leading Tomatis adherent and an expert in auditory impairment, "Poor listening can begin at any age and for any number of reasons. It might result from a health problem, an accident, a major lifestyle disruption, or from stress."[2] Among the symptoms of a degraded auditory function, says neurodevelopmental expert Doman, are "disorganized neurological function—affecting the ability to perceive, assimilate, process, and retrieve data—and emotional overreactivity."[3]

Additionally, when we can no longer tolerate a parent, sibling, spouse, boss, or the like, we begin to "shut down" the mechanism of the middle ear. This has the effect of eliminating the vocal frequencies we reject. Such psychological muting becomes a reflexive and subconscious action. As we shut out sounds, however, we also decrease the audio frequency spectrum.

The net effect of hearing loss, be it noise or stress induced, is that a vital energy source for the brain and nervous system is diminished. Additionally, the degradation of auditory function can result in muddled thinking and out-of-balance emotions.

Stress-induced auditory dysfunction affects the muscles in the middle ear. (The tensor tympani and stapedius muscles become flaccid; this causes the ossicles—the three tiny bones of the middle ear—to work less efficiently in protecting the eardrum from excessive sound and in transmitting a full spectrum of sound.) This form of hearing and listening loss can be addressed, to differing degrees, with sound stimulation auditory retraining programs. While inner-ear damage from noise cannot be *repaired*, auditory retraining of the middle ear allows for better use of what hearing remains.

Stress-induced auditory dysfunction is the psychological equivalent of physiologically based NIHL. Our current growing awareness of SIAD has evolved from the work of Tomatis, Doman, and others over the last four decades. Most healthcare professionals know little about SIAD. Those who recognize and treat the auditory results of stress are reluctant to discuss it due to a dearth of research data. However, many practitioners in neurodevelopment, psychology, psychiatry, speech and language, and occupational therapy acknowledge the SIAD they see repeatedly in their patients. Is the troubling rise in prescriptions of antidepressants and other psychiatric drugs for children and adults masking problems that could be adjusted through remediation of the ear? The auditory response to stress deserves discussion and research. Clinical observations abound, but the neurobiological underpinnings are lacking.

SONIC RESPONSIBILITY

What can be done about this epidemic in noise- and stress-induced auditory dysfunction? you might ask. Begin by establishing a new sound awareness. Assert your sonic rights. Take appropriate precautions and protect your ears. Become proactive in auditory health and restoration. Learn to create sound space conducive to the needs of your nervous system.

We all have the same equipment—two ears. The conscious use of sound comes down to understanding how sound affects us. Then we can apply positive psychoacoustic principles to our situations and environments. This is sonic responsibility.

Sound can be used as a tool to de-stress, improve mental productivity, accelerate learning, minimize pain, and facilitate healing. It is time to take back the space around our ears, to learn to govern our sonic environments or create new and better ones. With the information presented here, you will be able to take charge responsibly, according to your individual needs.

WHAT THIS BOOK CAN TELL YOU

The Power of Sound is divided into three parts.

Part 1 examines the physics of sound and the mechanics of hearing. It also discusses resonance, entrainment, the groundbreaking work of Alfred Tomatis, and Robert Doman's unique theories of neurodevelopmental auditory training.

Part 2 explores sound awareness and looks at current research into the personal applications of psychoacoustic principles.

Part 3 is a guide to soundwork techniques, the therapeutic uses of sound, and sonic neurotechnologies.

The appendices include interviews with three leading sound practitioners, explanations of psychoacoustic techniques in music production, a guide to the enclosed CD, and lists of helpful resources, recordings, and Internet sites.

The enclosed CD, *Music for The Power of Sound,* is comprised of specially orchestrated classical music performed by the award-winning players of The Arcangelos Chamber Ensemble. These beautiful pieces indicate the music of the future—intentional soundscapes for the enhancement of human function. Techniques used in these recordings are discussed in Appendix A, "The Anatomy of Psychoacoustic Music Creation."

I hope that *The Power of Sound* will serve as an introduction for the uninitiated and a further exploration for those already called to a deeper listening. Special sections should be of value to healthcare professionals and musicians.

PART I

Sound

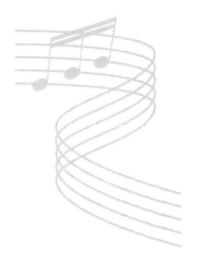

1 What Is Sound?

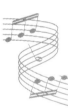Sound is vibratory energy. Sound touches us and influences our emotions like no other source of input or expression. It is the stuff of tone and timbre, silence and noise. It is a frequency of vibration that we audibly hear between 20 and 20,000 Hz. Traveling through the air at 770 miles per hour (its exact speed depends on temperature, humidity, and wind), sound moves almost a million times slower than the speed of light.[1] We perceive it primarily through our ears, where it is transformed into electrochemical impulses sent to the brain. It is also perceived through the skin. Like air and water, sound is ubiquitous. It can be a great thing . . . or it can really be a problem.

Ancient cultures knew about the power of sound long before the term *science* was coined. The spiritually wise men of India knew that the world *is* sound. From India's Vedic scriptures comes the term *Nada Brahman*—"the primal sound of being" or "being itself." Even four thousand years ago, India's scholars and religious leaders understood that we live in a state of vibration from which sound derives and on which sound has profound influences.[2]

Philosophers and prophets of old shared a common belief in the divine origin and nature of sound. In ancient philosophies and religions, sound (vibration) is the lead character in creation myths. The genesis of the universe—or, thinking locally, our planet Earth—is ascribed to the "Word" or the "One Sound." Cutting across historical, religious, and political lines, Egyptians, Hebrews, Native Americans, Celts, Chinese, and Christians all have spoken of sound as a divine principle.[3]

The roots of this belief in the power of sound can be found in the ancient cultures of the Ethiopians, Hopi, and Aborigines, as well as the temples of Greece and Rome. Many of the musical philosophies of Pythagoras have withstood the test of time. In *The Secret Power of Music*, however, David Tame states, "Almost three thousand years before the birth of Christ, at a time when the music of European man may have amounted to no more than the beating of bones on hollow logs, the people of China were already in possession of the most complex and fascinating philosophy of music of which we know today."

The Chinese dynasties compared music with a force of nature and held it in that level of awe. "The Chinese understood the power within music to be a free energy, which man could use or misuse according to his own free will."[4] The rulers and their philosophers believed that in order for their citizens not to misuse music—and for all to benefit from its optimally beneficent use—only the "correct" music could be played. Beyond entertainment, Chinese emperors believed moral influence was the major effect of music that they needed to control. And revere and harness the power of sound they did, for four and a half millennia, until the Ch'ing dynasty (1644–1912).[5]

Worldwide, powerful shamans cured disease and mental anguish by coaxing evil spirits into leaving their victims through the power of chanting. Today entire villages, from Africa to Alabama to the Arctic, continue to drum, sing, or dance themselves into states of spiritual ecstasy.

The entire planet vibrates to the rhythms and sounds of music. No matter how primitive or advanced, music plays an inclusive and vital role in every country. It is an inescapable part of life: of spiritual ceremonies, social celebrations, child rearing, armies marching off to war, initiations, funerals, harvests, and feast days.

Music strikes a chord within that cannot be expressed easily in words.

It soothes and excites us. We resonate with its rhythms, harmonies, and tones. It *feels* good. What is so deeply familiar about tone and rhythm that we can close our eyes and drift away, trusting we are safe in the timelessness of music's embrace?

I believe the answer to this question lies with resonance and sympathetic vibration.

VIBRATION AND RESONANCE

Virtually everything on earth vibrates. The planet itself vibrates. All matter consists of atomic material: molecules, atoms, electrons, protons, neutrons, and subatomic particles. Each atom consists of a nucleus surrounded by electrons, revolving at the speed of six hundred miles per second. It is an accepted construct of physics that motion creates frequency and frequency creates sound.

Whether or not we hear it, *everything* has a sound, a vibration all its own. The velocity (frequency) of the movement determines the specific sound. While we hear the sound of a fan moving the air, we cannot hear the sound of an electron. The speed of an electron is so fast that it creates a tone outside our human range of hearing. Nonetheless, the "sound" is there.

The fact that sound waves* are everywhere is an important point of reference in building conscious sound awareness. And to help you reawaken awareness of sound and the role it can play in your life, add the phenomenon of resonance.

Resonance can be defined as "the frequency at which an object most naturally vibrates." For example, a tuning fork that is tuned to 440 Hz (cycles per second) will, when physically struck, vibrate at 440 Hz. This frequency is known as its *resonant frequency*.

If you have two identical tuning forks manufactured to vibrate at 440 Hz, an interesting example of resonance occurs. Strike one of the forks to produce a sound and the second one—which has not been physically struck—will spontaneously vibrate, or sing along, with the first tuning

---

*_Sound waves_ can be defined as "oscillations in pressure or longitudinal-wave disturbances in any compressible substance, especially air."

fork. It acts as if it too were physically struck—and it was, by the sound waves from the first tuning fork. If a fork tuned to 100 Hz is struck nearby, however, the 440 Hz fork will not respond. Thus, when two or more objects have similar vibratory characteristics that allow them to resonate at the same frequency, they form a *resonant system.*

Resonance is a natural ability; substances such as metal, wood, air, and even living flesh and bone vibrate to a frequency imposed from another source. This aspect of resonance is known as *sympathetic vibration.*

SYMPATHETIC VIBRATION

Imagine that I have two violins tuned alike. I place the first violin on a table and leave it there, then I move to the other side of the room. I take the second violin and bow a single open string (say, the D string) ten feet away from the first violin. What happens? The soundbox of the first violin will begin to vibrate as the sound frequencies of the second violin resonate the nonplayed instrument's D string. If I play the A string on the second violin, the first violin's A string will correspondingly resonate. If I play all four open strings on the second violin, likewise all four open strings on the first violin will vibrate. As with the tuning forks, this is the resonant phenomenon of sympathetic vibration.

Given that everything has its resonant frequency—I think of it as a "resident" (or home) frequency—we humans are no exception. That is why certain colors feel good to us and why we are attracted to certain instruments and sounds. The colors or sounds are within our resident frequency range and can make us vibrate from across the room. Our familiarity with their frequency has an effect on our mood.

Some people like the sound of the saxophone; for others, it is like fingernails on a chalkboard. Your teenager loves that electric guitar sound; it drives you to distraction because it grates on your nervous system. Different people, different frequency perception. The connotation of sound varies.

The concept of sympathetic vibration—the way an outside vibration can sympathetically vibrate another vibration—holds true with people, too. When you are around someone with a vibrational rate similar to your own, you feel comfortable and familiar. Likewise, you instinctively know when someone's energy field is totally different from yours.

So when it comes to music and sound, finding sources that resonate positively is a good and healthy thing. If you passively allow yourself to be surrounded by sounds that do not resonate well with you, however, you stand a good chance of creating nervous system friction, a loop of internal interference. Continued exposure over a long—or sometimes even a short—period can cause you to simply fall out of tune, out of harmony with your body's inherent wisdom state. Secondhand tobacco smoke has been proved to have deleterious effects; what about secondhand sound? The phenomenon of sympathetic vibration is contingent not on volume but on pitch. This means that even quiet home or office sounds—the hum of a computer, fluorescent lights, a refrigerator, or a television—may be resonating you.

We are constantly being vibrated, on a cellular level, by heard and unheard sound frequencies: electromagnetic fields of all kinds, microwaves, electricity, radar, jet planes, jackhammers, horns, sirens, and loud sounds of many kinds, including music. The increase in stress-related disease in modern society is of little wonder. Many things contribute to stress, which might be defined as an overamping of the nervous system. A jagged nervous system is a stressed nervous system. The food we eat, the people we are around, and the thoughts we think have a proven effect on our well-being. It is time to add sound to this list.

If you combine the universality of sound vibration with the idea that we can be affected by external frequency sources, you begin to glimpse the importance of sympathetic vibration.

The goal is to not become paranoid about every sound around you, wondering whether it is vibrating you into schizophrenia or cancer. While we do not have earlids to block incoming sound, the brain has a magnificent adaptive mechanism that allows us to shut down, closing out unwanted sounds—however, we pay a long-term price for doing so. I will discuss this in chapters 5 and 6 when I look at the work of Dr. Alfred Tomatis and of neurodevelopmental specialist Robert Doman.

As you develop a new sound awareness, the basic objective is to become conscious of the principles of sound so you can make informed and intentional choices about the frequency elements with which you surround yourself. In the following lighthearted chapter, I will explore the medium of sound from a physics point of view.

The Physics of Sound

The horizons of physics, philosophy, and art have of late been too widely separated, and as a consequence, the language, the methods, and the aims of any one of these studies present a certain amount of difficulty for the student of any other of them.

—Hermann Helmholtz

 You might imagine that the complaint that heads this chapter resulted from recent trends toward specializing and compartmentalizing knowledge. The complainer, however—Hermann Helmholtz, a brilliant German physicist and philosopher and the author of *On the Sensations of Tone*—was in 1862 bemoaning the unbridgeable chasm between art and science that is still so commonplace today. Perhaps this fragmentation of knowledge explains why Helmholtz spent many years building and studying instruments, compiling all known sound data, applying intricate mathematical and physics formulas to harmony, and investigating the effects of tone on the nervous system.[1]

As a scientist, philosopher, and psychoacoustician (long before the term was first enunciated), Helmholtz researched the human perception of sound. He attempted to bring together two diverging systems to bridge the gaps in human understanding. His work reflects a common desire to reunify mind and body, heart and soul—and, most specifically, art and science.

In my undergraduate studies, I came across a wonderful text titled *Conceptual Physics*. In its author, Paul G. Hewitt, I found a lover of science who also possessed a sense of poetry and humor. Hewitt's discussion of sound includes this delightful passage:

> *Many things in nature wiggle and jiggle.*
> *We call a wiggle in time a vibration.*
> *A vibration cannot exist in an instant,*
> *but needs time to move to and fro.*
> *We call a wiggle in space and time a wave.*
> *A wave cannot exist in one place,*
> *but must extend from one place to another.*[2]

Hewitt has skillfully refined the physics of sound into five concepts. Let's take a closer look at what this poem says about the building blocks of sound.

"MANY THINGS IN NATURE WIGGLE AND JIGGLE."

Frequency is one of the most important elements in any discussion of energy, be it molecular, light, or sound. The term *frequency* refers to how often any regularly repeated event occurs in an assumed unit of time. Therefore, we can refer to the frequency of atomic vibration, of planets around the sun, or even of a heartbeat. For each of these events, a scale of measurement has been devised. In sound and light, we refer to the frequency of vibrations. This unit of frequency is measured in hertz (Hz), the number of vibrations or cycles per second (cps).

"WE CALL A WIGGLE IN TIME A VIBRATION."

Vibration is defined as a "rapid alternating motion to and fro, or up and down." This vibrational motion can be produced in any medium made up of molecules—earth, water, air, metal—if there is a disturbance of that medium's equilibrium. If the vibration occurs among particles of anything other than a vacuum, sound will be produced.

What causes the disturbance of equilibrium? The answer is any vibrating source. This could be a saw cutting wood, a hammer striking a nail, the strings of a guitar, the reed of a wind instrument, or the fluctuation of vocal cords.

"A VIBRATION CANNOT EXIST IN AN INSTANT,
BUT NEEDS TIME TO MOVE TO AND FRO.
WE CALL A WIGGLE IN SPACE AND TIME A WAVE."

Using physics as our guide, *waves* are defined as "rhythmic alternations of disturbance and recovery in successively contiguous portions of a fluid or solid mass." This is true, but what does it mean? Essentially, a vibration needs something to carry it along. The wave is the vehicle, so to speak, on which the frequency of vibration travels. But an important distinction needs to be made here. The image of a vehicle conjures up, say, a bus, picking up a bunch of waves and delivering them somewhere. At the same time, I have always thought that a sound wave was like a ribbon of energy that, in its entirety, started one place and went somewhere else. Both images are common misconceptions. A wave does indeed carry energy outward from the source. But instead of this energy getting on a single bus and later getting off, it is actually transported by millions of buses—molecules.

Let's use this image instead: You are stuck in miles of bumper-to-bumper traffic and you are hot, cranky, and holding a big secret—which happens to be nothing less than *the original impulse of sound!* Now imagine getting out of your car and, after exchanging a few pleasantries, getting into the car in front of you and telling that driver your secret. He says, "Good grief! Does anyone else know?" and gets out of his car and into the car in front of his, telling the next driver your original secret. This driver then gets out of her car and goes to the next—and the routine goes on and on and on. In the meantime, you are still sitting in the first car while the secret has been passed along by others.

Fortunately, waves don't have to open and close car doors. And instead of having to ride in zillions of cars, the original vibration hitchhikes on molecules. This is basically how energy travels: The original sound impulse moves while the molecules stay put. Molecules, like bumper-to-bumper cars, remain in the same place after the impulse has passed through.

Almost all information comes to us in the form of some kind of wave—of which there are many: the waves on the surface of water, the waves of the air that convey sound, and the waves of ether that are concerned with the transmission of light, heat, and electricity.

"A WAVE CANNOT EXIST IN ONE PLACE, BUT MUST EXTEND FROM ONE PLACE TO ANOTHER."

Wave motion is the phenomenon of a transfer of energy (or information) from one source to another. The vibration is the information. The wave is the impulse that carries the information outward. The wave motion is the propulsion of that information out into the world. This propelling of the wave is accomplished through what is called *compression and rarefaction*, a process involving the alternating density of molecules in the air and how information is passed.[3] It is through compression and rarefaction that the actual energy of sound is transmitted.

The study of physics tells us that what is transported from one place to another is a disturbance in a medium but not the medium itself. The medium carrying the wave returns to its initial condition after the disturbance has passed.

When air blows over a field of tall grass, we see the movement of each blade as it bends and then returns to its original state. Likewise, as waves move through water, a rubber duck will bob and dip in response to each one that passes, but after it has passed, both duck and the particular batch of water it sits in will be in roughly the same place. The same holds true for the molecules in the air, but because air is invisible, we don't see this springy, to-and-fro movement. In the movement of sound waves through the air, it is not the air that travels; rather, it is the impulse, the wave, using the air as the medium in which to travel (think of hitchhiking molecules).[4]

THE COMPONENTS OF SOUND

Let's put together the components of sound:

- *Sound* is a sensation caused by an object or objects that vibrate.
- When we put out a sound, a *vibration* at a certain rate *(frequency)* is created.
- This vibration then becomes a sound *wave* if it is in a medium that allows it to travel (that is, a medium in which the molecules are not too dense, as they are in rubber or putty, or where there are no molecules at all, as in a vacuum).
- This information is then transported by molecules *(wave motion)*.

The molecules themselves are not traveling with this information; they are essentially handing it from one to another. They are serving as transfer points for information, and the way they do this is by taking on the vibration of the initial pulse and handing it over to their neighbor as they spring back into place to receive the next impulse (compression and rarefaction). It is essentially a game of molecular baton-passing.

SOME FURTHER PROPERTIES OF SOUND

Knowing some of sound's special properties will enlarge your comprehension of the nature of sound.

As I previously stated, a *sound* can be defined as "a sensation caused by an object or objects that vibrate." A *noise* is any unwanted sound; the term is obviously very subjective. *Pitch* signifies how high or low a tone sounds to the ear; this is also a subjective impression. We say a piccolo sounds high and a tuba sounds low. In fact, the piccolo is vibrating at a high frequency and the tuba at a lower and slower frequency. Pitch is any periodic frequency between 20 and 20,000 Hz. The lowest note on a full-sized piano is A0, with a frequency of 27.5 Hz, which means this tone is vibrating 27.5 times per second. The highest note on this piano is C8, with a frequency of 4,186 Hz; this tone is vibrating 4,186 times per second! *Tone* can be defined as "a sound of definite pitch and duration."

We hear the pitch of a tone only if it possesses *periodicity*, which means that the vibration repeats precisely the same pattern on a regular basis.* Only if something repeats at the same frequency will it produce a steady tone. With the exception of percussion, music is made up of tones. For example, orchestras tune to the pitch of A = 440—an A tone vibrating at 440 cycles per second. However, another example of a tone is the sound of a jet engine. It may not seem musical, but it does have a pitch because it is vibrating with regular periodicity.

If a sound is *nonperiodic*, which means it has no regular pulse and frequency, it will not produce a tone. Rather, we will perceive the sound either as percussive or as noise. In terms of percussiveness, nonperiodic sounds can be rhythmic in nature and are most often of short duration. In terms of noise, the sound of traffic and the crunching of a newspaper are nonperiodic sounds; they have changing frequencies and irregular patterns.

Concepts, as we know, are not fixed in stone. To say that periodicity or nonperiodicity determines the difference between tone (music) and noise would be misleading, albeit often true. A musical note is periodic, whereas a handclap is nonperiodic. Yet if the handclapping is performed in a repetitive periodic fashion, while not tonal, it is musical. A jackhammer is very likely periodic and very definitely noisy. And a conga drum solo is nonperiodic and quite musical. Helmholtz attempted to bridge the difference between periodic and nonperiodic vibration when he said, "The sensation of a musical tone is due to a rapid periodic motion of the sonorous body; the sensation of a noise to non-periodic motions."[5] As you have seen, in most cases this is true.

Continuing, a *sonorous body* is anything capable of producing sound, especially of deep and rich quality. All musical instruments—the body of a cello and the sounding board of a piano—are sonorous, as are the rib cage of a soprano and an apple juice jug. These sonorous bodies are the containers of the vibration; it is the molecules inside the wood of a violin that are set into vibration by the bowing of the string; in turn, the air inside the soundbox amplifies the vibration.

As I noted, the parameters of the normal human *hearing range* are

---

* A *pattern* is "an arrangement of form, a definite direction, tendency, or characteristic."

between 20 and 20,000 Hz. Some creatures, however, can hear outside this range. Dogs hear above 20,000 Hz, as do dolphins, elephants, and alligators, among others. Because of normal physiological processes, as we age the highs and lows that we hear begin to diminish.

Sound waves above 20,000 Hz are called *ultrasonic. Infrasonic* waves are those below 20 Hz, which are perceived as rhythm, if they can be heard at all.

Timbre is the tone color or characteristic quality that distinguishes one voice or musical instrument from another, determined by the harmonics of the sound.

Like pitch and timbre, *loudness (amplitude)* is actually a psychological impression. Loudness is a perception of sound strength; what may be offensive to one person is comfortable to another. Loudness is also a function of intensity. Vigorous vibrations produce more-intense sound waves, which cause larger air pressure variations that then have an impact on the eardrum.[6] *Volume* can be defined as "the quantity, strength, or loudness of sound." In the world of sound, *volume* is synonymous with *loudness* or *amplitude.*

Loudness is measured in *decibels* (dB). A falling pin measures 10 dB, a whisper 30 dB, a quiet conversation 40 dB, a subway train 90 dB, amplified rock music 110 dB, a jet engine at ten feet 130 dB. For most people, pain begins at 110 to 120 dB. Levels above 100 dB not only are unpleasantly loud but also can cause ear damage, which gets progressively worse with prolonged exposure. Ear damage can actually begin with lengthy exposure to noise levels above 85 dB.*

Sound must have a medium in order to vibrate. If there is nothing to compress and expand, there can be no sound. Any elastic substance can transmit sound, be it liquid, gas, solid, or even plasma. Professor Hewitt says that "compared to solids and liquids, air is a relatively poor conductor of sound"—yet it is our primary medium for receiving sound. Hewitt goes on to describe how the sound of an approaching train can be heard sooner if you put an ear to the rail. This is because the vibrations are moving fifteen times faster through the metal than through the air. In water, sound travels about four times as fast as in air.[7] Much like listening to

* See page 95 for a chart of noise and safety levels.

sound through a metal rail, indigenous warriors or hunters often put an ear to the ground to hear sounds that were not yet audible in the air.

The transmission of vibrations from a vibrating body to another body is, again, called resonance. This phenomenon takes place only when the two bodies are capable of vibrating at the same frequency.

It is from resonance that sympathetic vibrations come. A bowed note on one violin's open string will make the same string vibrate on another unplayed violin if it is in the vicinity. The second instrument is playing sympathetically. A violin, however, could not make a rock sing; their two bodies are too different. Resonance takes place frequently with pianos and tuning forks. In this book you will also learn about the direct application of resonance to people.

A NOTE ON LIGHT AND SOUND

A common misunderstanding regarding the relationship of light and sound is the notion that because both are by-products of frequency, it is just speed and perception that separate them. This being the case, it would seem reasonable to say that sound is actually slow light—and, conversely, that light is fast sound. Taking this concept of a single large spectrum of vibration even farther, you could say that all the sensory receivers located in our heads—eyes, ears, nose, and mouth—are there to perceive the frequencies of light, sound, smell, and taste, each being calibrated to a different segment of the same frequency spectrum.

It's a great concept, but it's not true.[8]

This is how light and sound are similar:

1. They both move through space very rapidly as waves.
2. They are both perceived by sense organs in our heads.
3. They both have the same source—vibrations.
4. They both are measured in Hz.
5. Physicists and other beings love them both.

This is how they are different:

1. *Speed.* Light moves at the unbelievable rate of 186,000 miles per second! Sound looks like a laggard at only 1,100 feet per second. Therefore, in five seconds sound has traveled only 1 mile while light has traveled 930,000 miles (equivalent to thirty-seven times around the globe). This is why you see the lightning long before you hear the thunder even though they happen simultaneously.

2. *Waves.* Light moves on a transverse wave (crossing side to side) in direct lines; sound moves spherically on longitudinal waves.

3. *Material.* Light depends on an electrical exchange of energy. It is not dependent on any physical matter. It does not need molecules to push around; it travels through the vacuum of space! Sound, however, depends on the molecules of physical matter being displaced. For its waveform to exist, sound requires solids, gas, liquids, and so on, or else it won't play.

4. *Constancy.* The speed of light rarely changes. The speed of sound absolutely changes based on the environment.

5. *Consistency.* Light is an electromagnetic force. From the slowest frequencies to the fastest, its frequencies are: radio waves, microwaves, infrared, and ultraviolet. Sound is a grosser phenomenon involving physical matter.

   While our human bodies are made up of the same basic components of light and sound—light is electromagnetic and sound is physical matter (atoms and molecules)—it seems that we are tuned to handle the vibrations of sound more easily than those of light. Perhaps we can vibrate with sound because each of us can produce and hear sound, whereas making discernible light—from our minds and bodies—is a fairly advanced art form.

   We can also make sound from our bodies; it is a part of us! With sound we have a tool to merge with the greater sonic stream and be resonated by it. Sound may be an interconnection to realms previously inaccessible without our conscious awareness. Sound is available for us to play with, manipulate, mold, swim in, ride on. At 770 miles per hour, sound is within our conceptual and practical reach.

The 3 Mechanics of Hearing

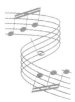It is often said that the primal instinct of all animals is twofold: survival and reproduction. Human beings are no exception. Our sensory organs are barometers of conditions outside the body. Is it safe? Do we need to run away? Can we relax? Can we sleep? The eyes, ears, nose, mouth, and skin are essentially body scouts, constantly surveying the outer scene and sending reconnaissance reports to central headquarters.

Our eyes—the sensory organs to which most attention is paid—perform one function brilliantly: the detection of the presence of light and image. The ears, mostly relegated to a secondary role, serve multiple purposes: They convert sound into electrical energy that charges the brain; they keep our physical equilibrium; and they analyze acoustic information, thereby allowing us to communicate.

The focus of this chapter is what takes place once sound waves enter the outer ear. I will examine the steps that occur as the incoming air fluctuations of sound convert into electrochemical impulses that are processed by the brain. The understanding of how we hear

brings a deeper awareness of the impact of sound, and with this understanding we can assess the value of the sounds around us. As our eyes see
what is in front of us, so our ears hear what is around us. And just as we can
sometimes choose what we wish to see, we can also exert our power of
choice on what kinds of sounds we are willing to let bathe our psyche.

The emerging field of soundwork or sound therapy, which is different from music therapy, is based on the theory of vibration: how frequency resonates and affects our nervous system. Soundwork is
neurological in nature, working with vibrations to create a charge in the
brain and nervous system.

Through the understanding of what happens to sound once it enters
our heads, we can more easily ascertain which sounds actually strengthen
us, as well as which frequencies weaken us. The power of sound is often
subtle and therefore easily ignored. But it is through this subtlety that
sound surreptitiously influences our energy, our health, our entire ability
to stay in balance. As with so many kinds of sensory input—food, aroma,
fitness, sound, image—we have a choice as to how and what we ingest.

THE JOURNEY OF SOUND

From the study of physics, we know that audible sound creation and
transmission consists of four basic stages:

- Something vibrates.
- This disturbance creates a wave, spreading out to all molecules
  around it.
- The pulse of the wave rapidly passes from molecule to molecule.
- The pulsing molecules nearest the ear vibrate the eardrum.

But what happens then?

THE EAR

The ear itself is a funny slab of skin extending from the side of our head
like a primordial radar dish. And much like its technological emulators,
the ears simply hang out, dutifully awaiting information. In this case the

data come in the form of fluctuating air waves. In the world of physiology, function defines form. And the function here is to scoop up sound and transfer it inward.

In order to accomplish this "recycling" of sound, the mechanism of the ear is highly sophisticated. Its circuitry is miniature and delicate, hidden from view and protected inside the recesses of the temporal bones of the skull. Conventional wisdom has long believed that the ear is divided into three parts: the outer, middle, and inner ears.

The outer ear or external ear. This consists of the pinna (auricle), auditory canal (meatus), and eardrum (tympanic membrane). The *pinna* is the corrugated flap of skin on either side of the head. Its broad function is to corral sound waves and funnel them through the external auditory canal toward the eardrum. The *auditory canal*, about one inch long in adults, allows the delicate eardrum to be set inside the skull, where it is safely protected. The *eardrum* is a thin disc of fibrous tissue. It vibrates with the sound waves; the alternations of air pressure cause it to bulge inward and outward.

The middle ear. This is the small, connecting section of the sound highway. A hollow region directly behind the eardrum, the middle ear is only about two milliliters in volume. Here are located the *hammer* (malleus), *anvil* (incus), and *stirrup* (stapes) we all remember from physiology class. The middle ear houses these three small bones, collectively known as *ossicles.* Conventional wisdom asserts that the job of the ossicles is to transfer sound vibration from the eardrum (outer ear) to the cochlea (inner ear). Working together, these bones form a lever system. The handle of the hammer sits against the inside of the eardrum. The anvil rests between the hammer and the stirrup. The foot of the stirrup presses against the *oval window,* which is the opening in the bony process surrounding the cochlea. As the eardrum fluctuates, the ossicles are the bridge on which the mechanical vibrations cross over.[1]

Dr. Alfred Tomatis has proposed an alternative concept about the pathway of sound and the role of the ossicles. He believes that sound is *not* transferred through the ossicles, as is the common belief—referred to as the Helmholtz-Bekesy concept. Tomatis states that "the peripheral bone that surrounds the tympanic membrane, especially in the lower area, conducts the sound toward the inner ear." Essentially, it is the entire bony structure of the middle-ear chamber—not the ossicles—that transfers sound vibrations to the inner ear; the primary function of the ossicles is a protective muting device to protect the inner ear from dangerously loud sounds. (For more about Dr. Tomatis, see chapter 5.)

The middle ear also contains two small muscles that are quite often ignored (a current physiology text does not even bother to mention them). The *tensor tympani* is attached to the hammer and increases the tension in the eardrum. The *stapedius* pulls the stirrup sideways. The effect of this counterlevering is to reduce the mobility of the ossicle chain, thereby reducing the sound transmission through this middle chamber. This protects the inner ear from damage from very loud sounds.

The role of these two tiny muscles, however, goes much farther than this. In fact, they are of major importance in the groundbreaking auditory retraining work of Dr. Tomatis and his Electronic Ear. According to Tomatis, the tiny stapedius muscle is the only muscle in the human body that never rests. It constantly regulates our perception of sound from the sixteenth week in utero until the moment of death.*

The inner ear or cochlea. Like an alchemist's laboratory, this sacred sanctum of hearing is where transformation takes place, for it is here that the vibration of sound is converted into electrical signals. It is also in the inner ear that the vestibular system resides. The *semicircular canals* and the *vestibular sacs* are the upper part of what is known as the *bony labyrinths of the inner ear.*

The cochlea is the bottom part of this labyrinth. The function of the vestibular system includes balance, maintenance of the head in an upright position, and adjustment of eye movement to compensate for head movements.

---

* In reference to this statement, questions have been posed regarding the heart. Wouldn't it fit into the same category as the stapedius—as a muscle that never stops? According to Dr. Bradford Weeks, though, "The heart pulsates, a motion which involves periodicity and therefore a rest of sorts."[2] Still, the point of great interest is that a muscle in the middle ear never stops. According to Dr. Weeks, "This constancy has significance as regards cortical charge." Whether it is the only muscle to make the claim of perpetual motion is actually immaterial. What is of note is that sound information is being processed nonstop without even the gap of a normal muscle's rest cycle.

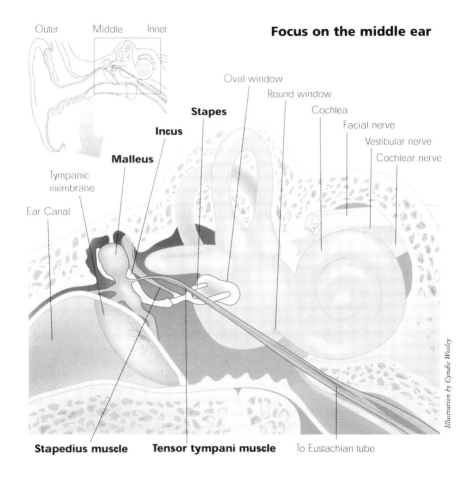

Outer   Middle   Inner

Oval window
Round window
Stapes
Cochlea
Facial nerve
Incus
Vestibular nerve
Cochlear nerve
Malleus

Tympanic
membrane

Ear Canal

Illustration by Cyndie Wooley

Stapedius muscle   **Tensor tympani muscle**   To Eustachian tube

The cochlea houses the intricate mechanisms for this alchemical transaction and will be the focus of my inner-ear exploration. The word *cochlea* derives from the Greek word *kokhlos*, meaning "land snail." Indeed, the shape of the cochlea is similar to the shell of a snail; it is a gradually tapering cylinder of two and three quarter turns. Unrolled, it would be about an inch and a quarter long.

For the purposes of visualization, imagine the cochlea unfurled. The cochlear shell is divided longitudinally into three sections: The *scala vestibuli* and the *scala timpani* are chamberlike areas, filled with a fluid called *perilymph*. These regions are divided by a very complex structure called the *cochlear duct (scala media)*. The cochlear duct is hollow and filled with another fluid, *endolymph*. It is in and adjacent to this cochlear duct— which is actually the middle and smallest chamber of the three—that the major transformational activities of converting wave motion to electrical impulses take place. Herein lies a section of the inner ear called the *organ of Corti,* consisting of three elements: the *basilar membrane, hair cells,* and the *tectorial membrane.*

At this point, with so many separate names and functions, mental overload can set in. Let's retrace the path of sound incorporating the information above.

Sound waves are funneled via the outer ear through the auditory canal to vibrate up against the outside of the eardrum, which is like a taut drumhead. Pressing against the inside of the eardrum are the three tiny bones (hammer, anvil, and stirrup) known as ossicles. Their job is to transfer the vibration from the eardrum to the cochlea, intensifying the energy transmission.

Vibrations enter the cochlea through an opening of the bony structure called the oval window. These vibrations set the perilymph, one of the internal cochlear fluids, into motion. Interestingly enough, the sound waves in the air have now become liquid waves inside our heads. The low frequencies cause the wave motion to move all the way up and around the cochlea and come back down the other side. Higher frequencies take a different route. Because they create much faster waves, there is not enough time for them to traverse the upper and lower chambers without causing excessive compression. Therefore, high-frequency waves essentially recirculate by going a very small distance up one side of the top chamber, flexing the basilar membrane, which lies between the upper and lower chambers. This in turn creates wave motion in the lower chamber. So, having traveled this far, what happens in the movement of fluid that now transforms sound into electrical energy?

In the middle chamber of the cochlea is the alchemist's workbench, the organ of Corti, made up of the basilar membrane, 15,400 hair cells, and the tectorial membrane. The basilar membrane rests just between the lower and middle chambers. Anchored on this membrane are *hair* cells, with fine, hairlike appendages at the top of the cell similar to eyelashes; these are known as *cilia.* The cilia are stiff and rigid, arranged in rows according to height. Anchored to the basilar membrane, many of the hair cells also attach to a parallel membrane known as the tectorial membrane.

The motion of the sound waves causes the basilar membrane to move relative to the tectorial membrane. This bends the hair cells' cilia, and this back-and-forth bending of hairlike auditory receptors initiates signals on the individual fibers of the *auditory nerve*. In other words, the cilia are like a trip-switch: Once they are set in motion, chemical actions are induced, sending electrochemical activity through neurons, the nerve cells of the brain. Before we know it, sound is on its way to numerous auditory centers in the brain.

Let's trace these new stages:

- Vibration hits the eardrum; it is passed along by the ossicles and introduced into the cochlea, where it becomes sound waves.
- Waves, circulating around the cochlea, move the basilar membrane and cause the cilia to bend.
- This movement of hairs stimulates neuronal activity beginning an electrochemical journey into the brain through the eighth cranial nerve. Ultimately, it is both the vibration of the basilar membrane and the actions of the brain that determine our perceptions of sound.

THE AUDITORY PATHWAY

The bending of the cilia at the tip of a hair cell causes a series of reactions inside the cell. Chemically stated: Ion channels open and close, potassium flows in and out, and neurotransmitter substances increase and decrease.[3] You can see the ebb and flow of reactions tied to the movement of the sound waves inside the cochlea. Imagine the speed at which this all transpires; each of these reactions occurs multiple times for every slight segment of sound we ingest. The inner ear, not unlike other parts of the body, is a high-speed processor of information. It essentially digests megabytes of sound before sending sonic nutrients to the brain. Recall that *the primary function of the ear is to charge the neocortex of the brain with electrical impulses.**

---

* Much of the theory in this book is based on the discoveries of Dr. Alfred Tomatis. Dorinne S. Davis—an audiologist, a sound therapist, and the director of the Davis Center for Hearing, Speech, and Learning in Budd Lake, New Jersey—makes an observation about the statement that "the primary function of the ear is to charge the brain with electrical impulses." She points out that to those who study the science of *hearing* (as distinguished from *listening*), the primary function of the ear is to register sound. The Tomatis circle of influence is small within the general audiology community at this time.

Most sounds will accomplish this—some more effectively than others.

You can see the pivotal role that auditory hair cells play in the transmutation of sonic information. But beware! The sensation of loudness is a factor of how many cilia are brought to excitation; these cells can be permanently damaged when the ear is exposed to extremely loud sounds. If you were a fish, bird, or amphibian, broken hair cells would regenerate. Unfortunately, humans cannot repair these damaged cells.

The anatomy of the auditory pathway—and what takes place once the stimulus arrives in the auditory cortex of the brain—is even more complex than that of the visual system. Consider the following:

The neuron is the information-processing and -transmitting element of the nervous system. Each neuron receives information through its branchlike dendrites and transmits it to other neurons through synaptic connections. The average neuron links up with sixty thousand other neurons—with a capacity of two hundred thousand connections or more! There are more than ten billion neurons in the brain.

None of the auditory neurons goes directly to its final destination in the *primary auditory cortex*. Instead, auditory signals mix and get processed at several stations along the way. They visit numerous places in the *medulla* (lower brain), then make stops in the *midbrain* and *cerebrum* before arriving at the auditory cortex. This area is located on both sides of the brain, tucked away inside the *Sylvian fissure*. Signals come from both ears, traveling separate pathways. Each hemisphere of the neocortex receives information from both ears, but its primary source is the opposite ear (that is, the auditory cortex in the left hemisphere receives most of its information from the right ear). It should be noted that the maze of the brain is so complex that the above-stated routing of auditory signals should be considered only a simplistic generalization.

The transference of electrochemical signals pertains to the sound coming from the auditory nerve—out of the cochlea—and up into the medulla, located in the brain stem. But the fact is that sound is actually collected and disseminated throughout the body by numerous nerves and by bone conduction.

The Ear and the Body

Because most cranial nerves lead there, the ear has been called "the Rome of the body." According to Dr. Bradford Weeks, ten of the twelve cranial nerves are affected by the ear. Most of the cranial nerves regulate the motor functions of the head and neck area, including all the sensory organs located in the head. Weeks adds that all motor functions in the head—except smell, the tongue, and the neck muscles—are affected by the ear. This includes vision, eye movements, facial sensations, chewing, taste, and head and neck muscles.[4]

One of the most fascinating facts about hearing is the relationship of the ear to the *pneumogastric*, or tenth, cranial nerve. This nerve is also called the *vagus* (wandering or vagabond) *nerve* because it meanders through the thoracic and abdominal cavities. The enormous task of the vagus nerve is the functional regulation of a host of organs, from the larynx, heart, lungs, stomach, liver, bladder, kidneys, small intestines, and colon all the way down to the anus. And the vagus nerve attaches the outer and inner eardrum on its way south from the brain. What is the significance of this interconnection? An important conclusion asserts itself: Vagus nerve communiqués to the rest of the body are affected by the ear! This vagus nerve–acoustic interaction means that mixed into the parasympathetic instructions to our major organs are vibrations from the eardrum. And what makes the eardrum vibrate? Sound. And who determines the sounds we put into our ears? Or, getting specific, who determines the vibration we put into our internal organs? Clearly, the effect of sound can no longer be simply measured by how our ears feel. The ear brings in energy that touches us from top to bottom. Sound is not just vibrating the eardrum. It is actually resonating the entire being.

Having discussed the nature of sound, the physics of sound, and the mechanics of hearing, let's turn our attention to the fascinating world of resonance—the impact of one vibration on another. Given that sound is a vibration and that we have an extraordinary system designed to perceive and translate sound vibrations, the question arises, *What effect does resonance have on you and me?* Read on.

4 Resonance and Entrainment

Resonance can be broadly defined as "the impact of one vibration on another." Literally, it means "to send again, to echo."

I mentioned an example of resonance in chapter 1: The open string of an untouched violin sounds when a similar string on another violin is played across the room. The untouched violin is responding to the similar frequency of the violin that is actually played. The frequency that is causing the string of the untouched violin to sound—the resonant frequency—is the frequency at which the unplayed string most naturally vibrates.

To *resonate* is to "re-sound." Something external sets something else into motion, or *changes* its vibratory rate. This can have many different effects—some subtle and some not so.

The term *sympathetic vibration* refers to the phenomenon of resonance whereby one object's vibration alters that of another object. If you can match the vibratory rates of another object, it will "sympathetically" change. Matching vibratory rate creates a resonant system. For example, a stationary rock won't cause a nearby table to vibrate sympathetically; their vibratory rates are very different, and they don't share a resonant system. But place a struck tuning fork on a table and the sound will be much louder than the fork would make by itself. This is an example of *forced vibration*. The sound of the tuning fork is louder because the table is forced to vibrate by the vibrations of the tuning fork and, with its larger surface area, sets more air in motion.[1]

The principle of resonance holds true with people as well as tuning forks and violins. When we find ourselves feeling good around somebody, we actually use the phrase *good vibes*. Sharing both metaphorical and real sensitivities, we feel good because someone with a similar frequency "feels" familiar. Familiarity brings a sense of safety and security. These comfortable feelings allow us to be natural and unguarded. Soon we actually resonate with the other person. It is a close feeling, be it on a mental, physical, or emotional level. However, if people resonate in a way that offends or disturbs our resident frequency rate, we move away from them because we do not want to be affected by the vibrations they emit.

Opera singers and crystal glasses are a common example of resonance in acoustics. Here's how it works: The singer taps the glass lightly and hears the sound that it emits. This sound is the glass's natural frequency. By then singing a very pure and steady tone at that same frequency, the singer builds up a strong resonant response, a vibration with amplitude large enough that it may exceed the breaking strength of the glass.[2] Another example of over-amping resonant structures: Soldiers "break step" when marching across a bridge. There has been at least one instance—on a footbridge in Manchester, England, in 1831—in which soldiers' combined rhythmic marching matched the natural frequency of the bridge structure and caused it to fall apart. Unintentionally, the soldiers created a resonant system.[3]

Resonant systems occur in nature as well. In 1940 the Tacoma Narrows bridge in Washington State was destroyed by wind-generated resonance. According to Paul Hewitt: "A mild gale produced a fluctuating force in resonance with the natural frequency of the bridge, steadily increasing the amplitude until the bridge collapsed."[4] Research suggests that giant icebergs are splintered by the resonant force of constant gently lapping waves.[5]

The concept of resonance plays heavily in the construction of airports. Certain materials sympathetically resonate with the sound of the jet engines and, like the bridges, will dissolve. Therefore, materials that will not form a resonant system have to be used. Another aeronautical story of resonance: The ill-fated Electra prop jet had a habit of falling apart when rotating propellers matched the natural frequency of the wings.[6]

In medicine the noninvasive practice of lithotripsy is becoming standard procedure. Pancreatic and kidney stones are being dissolved with acoustic waves. French sound researcher Fabien Maman—director of the Academy of Sound, Color, and Movement—has scientifically documented the effect of sound on cancer cells. Fascinating photographs of microscope slides show healthy cells expanding and contracting at the sound of a nearby xylophone. You see the cells enlarge as they absorb the sound waves, then return to normal size as the sound dissipates. Cancer cells do not have enough flexibility to expand, however, and they explode as the sound waves impact. Healthy cells resonate; unhealthy cells don't.

If concrete and cement can be made to dissolve by sound and rhythm, what about the effect of sound on tissues and organs? The tenth cranial nerve, or vagus nerve, attaches to both sides of the eardrum before traveling down the torso and attaching to every organ but the spleen. Every sound that we hear affects—to whatever degree—the organs of the body through this nerve. To this, add the effect of heard and unheard sound waves against the entire body.

Resonance is the single most important concept to understand if you are to grasp the constructive or destructive role of sound in your life. Entrainment, sympathetic vibration, resonant frequencies, and resonant systems all fall under the rubric of resonance.

NATURAL AND FORCED RESONANCE

Resonating substances can be divided into two types: those that vibrate at their own characteristic frequencies, their natural frequency, such as tuning forks and bells,* and those that have the ability to resonate at a variety of frequencies. The first is a free or natural resonance; the second is referred to

* Factors such as shape and elasticity have a bearing.

as *forced resonance* because the sounding frequency forces its tone on the resonating body.[7] Paul Hewitt points out that "most things from planets to atoms and almost everything else in between have a springiness to them and vibrate at one or more natural frequencies."[8] Forced resonance is by far the more important of the two for musical purposes.

In listening to music—or, for that matter, any sound—our eardrum (tympanic membrane) responds to the principle of forced resonance. If our ears worked solely to free resonance, then we would hear only certain frequencies that approximate our own.

Many physicists use the example of a child on a swing as an illustration of resonance. The thrust of the pump has to coincide with the natural rhythm of the swing.[9] The trick is in the timing. Pushing or pumping at the wrong time gets the swinger nowhere, but a few well-placed pushes by a parent or friend—at the exact right time—effortlessly propel the child.

On a recent trip to Germany I was taken to the Institute for Stress Research in Berlin. In what was once East Berlin, I met with a physicist who used to work with the Russian space program. Now that he was no longer obligated to the Soviet Union, he was applying his expertise to research into stress. He spoke excitedly to me about the swing-set example and how similar principles were used in the space program. Knowing the ideal moment to apply propulsion, exert pressure, or create release led to optimal results with minimal exertion. His team of researchers now exercises these concepts of resonance in relationship to stress, a malady regarded with utmost seriousness and concern. They call their work Chronobiology, and the major influence they now study is music. These German doctors and physicists believe that with the application of the right music (or musical tones) at precise times of the day—matching the circadian rhythms of the body—they can accomplish tremendous things in the reduction of stress. Like pushing a swing at the exact right moment in the cycle.

Rocket scientists and composers joining forces to create resonant health with quarter notes: The twenty-first century has arrived!

Understanding that all matter vibrates, vibrations have frequency, frequencies produce sounds, and sounds resonate each other propels me into a sonic activism. The more I know about sound, the more I aggressively advocate intentional soundscapes.

ENTRAINMENT

Another fascinating and important aspect of resonance is the process of entrainment. *Entrainment,* in the context of psychoacoustics, concerns changing the rate of brain waves, breaths, or heartbeats from one speed to another. The very sound of the word, *en-train-ment*, implies transportation—to embark on a train. The "train" in this instance is rhythm. Our major body pulses can voluntarily ride periodic rhythms to Fasterville or Slowertown.

The most common example of entrainment is tapping your feet to the external rhythm of music. Just try keeping your foot or your head still when you are around fun, up-tempo rhythms. You will see that it is almost an involuntary motor response. The natural interconnection between the body's motor skills and external rhythms is one of the most highly researched phenomena in the field of rhythmic entrainment. Rhythm is successfully used as a complementary therapeutic technique for stroke patients, as well as for brain injuries, Alzheimer's disease, autism, and more. It has been ventured that one of the reasons for our easy auditory–motor arousal connections may have to do with adaptive evolutionary processes related to survival—fight-or-flight reactions. Michael Thaut, the scientific director of the Center for Biomedical Research in Music (see "Soundwork Resources"), says, "It is well known that the auditory system is an extremely fast processor of sensory information." This is because it must capture and extract meaning from sensory information that comes and goes very quickly. Unless you have a tape recorder at hand, what you hear is gone as soon as the sound waves dissipate. Visually, you can stare at a mountain; you can't freeze-frame a sound. Because of this, continues Thaut, "an interesting dynamic parallel between the temporal nature of auditory information and movement performance arises." This is confirmed in the speed of our reaction to sound. Says Thaut, "Auditory cues create consistently 20–50 milliseconds faster physical reactions than do visual or tactile cues."[10] We respond faster to sound than to sight or touch.

On a lighter level, tapping your feet or bopping your head to external rhythms is just the tip of the iceberg. While your feet might be jitterbugging, your nervous system may be getting a terrible case of the jitters! Rhythmic entrainment is contagious: If the brain doesn't resonate with a rhythm, neither will the breath or heart rate. In this context, rhythm takes on new meanings. Not only is it entertaining, but rhythmic entrainment is a potent sonic tool as well—be it for motor function or other autonomic processes such as brainwave, heart, and breath rates.

The effects of rhythm on the body can be observed in two ways. On an *internal-to-internal* basis, our pulse systems naturally synchronize with each other. The heart rate entrains, or locks in, with the breath rate. If the heart speeds up, it naturally causes the breath to do the same. On an *external-to-internal* basis, our brain waves can be entrained to musical rhythms or the pace of a minister's sermon. In the context of external-to-internal entrainment, sound is the vehicle through which change takes place. Alter one pulse (such as brain waves) with music, and the other major pulses (heart and breath) will dutifully follow.

The focus of this book is the intentional application of music and sound to enhance our daily lives. Therefore, my explorations of entrainment will center on the external-to-internal process in which we use external rhythms to influence the interior landscape.

A generalized scientific definition of *entrainment* is "the effect of one system on another." While the process of entrainment is referred to often in medicine, biology, and other "hard" science disciplines, very little research has been done on the perception of external rhythm by the autonomic nervous system. Psychologists and physiologists rarely consider this—despite the fact that physicists have long known that any atomic matter can be affected by external pulses.

When it comes to the intentional applications of music, the entrainment effect completes the circle of the chain of vibration: atomic matter → vibration → frequency → sound → sympathetic vibration (resonance) → entrainment. *Music alters the performance of the nervous system primarily because of entrainment.*

ENTRAINMENT: RESONATING WITH A RHYTHMIC TWIST

Understanding the interlocking concepts of resonance and entrainment enables us to grasp the way external tone and rhythm can heal or create havoc. Sound affects glass and concrete as well as brain waves, motor response, and organic cells. As I discussed earlier, a structure's resonance may be thought of as that frequency of vibration most natural to it and most easily sustained by it.

Entrainment is part of resonance—but with a twist. There is a subtle but important distinction here. Entrainment is the rhythmic manifestation of resonance. With entrainment, a stronger external pulse does not just activate another pulse but *actually causes the latter to move out of its own resonant frequency to match it.* Entrainment is a classic example of the principle of forced resonance. When you play music at 140 beats per minute and your heart rate increases over time, you are actively changing your frequency.

According to sound researcher Jonathan Goldman: "Resonance is a cooperative phenomenon between two different objects sharing the same frequency." Stimulate the natural vibrations of an object with its own frequency and resonance is set in motion. However, Goldman sees entrainment as the imposition of another frequency onto the weaker vibration. With entrainment, he says, "you are actively changing the vibrations of one object to another rate." Goldman thinks of resonance as passive in nature, while entrainment is active.[11]

The concept of entrainment was first noted in 1665 by Christian Huygens, the Dutch scientist. Huygens noticed that two pendulum clocks, mounted side by side on a wall, would swing together in precise rhythm. They would hold their mutual beat, in fact, far beyond their capacity to be matched in mechanical accuracy. It was as if they *wanted* to keep the same time. Huygens assumed a sort of sympathy between the two of them and conducted experiments to learn just how the interaction took place—whether they were linked through the air or through the wall on which they hung. From his investigations (the pendulums, he found, were synchronized by a slight impulse through the wall) came the first explanation of what scientists were to call "mutual phase-locking of two oscillators" or simply "entrainment."[12]

The scientific explanation for entrainment is that any two vibrating bodies will try to synchronize with each other. Why is that? One theory is that entrainment is nature's form of energy ecology. Scientist Itzhak Bentov, a proponent of this view, says that asteroids and planets are actually rhythm-entrained to the gravitational fields of the sun and other planets. Bentov explains that asteroids, which are minor planets, actually develop resonances in their orbits as a reaction to the combined gravitational pull of nearby planets and the sun; they "must dance to the tune of two masters."[13] He continues, "It seems that nature finds it more economical in terms of energy to have periodic events that are close enough in frequency to occur in phase or in step with each other. This is the meaning of rhythm entrainment."[14]

External periodic rhythms—*periodic* defined as "regular" or "ongoing"—cause our major body pulses to change. In the case of two tuning forks tuned to different pitches, one fork cannot entrain the other; the density of the metal will not allow it. But the more mutable rhythms of nature are very entrainable. This includes human rhythms. We pulse, vibrate, and resonate; these are perfect materials for entrainment. Resonant entrainment of oscillating systems is a well-understood principle within the physical sciences. And because human bodies are oscillators—moving in a periodic, repetitive fashion between two points of rest—the laws of entrainment apply.

F. Holmes Atwater, a scientific investigator, behavioral engineer, and consultant with The Monroe Institute, posits three basic rules of the physics of entrainment:

1. *The resonance rule.* For one system to entrain another, the second system must be capable of achieving the same vibratory rate. In other words, a human being could not entrain with a rock—but he or she would entrain with another person.
2. *The power rule.* For one system to entrain with another, the first must have sufficient power to overcome the second. Therefore, proximity is an important consideration. If the systems are far away from each other, the power is diminished with distance.
3. *The consistency rule.* For one system to be capable of entraining another, the first must be at a constant frequency or amplitude. This is where periodicity comes into play: Rhythms must be constant and regular.[15]

RHYTHM, THE PULSE OF LIFE

Rhythm, or periodic movement, is an integral part of life. It determines if sound is a beat or a tone; it provides the contours of speech and melody. In the case of energy, sound, and light frequencies, the rhythm of the waveform distinguishes each.

Rhythm means many different things. To a musician, it is a tool to mark time. To a doctor, the periodic pulse of the heart or brain determines the health of the patient. To an astronomer, planetary gravity fields are critical in the planets' interrelationships. And to the mother and unborn child, rhythms of breath and blood flow provide the womb sounds with which they bond and the baby forms.

Without rhythm there would be no life. While this is a broad and simple statement, its truth is absolute. Nature could not exist without its interdependent as well as independent rhythms. The dance of day and night, summer and winter, outward blossoms and inward renourishment—graceful acts of balance, all. Too much rain and we flood. Too much sun and we bake. Can you imagine the ebb and flow of the ocean wave if the rhythm of balance went awry?

The independence and interdependence of the multiple rhythms of the human body are vital: molecular rhythms, action potentials, cardiovascular and respiratory patterns, even the monthly cycles of menstruation and pregnancy. These are examples of the internal periodicity carried on against the external rhythmic clocks and calendars of seconds, years, and millennia.

From the orbit of stars down to that of an electron in an atom, *periodic rhythm*—the activity of something occurring in cycles—is considered a stable and good thing. It is common knowledge that arrhythmias in the heart, in a planet's rotation, or in a global weather pattern are cause for tremendous concern. Erratic rhythms are highly problematic because they offset the consistency necessary for interdependence to take place. The planet and its people do better with stable, periodic rhythms—internally and externally.

Fortunately, periodic rhythms are everywhere. In water, air, solid matter, and organic life cells, vibrations are twirling, pulsing, pushed, and pulled with an ongoing, steady tempo. Anything that vibrates is susceptible to the influence of the external rhythms around it. This is what makes entrainment so powerful.

COMMON APPLICATIONS OF
RHYTHMIC ENTRAINMENT

Strong communication between individuals or among groups may cause entrainment of brain waves. This can sometimes be seen between professors and students, preachers and congregations, and therapists and clients. Audiences entrain to performers, while marching teams and choir members entrain to their compatriots. Other examples of entrainment can be seen in flocks of migrating birds flapping in rhythm and gliding at the same time, fireflies blinking together, college roommates having similar menstrual cycles, and lovers sharing a synchronized heartbeat as they move closer together.

Individually, we entrain to the rhythms around us, be they ocean waves, music, the periodic sounds of machines, or electromagnetic frequency fields. Some nonperiodic rhythmic elements such as traffic, however, do the opposite of entrainment. They jangle our nervous systems, because the brain tries to categorize them. It is looking for the periodicity, or regularity, of the traffic patterns. When it cannot find this neat, organized auditory tonal processing, it acts like a hard drive that can't find a file: It just keeps on searching. This prevents the brain from paying full attention to other sequential functions, such as concentration.

Because we lack full awareness of the effects of all such external rhythms on our systems, our urban sonic environments are generally not the most conducive to health or productivity. Indeed, there are very few places—outside our own homes or cars—where particular attention is given to the rhythms that surround us. The goal of this book is to equip you with the knowledge to create your own healthy sonic environments.

CONCLUSION

Resonance can be thought of in terms of tone: *What is the effect of one pitch on another?* Entrainment is essentially the resonance of rhythm: *What is the effect of external rhythms on our internal rhythms?* Using both tone and rhythm gives us naturally effective, inexpensive tools. The conscious use of rhythm can alter major body pulses, allowing us to be in states most conducive to specific activities. Whether mental productivity, emotional release, or physical sleep is your goal, rhythm is a noninvasive way to wind up or lay back. If you feel out of sync, rhythm can help you find your center and begin again.

After I concluded a recent lecture in Germany, I was approached by a woman with a very worried tone in her voice. She asked if I wasn't concerned about the misuse of the power of resonance and entrainment. This is a reasonable concern, especially coming from a region where sound was used by Hitler to manipulate the psyche. My response to her concern was that any element can be misused or abused. Unlike processes in the motor system, which can be therapeutically aided by external rhythm, however, many other physiological processes cannot be entrained as effectively by external sensory stimuli. According to Dr. Thaut, there is probably a very good protective reason why other cyclical physiological processes (autonomic processes such as heart rate) have only very limited capacity to entrain to external rhythmic cues.[16] If this were not the case, anyone exposed to fast rhythms for a long period would suffer from an overexcited pulse system and drop in his or her tracks. We know that this does not happen.

Look at the example of a dance club or disco. Depending on your mood and state of health, fast and loud rhythms will do one of two things to you—either energize you to dance up a frenzy, sweat a lot, and release endorphins from the exercise or give you a headache or stomachache and ringing in the ears from overstimulation of the auditory system. You can choose either to stay and be exposed to loud, fast music or to leave. The body has an inherent wisdom that was originally smart enough to grow from two tiny cells. The built-in protective mechanism that I mentioned previously is there to keep your autonomic nervous system somewhat sheltered from external influences. This does not mean that rhythmic entrainment cannot penetrate; what it means is that some things influence you on a gross level, others more subtly. Music, sound, resonance, entrainment: subtle influences with powerful possibilities.

Resonance, in all its forms, is the overarching theme of all sound technologies intended to affect your psyche and body. Whether simple or complex, binaural beat frequencies, Tomatis-oriented filtration and gating techniques, pitch, timbre, lyrics, or rhythms . . . their effect is based on how they vibrate your nervous system.

5 Frequency Medicine: The Work of Alfred Tomatis

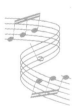 Any discussion of the effects of sound would be noticeably incomplete without an exploration of the work of Dr. Alfred Tomatis, the leading figure in the field of therapeutic music and sound. Some would call him an ear specialist, but Tomatis is really a frequency researcher, working in the subtle yet powerful domain of vibration and resonance. He prescribes sound frequencies in lieu of pharmaceuticals. His sonic solutions consist of specially reinforced and filtered music and sounds. Most impressive of all, the results achieved by hundreds of busy Tomatis Listening and Learning Centers around the world are startling!

The name *Tomatis* may someday be a household word like Schweitzer, Freud, or Jung. Over the last fifty years, this French surgeon, ENT specialist, psychologist, and inventor has developed a method of retraining the muscles of the middle ear through noninvasive listening techniques. This is so innocent-sounding that it is enough to elicit a yawn. But to those who have suffered from the debilitating effects of learning disabilities, autism, depression, chronic fatigue, or immune system disorders—or for anyone who wants to learn foreign languages faster, communicate better, or improve creativity and on-the-job performance—Tomatis is a lifesaver.

Dr. Timothy Gilmor is a Toronto psychologist who has been actively involved in Tomatis research, evaluation, and clinical application since 1979. Paul Madaule—who with Gilmor founded the Listening Centre—was diagnosed as dyslexic at an early age. He made a remarkable recovery with the help of Dr. Tomatis and went on to become a Tomatis practitioner who has helped thousands of people. In their book *About the Tomatis Method*, Gilmor and Madaule state, "This Method provides a comprehensive approach to communication, language, and the learning process which is based on listening. Dr. Tomatis defines listening chiefly as a process of focusing the ear."[1]*

Tomatis's basic premise is that the primary function of the ear is not communication but, rather, to charge the brain's neocortex with the electrical impulses of sound. He also discovered we can give voice to only the sounds we can hear. If we retrain the way we hear, the result, in simple terms, is a refurnishing of the brain with missing frequencies. These frequency deficiencies are often the root cause of many life-robbing afflictions.

According to Tomatis, the ear is the first fully functioning sensory organ in a fetus; it begins charging the brain—thereby *growing* the brain—by week eighteen in utero. Tomatis also came to understand that we perceive sound in many ways. Not only do we hear with our ears through air conduction, but we hear through bone conduction as well. Tomatis makes the distinction that the ear is not differentiated skin—rather, the skin is differentiated ear. In other words, we hear with the whole body.[2]

* I'm extremely grateful for the investigative work of Paul Madaule in relation to the effects of the Tomatis Method for musicians. As a Frenchman and Tomatis colleague, fully versed in both language and practice, Mr. Madaule compiled and translated numerous writings by Tomatis concerning the subject. It appears as a chapter, "The Tomatis Method for Singers and Musicians," in his book *About the Tomatis Method*. Prior to Madaule's work, none of this information was available in English.

THE EAR IN UTERO

Tomatis discovered that the ear is functioning four and a half months before birth, and that listening is the first sense we develop. Intermixed with the organic sounds of a mother's heartbeat, circulation, gastrointestinal rumblings, and breath, the unborn child distinctly hears the mother's voice through the fluids of the amniotic sac. Researchers have verified that long before infants speak, they recognize sounds heard prenatally.

Tomatis has stated that while in the womb, the higher frequencies of the mother's voice actually nourish the fetus. A pattern establishes itself very early—waiting for this sound, being gratified when it comes, waiting, being gratified, and so on—a process Tomatis calls the uterine dialogue. It is with this process that listening begins, and it carries on into childhood. The later development of communication skills, language, learning ability, and (in particular) social adjustment depends on the quality of this early listening. But for a variety of reasons, such listening can be obscured, impaired, or shut down altogether. The Tomatis Method presents a means of retrieving the "open" listening that is our birthright.[3]

If we are robbed of the ability to communicate easily, then learning impairment and social maladjustment are likely. It is well known that learning disabilities are prevalent in the American prison population. Given that methods of early detection and correction of learning disabilities have been inadequate, is it possible that children from stressed or difficult pregnancies who did not establish the "loop of gratification" fall through the cracks? If indeed the seeds of social behavior are planted in utero, is it any wonder, then, that given the current high percentage of disintegrating family units, we are seeing gangs, violence, and illness like never before?

What does Dr. Tomatis suggest we do to remedy this? "I do not treat the children who are brought to me," he says; "I awaken them." He believes that it is a problem not of *hearing* but of *listening*. While there may be physiological problems that hinder the ability to focus on sounds, the Tomatis Method concentrates on the numerous psychological and social factors that bear on listening, including the family system and emotional background. According to Gilmor, "A child with a reading problem very often presents myriad other difficulties such as short attention span, poor concentration, weakness in oral language, poorly articulated speech, poor vocabulary. Such children are also often immature, with a poor self-concept and sense of self-confidence. They have difficulty adjusting socially to their families and peer groups. Many of these problems affect adults as well."

Listening-related difficulties in children and adults often manifest in diminished learning, speech, language, or communication skills. Difficulty with attention and musicality may also result from listening-related problems.

The Tomatis Method is currently used in more than 250 centers and schools across Europe and North America. Children as well as adults access this revolutionary process of auditory refocusing. Both educational and emotional imbalances are addressed through the unlikely portal of the ear with the music of Mozart. How did this unlikely process come about? The story begins in Paris in the 1940s.

A BRIEF HISTORY

Alfred Tomatis was born in Nice, France, on New Year's Day 1920. His sixteen year-old mother did not carry the pregnancy with pride. To the contrary, she went to much trouble to prevent her pregnancy from being noticed. Consequently, Tomatis was born two and a half months early.

"It is useless to bother with him, he's dead," were the first words spoken when he was born. Three-pound Alfred was discarded in a basket, left to perish. Had it not been for his paternal grandmother—who had borne twenty-four children herself—Tomatis would have died. The rough start with his mother plagued their relationship for the course of her full life. Fortunately, Tomatis had a strong, loving relationship with his father, Umberto, who was a successful opera singer.

A very sickly child, Tomatis was affected by one particular doctor who was called on to treat him. When faced with a tricky diagnosis, this doctor exclaimed, "I don't know what is wrong with him. I must search for the answer." This level of dedication so impressed the young Tomatis that he decided to become a doctor himself and to search for what he did not know. Unbelievable as it may sound, Umberto Tomatis procured an apartment for his eleven-year-old son. Living completely alone, Tomatis began his studies in Paris. At age nineteen, while a first-year medical student, he was drafted into the French army. The year was 1939. He completed his medical studies in wartime hospitals and clinics and began his first civilian practice in 1945 at the age of twenty-five.[4]

Tomatis's early-childhood experiences motivated and defined his lifework. The trauma of his birth led to his exploration of the critical role of sound in the development of the unborn child. His struggle with his mother brought him to understand the lifetime effect of the mother's voice on the fetus and young child. And as the son of a widely acclaimed opera singer, Tomatis was drawn to applying his theories to musicians.

Umberto Tomatis sent many distressed musical colleagues to his young son, Alfred, the new ear, nose, and throat doctor in Paris. After long operatic careers, these singers were experiencing difficulty staying on pitch or producing certain sounds. In the 1940s the standard prescription for most singers' problems was to treat the larynx with strychnine. Tomatis initially followed this procedure but with no success. In a fit of frustration, he administered the same audiometer tests he had used with munitions factory workers after World War II. To his amazement, he discovered that both singers and arsenal workers showed diminished hearing at the same frequency level. Clearly, the factory workers' occupational deafness could be attributed to long-term exposure to violently loud explosions. The singers, however, were surrounded by the beautiful sounds of arias and orchestras. Yet the audiometric curves of both groups were stunningly similar and perplexing.

To gather additional information, Tomatis actively sought out and examined as many singers and musicians as he could. A surprising correlation emerged: The amount of time a singer had practiced was directly proportional to the amount of damage to the ear. This manifested in the inability of the singer to hear certain frequencies. It appeared that the longer a singer was at the profession, the worse his or her hearing became. Tomatis's observations were impossible to ignore. Prominent singers were damaging their hearing with the sounds of their own voices!

These findings flew in the face of conventional wisdom, and Tomatis suffered scathing criticism from his medical peers. It was commonly believed that a singer's volume reached no more than a gentle 80 dB; certainly no harm could come to a singer from his own voice. But Tomatis's audiograms were irrefutable—the opera singers and munition workers both suffered from high-volume occupational hazards.

Faced with this anomaly, Tomatis said, "I did what all researchers do: I ignored all previous discoveries and started from scratch." Again employing a sonometer—the audiometric tool he had used in the munition factories—Tomatis was able to measure the intensity of sound. To his amazement, he found that professional singers were putting out 80 dB at only half strength! At full vocal power, they could emit between 110 and 140 dB. Tomatis noted that "130 decibels represents 150 decibels inside one's skull. By comparison, a jet engine registers only 132 decibels on the ground." He points out that these figures are all the more extraordinary because decibels are logarithmic—that is, 90 dB is ten times louder than 80 dB. "Though the energy of a singer is not comparable to that of a jet engine," he says, "the intensity of the sound is the same."[5]

While conventional medicine treated pitch difficulties as the result of an overstretched larynx, Tomatis came to see that the problem was in the ear itself. Opera singers were going partially or fully deaf due to the excessive volume of their own sounds. He reasoned that "if they were singing poorly, it was because they were hearing poorly. Because of this, they were no longer able to control themselves. . . . To sing well, the subject must have a special perception of the sound being produced. The poor quality of this 'self-listening' was responsible for everything." Based on this belief, Tomatis abandoned the prevailing theory that the larynx was the primary instrument of singing; rather, he came to see the ear as "the fundamental instrument of utterance."

Tomatis became so adroit at the interpretation of audiometrics that he could pinpoint the range of frequency loss in a subject's hearing by that person's inability to produce sounds in the corresponding frequency range. At this point, Tomatis formulated a concept that was to become the cornerstone for all his subsequent discoveries: "A person can only reproduce vocally what he is capable of hearing." Put more simply, and as Tomatis prefers to say, "One sings with one's ear."

THE NECESSITY OF SELF-LISTENING

Tomatis's breakthrough was to link the psyche to the ability to hear. Not hearing because of difficulty in listening is universally applicable. It seems that the quality of our self-listening determines the quality of our existence on all levels. We cannot reproduce a note that we cannot hear; it follows that if we cannot hear ourselves, we cannot authentically present ourselves to the rest of the world.

Tomatis maintains that sound is a vital nutrient for our nervous systems. As unborn babies, vulnerable children, or sensitive adults, we unknowingly have the psychological capacity to slowly block out sounds that are displeasing, offensive, or hurtful. This damping is manifested physiologically by a relaxation of the tiny muscles of the middle ear. The net result is a diminution of our ability to hear specific frequency ranges corresponding to the sounds we essentially lock out. This survival mechanism is available to us all, and in most instances we use it unconsciously.

THE TOMATIS METHOD:
FOCUSED LISTENING

The Tomatis Method—consisting of sound stimulation, audiovocal activities, and consultations with a trained professional—can be used to enhance abilities or overcome problems that are listening related.[6] The goal of the method is to achieve the ideal listening ear. Retraining the auditory mechanism of the middle ear may result in focused listening skills.

The retraining is accomplished by listening to specially filtered recordings of up-tempo Mozart and, if possible, the recorded sound of the mother's voice. These sounds come through earphones that have been modified to deliver through bone conduction as well as through air conduction—the ear. (In addition to the two transducers for the ears, a third transducer is placed either on top of the head or behind the lower right ear, pressing against the occipital bone of the head.) The special music, the client's own voice, and Gregorian chants are fed through a Tomatis invention known as the Electronic Ear (EE). At the heart of the method, the EE is a device connected to tape cassettes or CD players that allow frequencies of 16,000 to 20,000 Hz to be heard.

Drs. Billie Thompson of Arizona and Susan Andrews of Louisiana are part of a small group of Americans who have been trained by Dr. Tomatis. Thompson comes from an educational background; Andrews had clinical expertise in developmental neuropsychology. Individually, they recognized the intrinsic value of sound stimulation auditory training. After a decade of working with the Tomatis Method in separate listening centers, they describe the function of the Electronic Ear as follows: "The EE can filter recordings of music and voice, and the sound travels through two channels, with different settings. A gating mechanism alternates the sound between the channels when it reaches a specific intensity. The EE is designed to educate the ear to its full functions as a receptor, a mechanism to make subtle discriminations, and an energy generator. The right ear is trained to be the leading or dominant ear, to make for the most efficient processing of speech directly by the speech center in the left hemisphere of the brain."[7]

Through highly specific filters and gating mechanisms, the sounds of the Tomatis Method tonify the muscles and bones of the middle ear, thereby enhancing the ability to focus auditorily. Tomatis believes that "focused listening" is a state preferable to "passive hearing." Hearing is different from listening just as casual looking contrasts with actively seeing.

According to Thompson and Andrews, "Hearing is the passive reception of sound, while listening is the active motivated tuning in and tuning out at choice. Good listening results in well-organized auditory processing and vestibular control of information. Listening plays the fundamental role in processing all language information. The motivational and emotional need for communication begins with listening." Without easy communication, our lives, and those around us, suffer.

Beginning with a battery of diagnostic procedures consisting of listening tests and interviews with certified Tomatis practitioners, a typical application of the method involves sixty to seventy-five hours of listening, in daily sessions of one to two and a half hours.

First intensive: Two full weeks of listening.
Three to six weeks off.

Second intensive: One full week of listening.
Three to six weeks off.
Third intensive: One full week of listening.

The time off between the three listening intensives allows the client the necessary space to experience, integrate, and habituate the new listening patterns.[8] The program is highly individualized and flexible, with the length of each phase and daily listening determined by the client's goals and progress. Both counseling and specialized listening tests note the changes in ear, psyche, and body. According to Dr. Thompson, the listening test has parameters and protocols different from those of standard audiology hearing tests. The Tomatis listening test charts air, bone, and spatial perception of sound. Its specific purpose is to assist the practitioner in determining how to work with the client using the Tomatis Method.

There are five basic phases to the method, three considered passive, the other two active. Simply put, the passive phases consist of listening to music and sound with increasing amounts of filtering and processing by the Electronic Ear, then a decreasing of the same process. The purpose is to adjust to the presentation of filtered sound on a gradual basis, develop the focusing response, and stimulate the desire to communicate. Additionally, a "sonic birth" is replicated in order to simulate the transition from the liquid prenatal acoustic environment to the airy postnatal acoustic environment.

In the passive phases, the individual merely listens to sound. In the active phases, the individual participates more fully in the sound training process. This is done by humming, singing, reading aloud, and repeating specific sentences through a microphone into the Electronic Ear. These sounds are then fed back to the ears via earphones. The purpose, according to Gilmor, is to introduce spoken language in the prelinguistic and linguistic stages. Depending on the individual, the tones of the voice may be filtered and gated in the same way that the music was in the passive phases. Additionally, increased stimulation is given to the right ear in order to enhance its dominance: Right-ear dominance is a preferred state for audiovocal control.

Dr. Tomatis believes that music and vocal sounds rich in high frequencies have an energizing effect. This corresponds to the effect of the mother's voice on the development of the fetal nervous system. What the unborn child hears are the highest frequencies of the mother's voice, which nourish the fetus in the womb. Consequently, high frequencies still affect us as adults. This is why filtered audiotapes are the backbone of the listening training process. These recordings have all but the high end of sound rolled off; the net effect is listening to the ghost of a musical phrase, replaced with the sounds of sibilants.

One of the foundation concepts of the Tomatis Method is a hypothesis known as the Tomatis Effect, independently confirmed at the Sorbonne in 1957. This effect holds that the voice can produce only what the ear can hear. Therefore, if I sing off-key or speak in a flat, monotone voice, chances are I am unable to hear specific frequency ranges. Thompson and Andrews state, "Two corollaries to the Tomatis Effect led to the development of the Tomatis Method: 1) if the sounds are restored to the ear, they will be immediately restored to the voice, and 2) with sufficient conditioning of one's ear to one's own voice heard with good quality, the changes can be maintained and strengthened."

Additionally, just as there are "charging" sounds that energize the nervous system, there are "discharging" sounds that tend to weaken and fatigue it. Tomatis believes high-frequency sounds—the overtones of music and the voice—energize because of the preponderance of specific cells in the inner-ear membrane that respond to high tones by sending electrical impulses to the brain. Indeed, the number of nerve cells in the cochlea that respond to high-frequency sounds is four times greater than those stimulated by sounds of under 3,000 Hz.[9]

Consequently, an abundance of lower bass tones may actually have the effect of overwhelming the system to the point of overload, causing mental and physical fatigue. Overwhelming low bass tones are a modern-day phenomenon, a result of improvements in amplifiers and sound systems. Prior to this, bass tones (long sound waves) in an open performance context had room to breathe, so to speak. This is very different from the effect of "boom cars" and small performance venues filled with large bass speakers.

The Tomatis Method is a powerfully effective process for change. Learning disabilities, depression, and immune disorders are not the only reasons people seek out Tomatis practitioners. Some go to correct a stutter, others to improve public speaking. Actors and musicians seek improved vocal and pitch control. Many have learned that foreign-language acquisition is a matter of retraining the ear. As public awareness of Tomatis's concepts grows, people are using this sonic process for reasons other than "fixing." Increasing numbers come to Tomatis for productivity enhancement or consciousness exploration.

It is odd to think that the ear and how we hear form a psychological portrait of our lives. Yet through the Tomatis tests, an experienced practitioner can tell which year you might have been sick, separated from a parent, incurred physical or emotional trauma, and much more. As amazing as it sounds, our emotional histories are reflected in our individual frequency spectrums.

The effects of deeper internal listening are uncharted. It seems remarkable that many problems and disabilities can be dissipated by listening to a full spectrum of sound. Yet in my own Tomatis experience, this has been the case.

DR. RON MINSON— A HEALER FOR THE FUTURE

I came from a household with a controlling, angry, and verbally abusive father. He traveled often, but when he was home, he yelled at his family a lot. As a child I learned essentially to tune him out. While I minimized the impact of his verbal assaults through the first part of my life, I have paid an adult price within my auditory system because of it.

I was lucky enough to meet Dr. Ron Minson in Denver, Colorado. Dr. Minson, a board-certified psychiatrist, had spent twenty-five years directing behavioral and therapeutic activities for major medical institutions, consulting for mental health organizations, and maintaining a large private practice. But when his adopted daughter became deeply despondent over the burden of learning disabilities and lifelong depression, Minson found his tools unable to quell her rapid and life-threatening decline.

Minson's daughter was suffering from symptoms endemic to some adopted children. According to Tomatis, when a baby is separated from its mother, the vital sound connection between the pair is severed. While outer nutrition can be supplied elsewhere, this sonic lifeline is a critical biological connection. Sometimes aural transference to another mother can take place; often it doesn't. Tomatis speaks of the *uterine dialogue*—a post-birth sonic connection between mother and child that has a tremendous effect on the psychological outreach of a newborn. These early tendencies to either reach out or pull in can then manifest throughout life, in learning disabilities, for instance, depression, poor self-esteem, or unstable health.[10]

In his quest for an effective treatment for his beloved daughter, Dr. Minson came across the Tomatis Method. He and his daughter simultaneously went through the process with Dr. Thompson at her Sound Listening and Learning Center in Phoenix, Arizona. Both daughter and father experienced such dramatic positive results that Minson shuttered his practice, hurriedly learned French, and went to Paris to study directly with Dr. Tomatis. On returning to Denver, Minson set up a Tomatis Listening Center in 1990.

As is so often the case with alternative therapies, the going was slow in the beginning for the new clinic. But as word spread of the success of its treatment programs, Dr. Minson's Center for InnerChange began to boom. A more gentle and respectful environment would be hard to find. Minson's marriage of traditional Western medicine with the breakthrough technology of the Tomatis Method and other modalities is not only effective but also, indeed, exemplary.

TURNING MY WORLD ON ITS EAR

When I underwent the Tomatis Method, my listening tests showed severe dips in the 1,500 Hz range. (Listening tests are conducted every four or five days to chart the progress of the Tomatis Method. Necessary sound processing changes—more or less filtration; quicker or slower amplitude gating—with music and voice are made based on these tests and on interviews with attending therapists.)

Among other things, this range corresponds to the frequency of an adult male voice. Not only had I auditorily locked out my father, but I had also shut down my ability to clearly hear anyone or anything in his range.

As I review my childhood and adult years, a long history of difficulties with male authority figures emerges as a significant pattern affecting decisions and choices. It stands to reason that not only could I not hear others in this adult male range, but that I have also had a problem hearing my own voice—literally and metaphorically.

By the end of the Tomatis program—and as my listening tests showed—the hearing dip at 1,500 Hz was basically gone. Since I've completed the method, I find that relating to my elderly father is no longer a problem. For the first time, I feel I can hear what he is saying when he speaks. Also, I notice that I now crave contact with male friends. And I am hearing myself more clearly than ever. This manifests as greatly increased clarity in professional and personal choices.

At the center, one of the things I hoped to remedy was a tendency to sing off-key in a certain range. As a musician, not to be able to hold pitch embarrassed me greatly. I had even stopped singing. What I didn't know was that I didn't hear the notes in this range because I had shut down that part of the frequency spectrum. After completing the method, I find my pitch is much improved; finding the time to sing may be my only remaining challenge.

Ostensibly, I came to the program out of professional curiosity. In truth, I was looking to see if this cutting-edge concept would help me break tired patterns—balance all my fairly common hang-ups. After some seventy-five hours on the Electronic Ear, I came out a changed man. Yes, I still have challenges, but something inextricably moved. Increased concentration, improved pitch, better memory, stronger language skills, and enhanced dexterity just scratch the surface of what I have experienced as the result of the method. Certainly after mainlining high-frequency matrices directly into my brain, I would expect greater mental agility. But to me, the real goods lie deeper. It has been five years now since I completed the program, and I am still awed by the depth to which this work goes. I don't think you ever *finish* Tomatis work, for it is actually a retooling of the human mechanism. Poor listening can begin at any age and for any number of reasons—major lifestyle disruption, extreme stress, a health problem, an accident. Auditory retraining and sound stimulation are ongoing tools for staying healthy and centered.

The Tomatis work has changed the way that I listen. And *listening—*

in the Tomatis context—refers to how I process the sonic nutrients around me and how I listen to myself. I am not referring to increased intuition, awareness of long-buried feelings, or receptivity to channeled beings from Mars. Rather, I refer simply to how I listen.

My inner and outer ears are now attuned in such a way that I notice *hearing* the energy behind words, feelings, and sounds. I have always been sensitive, but this is a quantum leap in perception. The power of the subtlety is immense. And the beauty of this process is that the more I listen to myself, the easier it is for me to really hear the truth of things. This sonic energy somehow allows a painless detachment to take place. I don't have to process my "stuff" inside and out. It seems that by hearing a fuller spectrum of sound, I can now hear a fuller spectrum of my internal engines. Thankfully, some of the things that used to be terribly painful in my life no longer hold such a charge.

By the nature of the modality of vibrational healing, subtle and obvious changes go hand in hand. All physical matter resonates, so using sound to reharmonize our systems is logical. There are still many things not understood about the medium and its varied effects, but its results are irrefutable—whether or not we rationally understand every detail.

Tomatis laid the theoretical foundation on which the emerging field of soundwork rests. His concepts and theories cause us to reconsider the awesome power of music and sound.

For more information on this pioneer, see appendix D, "Tomatis: Revising the Map of the Musician's Odyssey." Included are five interviews with musicians about their Tomatis experiences and the ensuing impact on their creative work.

6 Neurodevelopmental Auditory Training: The Work of Robert J. Doman Jr.

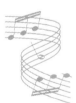 Robert Doman Jr. works with children and adults who have special needs. Crisscrossing America, sometimes three hundred days a year, he evaluates clients with neurodevelopmental problems. Sound stimulation, nutrition, movement, visual perceptual training, speech and language, and education are vital components of Bob Doman's eclectic and highly effective treatment programs.

Since the 1970s, Doman has become an internationally recognized educator and lecturer in neurodevelopmental programs. He is also the founder (in 1979) and director of the National Academy for Child Development (NACD), headquartered in Ogden, Utah. NACD is an international organization of parents and professionals dedicated to helping infants, children, and adults reach their full potential through home programs. Clients served by NACD arrive with labels including learning disabled, dyslexic, distractible, ADD, ADHD, hyperactive, Down syndrome, fetal alcohol syndrome, Williams syndrome, Tourette's syndrome, Rett syndrome, fragile X, developmentally delayed, pervasive developmental disorder, autistic, cerebral palsy, brain-injured, comatose, retarded, minimal brain dysfunction, normal, accelerated, and gifted. Families have traveled to NACD locations from all fifty states as well as Europe, Asia, Africa, South America, Australia, and Canada. Doman has personally designed individual home-based neurodevelopmental programs for more than twenty thousand infants, children, and adults. (See "Soundwork Resources" for more information.)

Robert J. Doman Jr. grew up in a family deeply committed to the treatment of neurodevelopmental problems. His father received his medical degree in 1946 with a specialty in physical medicine and rehabilitation. Dr. Doman Sr. served in many directorial capacities throughout his forty-year medical career, including director of the Center for Neurological Rehabilitation in Morton, Pennsylvania, and medical director of United Cerebral Palsy of Delaware County, Pennsylvania. He held positions with more than twenty other hospitals and rehabilitation facilities.

Upon rejoining his son in 1986 and becoming the medical director of NACD, Robert J. Doman Sr. wrote: "The National Academy for Child Development speaks of persons who ineffectively pass through or miss critical developmental brain levels as being neurologically dysorganized. This simply means they have a brain which is inefficient in its ability to receive, process, store and utilize information. Depending on which level or levels of the brain are involved, the individual may exhibit a number of problems in areas of learning, socializing and behaving."[1]

A child with a severe condition needs to be treated in the home on an ongoing basis. Consequently, families come for Bob Doman and his staff's evaluations, taking his training and programs back home. Working with seriously impaired clients, Doman is sensitive to the sober business of small and fragile bodies and the determined hearts of loving caretakers. A consistently large global client base attests to the success of his eclectic programs, which ignore diagnostic labels and instead implement alternative therapeutic prescriptions.

Bob Doman learned at his father's knee and continued to develop his own theories and innovate new treatments. As a second-generation neurodevelopmental specialist, Doman believes that sound is integral to the therapeutic process. How did this come to be? In his own words, Bob Doman explains the genesis of his groundbreaking work.

THE STORY OF DAWN

"It is said that one learns from his failures. At one point in my career, I had the opportunity to learn from some of the most magnificent of human beings I am sure I will ever meet. These people, these children, were the living, breathing (though not always satisfactorily) failures of the entire profession dealing with hurt children.

"In 1971 my position was that of clinical director of United Cerebral Palsy of Delaware County, Pennsylvania. This old Victorian building, located on a hill surrounded by four acres of rolling grounds, was the site of my education. UCP also ran the George Crothers Memorial School a few miles away, where I had spent the previous three years developing some of my educational and behavioral principles and techniques. As clinical director, I was responsible for the team of therapists and therapy programs carried out with each of the children in the school, as well as the academic programs.

"My learning experience as clinical director began on my first day in my new position. This experience, as well as many others, arrived in the form of a problem. This particular problem involved a severely brain-injured child named Dawn. Dawn had just entered her teenage years and was a lovely, blond, warm, loving, and happy child. Dawn also weighed only about thirty pounds. On a good day she could move some facial muscles and turn her head slightly. Dawn's immediate problem was that she had stopped breathing on several occasions. On that particular day, the staff was afraid to touch her for fear that it would happen again. They all felt that Dawn should be taken home until she was breathing better. Or until . . .

"I already knew Dawn's history because I had spent hours reviewing the children's charts prior to my first day as director. Reviewing histories of severely brain-injured children and their families is always a sobering experience, but Dawn's had been one not to forget. Dawn had been born a brain-injured child. Her parents eventually found their way to the Institutes for the Achievement of Human Potential, where she received a full program and made fantastic progress. At five Dawn could walk, looked beautiful, seemed healthy, and was obviously on her way toward becoming 'normal.' Evidently, not all miracles are meant to be, because after working so hard and doing so well, Dawn fell victim to encephalitis. Not once, but twice, leaving her severely brain-injured. The program was tried again, but this time without much success. She then made the tour of surgeons and specialists, finally arriving at UCP for what was termed a maintenance program. A maintenance program meant failure. Not the child's failure, for Dawn never failed, but our failure—the world's failure. When everything the world knows has been tried without success, there is nothing to do but try to maintain the child's condition, and wait. And hope that you, or someone, will find something to help the child.

"On the particular day while Dawn was having the difficulty, I was fortunate, because the medical director was in the building examining children. The founder and medical director of UCP was also a cofounder and medical director of the Institutes for the Achievement of Human Potential, the founder and director of the Center for Neurological Rehabilitation, the holder of many awards and certificates, and one of the few physiatrists (a physician with specialization and certification in physical medicine and rehabilitation) in the nation. He was also my father and my mentor.

"That day when I presented the medical director with the problem, I received a reply that I have heard in various forms many times since. 'Dawn is a severely brain-injured child. With what we know today, she is one of the few whom we are failing, and when we fail severely hurt children, they do die. They cannot breathe, they cannot digest or properly metabolize their food, their circulation is poor, and their sensory channels are often so involved that they cannot even perceive the world in which they live. They die, because they starve. Their brains are starved for information. They need stimulation.' When a child is doing poorly, she doesn't need less, she needs more, and it was our job to see that Dawn received it.

"I spent most of the rest of that day on the floor with Dawn. At first she was white as a sheet, and her breathing was so irregular and shallow that it could have easily stopped completely if Dawn had let it. She didn't. For perhaps the first half hour I just sat and watched her struggle to breathe, her tiny body rigid and her blue eyes closed in a half sleep, half coma. After that, I started to whisper to her and gently stroked and squeezed her arms and legs, without receiving any signs of response. Then I rubbed and squeezed harder. I turned on sound-effect records of jets and trains; turned on all the lights; turned off all the lights; put the most horrible odors I could find under her nose and the most obnoxious tastes into her mouth. I rolled her and turned her and whispered softly into her ear. Gradually, her color got a little better and her breathing became deeper. I could see some flicker of recognition in her eyes. Toward the end of the day her mouth twitched and her eyes opened. This time bright and alert, she broke out with the most beautiful smile I have ever seen—and a long healthy moan.

"Five or six times a day after that I would come down to see Dawn and we would talk, or at least I would talk, and Dawn would react with a combination of sounds and expressions that could communicate all her feelings.

"I learned a lot from Dawn. She gave real meaning to many of the concepts that my father and uncle had developed and utilized to develop a treatment philosophy for brain-injured children. Dawn taught me that even the most severely impaired child can be bright. In fact, very bright. Dawn taught me the fantastic need for stimulation to sustain life itself. But perhaps most of all, she taught me that within those incredible bodies lie real people. Loving, giving human beings who can give so much without even speaking a word. Real people that we must never give up on, and for whom we must always search for new answers."

SENSORY STIMULATION

Bob Doman continues, "That night after spending the day with Dawn, I stayed awake, designing a program and designing a new environment for Dawn, as well as other children in her group, and for our children in preschool programs.

"Designing a program for severely brain-injured children in a clinical or school setting is extremely difficult. There are just not enough hours and enough one-to-one time to really do the job that needs to be done for these children. In a clinical setting there is the problem of staff. Staff who must be paid. At UCP I had three children for each staff member on a good day, when there were also volunteers, and five children per staff member on a bad day. The children we were working with could not provide their own stimulation. If left alone for two minutes, they would fall into an almost sleeplike state. With a maximum of six hours per day, we could not afford to waste even a minute of their time.

"The next morning I called a staff meeting and made an announcement. 'No child shall be without stimulation for a single minute, from the time he enters the building until he leaves.' Within a week, what had been rather normal-looking clinical rooms were transformed into maximum sensory environments. The floors became a series of ramps and platforms covered with padded mats and textured carpets, as well as vinyl surfaces. Mounted on two walls and the ceiling of each stimulation room was the most exotic light-show equipment I could find, so we could produce vivid moving visual images in every corner of the room. We also mounted slide projectors that were synchronized with tape recorders that played into cordless headphones, so we could supply different auditory stimulation to different children at the same time, while allowing them movement throughout the room. Each room also had dozens of sponge balls scattered around the floor that the staff would throw toward and at the children. In addition, two staff members would constantly move throughout the room, changing body position, increasing movement, masking, stimulating taste and smell, and, in general, creating as much disturbance as humanly possible. This is where the children would stay when they were not being taken into one of the many individual therapy rooms where they received their specific individual programs in mobility, language, vision, auditory competence, manual competence, tactility, or academics. The children thrived in this new environment, and progressed at a rate that amazed me.

"The stimulation provided to the children in these high-stimulation environments was great enough to get through even the poorest sensory channel. The children were being provided with specific stimulation delivered with the greatest frequency, intensity, and duration possible within the economic and social parameters afforded.

"Dawn and I remained together for almost four years. Four years in which we had little to offer her except love and attention. No new miracles were found for her. During those four years, Dawn progressed ever so slowly. There was significant progress, but she had a long way to go. Her breathing became fairly stable. Her awareness improved about a thousand percent. Her eyes and face were alert and sparkling. She became less spastic and developed some controlled movements of her arms and legs. She developed a great sense of humor and without a doubt understood everything said around her. During those years, we employed the combined expertise of our team of therapists, our medical staff, and whatever could be picked up from the literature. Dawn made progress, but it wasn't sufficient, for Dawn was still dependent on the intense stimulation of the center environment to keep her going.

"Children like Dawn are either turned on or turned off. When they are turned off, everything turns off. The brain virtually shuts down. It is an oversimplification, but you are essentially either learning or forgetting. That is, if you are being stimulated, you are learning; if you are not being stimulated, you begin to lose what knowledge you have. The brain never remains static. In a very real sense, if you don't use it, you lose it."

APPROPRIATE EDUCATION

Doman continues: "In Pennsylvania in the early seventies, we at UCP worked hard at getting the first Right to Education law enacted. Prior to the enactment of the Right to Education, children who were classified below the level of 'educable' were denied access to public education funds. Programs such as we had were either funded privately, paid for by the family, or funded through specific government HEW grants. We saw the acceptance of the Right to Education as a giant step forward for our children with severe problems. With enactment of the new law, all children were entitled to an 'appropriate education.' The problem developed with the word *appropriate*.

"Having succeeded in getting state education monies for our children, we then came face to face with government controls and guidelines, and a basic dispute as to what constituted an appropriate educational experience for a severely brain-injured child. The traditional care for such children was, and still is, defined as 'custodial.' Custodial care involves changing diapers, feeding, and very minimal therapy. Therapy that rarely exceeds range of motion. Range of motion is moving or ranging the joints in an attempt to avoid contractures. Specific sensory stimulation, per se, does not fit into traditional custodial care. In fact, traditional custodial care generally produces a sensorially deprived environment.

"What constitutes an appropriate opportunity for any child? How much is enough? How much is too much? How much can we expect the government institutions to do for us?

"The Pennsylvania Department of Education moved into UCP with its funding, guidelines, and restrictions. Guidelines and restrictions with which I was in direct opposition. These restrictions limited the type and degree of stimulation and opportunities that could be provided for children in a state-run school. I lost my battle with the traditionalists. Our school thus became like the others. I could not see my role as running another school for the state, and I resigned my position.

"A few months later, while on a trip to Barcelona, where I was working as part of a team that visited Spain every three months to design in-home stimulation programs for brain-injured children, I received a call from the States telling me that Dawn had died. Within six months after having received an 'appropriate' education, Dawn and another child from that original group of six were dead.

"As stated earlier, the level of function achieved by an individual is a reflection of the stimulation and opportunities afforded the individual by his or her environment. Brain injury is in the brain. The goal of treatment must be either the creation of function where none exists or improvement of function where it is delayed or inhibited.

"Stimulation 'excites' the brain. What does excitement of the brain produce? Functional activity. What is functional activity? Breathing, metabolizing food, walking, talking, reading, etc.

"The goal of treatment is to produce functional activity.

"Stimulation that is produced in sufficient frequency, intensity, and duration excites the brain, improves the organization of the brain, and permits increased functional activity."[2]

NEURODEVELOPMENTAL
AUDITORY TRAINING

As Doman continued his independent research, learning from each child he observed, treated, and tracked for years, he solidified his belief that sound stimulation was key. "Neurodevelopmental auditory training" became the umbrella for his many sound therapies.

Even as Alfred Tomatis became aware of the significant relationship of the ear to the nervous system while working with munitions factory workers and opera singers, Doman, as he treated autistic and neurodevelopmentally delayed children, arrived independently at the same conclusions. The auditory pathway is a portal into the brain; sound stimulation excites the brain, creating functional activity; music and sound unravel disorganized neural wiring critical to unlocking human potential.

Neurodevelopment can be broadly defined as "the development and organization of the central nervous system." We know from Tomatis that the auditory system is functioning by eighteen weeks in utero and unfolds through childhood. According to Doman, when the natural neurodevelopmental auditory process is derailed, auditory dysfunction may manifest. Abnormal neurodevelopment can be caused by psychological, physiological, or environmental problems in childhood, or by trauma. Deviations in normal auditory development can also occur later in life due to stress or trauma.

According to Doman, "The most primitive nerve in the body is the eighth cranial nerve (also known as the vestibulocochlear nerve). The natural evolution of the human brain begins with this auditory nerve. The early development of the vestibulocochlear nerve and the stimulation that the brain receives through it are vital to the growth of the brain and the well-being of the maturing individual."[3] He continues, "As the brain forms, it is not only stimulated and activated by sound, *it begins the process of learning how to differentiate and apply meaning to sound.* Problems resulting from a lack of appropriate auditory input affect language recognition, thought, speech, overall neurological development, and functions ranging from balance to the formation of muscle tone. The unfolding health of the auditory system is vital to the complete development of the brain."[4]

The ability to process, understand, and communicate with the world is largely dependent on a delicate combination of auditory functions. The goal of Doman's evolving neurodevelopmental auditory training was to develop and—if necessary—remediate problems associated with these vital neurological, physiological, and psychological functions.

OPTIMAL ACOUSTICAL ENVIRONMENTS

Doman says, "To understand the significance of neurodevelopmental auditory training, we must look at an optimal acoustic environment for the developing brain and compare that to the realities of today. Remember that initial auditory input for the unborn child far transcends the mere act of hearing. Sound affects the entire well-being of the brain, mind, central nervous system, and body.

"Optimally the fetus is enveloped in an environment of natural tones," Doman continues. "This consists of the mother's voice, her heartbeat, and body sounds, as well as sounds from the environment that are transmitted through the mother's body. In the best of circumstances, external environmental sounds would include the voices of the father, siblings, and other family members, as well as the sounds of nature. Following birth, the infant's acoustic world, it is hoped, would not change significantly. It would remain natural and pleasant, void of excessive harsh or loud sounds, and consist largely of lighter, natural high-frequency sounds such as the wind blowing through trees, the sound of a babbling brook, or the song of a bird. Hopefully, this acoustic environment of the infant is relatively pure—free of extraneous sounds, particularly louder mechanical noise. This pure auditory environment would permit the brain to process individual tones, first within a comfortable frequency range, and expanding as the system matures."

Doman emphasizes that at birth, the brain already hears; sound is transmitted as electrochemical impulses to the brain. However, at this infantile stage the brain must learn how to differentiate, interpret, and process individual tones. Later, these tones will have meaning as individual sounds that are then grouped, processed sequentially, and finally develop meaning as language. According to Doman, the child's brain is not capable of all this at birth; at that point it merely receives unidentified and undifferentiated impulses.

"A significant part of early auditory development is learning how to process the tones in language. It is generally felt that a child learns, within the first two years, how to process the specific tones in the native language. Without specific acoustic intervention, most individuals have difficulty learning to hear (and thus speak) another language if they have not been exposed to that language within their first few years of life.

"Unfortunately, the realities of today's world bear little resemblance to our optimal acoustic environment. Consider the contrast of two people talking together in a meadow with today's urban world. Compare the natural, positive neurodevelopmental acoustic environment with the destructive acoustic environments in which most of us live. It is almost impossible to find a place on the planet where one is not constantly assaulted by environmental noise pollution. This can have adverse neurological, physiological, and psychological ramifications. In our homes, disturbing sounds can include appliances, fluorescent lights, the traffic outside, and the mentally destructive thumping of the bass speakers on our teenager's or neighbor's sound system. Outside the home the assault only worsens: planes, trains, automobiles, power tools, and all the negative acoustic trappings of our technological cultures.

"If one were fortunate enough to have spent the first few years of life in an acoustically favorable environment, our current environment would shortly undo the positive aspects of that beginning."[5]

THE NECESSITY OF HEALTHY TONAL AND SEQUENTIAL PROCESSING

Language—the ability to process and use tones, phonemes, words, sentences, thoughts, and feelings—is integral to that which makes us thinking social beings. According to Doman's approach, the neurodevelopment of language is dependent on three specific factors:

- Auditory tonal processing—the ability to differentiate among the tones used in the language

- Overall organization of the central nervous system—the establishment of hemispheric specificity and a language center
- Auditory sequential processing—the ability to link pieces of auditory information

Says Doman, "Intervention in the neurodevelopment of language involves assisting in the natural development of these critical pieces and remediation when this natural development has not occurred. In most instances, auditory tonal processing develops normally if the child is provided with good-quality auditory tonal input as afforded by an unencumbered natural environment.

"However, if the developing child is deprived of sufficient tonal input from his or her environment, the neurodevelopment of tonal processing is adversely affected. Proper development can also be stopped, or even undone, if the developing child or adult is deprived of input. Often this vital input is significantly hindered by ear infections (more specifically, fluid within the middle ear), a problem that appears to become more common every year. At any point in life, the effects of sound pollution can destroy healthy auditory tonal processing, produce hearing loss, and negate the positive neurological effects of healthy sound."

One of the goals of neurodevelopmental auditory training is to provide a full spectrum of sounds This helps reverse and negate the effects of sound pollution, resulting in improved auditory tonal processing.

Addressing the necessity of full-spectrum sound and healthy tonal and sequential processing, Doman has recently been involved in the creation of eight hours of simply structured classical music CDs. The Sound Health Series (SHS) contains rearranged and rerecorded baroque and other classical music. Because of highly specific psychoacoustic refinements, this series is designed to filter out noise pollution and to enhance health, learning, and productivity. The SHS is currently used in schools, hospitals, psychotherapeutic clinics, and businesses in America and Europe. (See "Soundwork Resources" for more information.)

Proper auditory tonal processing supports:

- Receptive language skills—the ability to understand more complex language when it is heard

- Expressive language skills—the ability to speak clearly, effectively, and spontaneously
- Auditory attentional focus—a better ability to filter out distracting background noise and focus on foreground sound
- A balanced and flexible auditory system—imperative for the peak performance of the central nervous system
- Improved auditory sequential processing—the foundation for conceptualization and one of the building blocks of all thinking

Again per Doman, "As previously stated, the auditory nerve—the most primitive nerve in the body—provides stimulation and organization to the entire central nervous system. A significant effect of this stimulation is to assist in the development and formation of a language center within the brain. *Sound stimulation provides positive sensory input.* This stimulation facilitates the growth of neuronal networks—the links that organize the brain."

The third component involved in the neurodevelopment of language and thought is auditory sequential processing. Doman has found that if an individual has good auditory tonal processing and the brain is receiving good-quality input, the brain has the opportunity to learn how to put pieces together. This is auditory sequential processing.

"One of the major goals of society during the next decade needs to be improving the sequential processing of the population," says Doman. "Normal auditory sequential processing for an adult is generally considered to be seven plus or minus two digits. This means that if someone were to tell you a sequence of numbers slowly, at a rate of one digit per second, you should be able to listen to and then repeat seven digits, plus or minus two digits, or a range of five to nine.

"However, if the processing is below seven, an individual is functioning not only significantly below his or her potential, but also with a handicap. A digit span of seven should be considered minimal for adequate processing, with a digit span of nine or above as being preferred. Your digit span determines how many pieces of auditory information you can take in or your ability to process and understand language. It also determines how many pieces of information you can control or manipulate in your mind, thus the complexity of your thought patterns and ability to understand concepts. And finally, it determines your ability to organize and express your thoughts."

Brain Builder, an innovative computer-training tool, has been developed from Doman's years of clinical research. This program assesses and exercises both auditory and visual sequential processing. (See "Soundwork Resources" for more information.)

While Doman has recognized the necessity for remediation of tonal processing problems for more than thirty years, when he first became aware of the problem he couldn't find effective treatment. "I couldn't even find anyone else who understood the problem!" he says. However, while working in Spain in the 1970s, he heard of the work of Dr. Alfred Tomatis. Doman located a physician trained by Tomatis in Madrid and was impressed with the results he observed. On returning to America, Doman began referring some of his clients to Paris to work directly with Tomatis.

Before I continue with Doman's story, it is appropriate to note a common perception that occurs independently for numerous healthcare practitioners: Professional clinicians and educators find their methods ineffective in many cases, and determine that the missing link in their work revolves around auditory function. Psychiatrist Ron Minson, educator Billie Thompson, psychologist Susan Andrews, neurodevelopmental specialist Robert Doman—each on his or her individual healer's journey comes to the doorway of Tomatis. Each then shapes Tomatis's pioneering concepts and practices into his or her own matrix.

In the case of Doman's work with neurodevelopmentally impaired children and adults, NACD has experimented with just about every known formal sound stimulation therapy available—all offshoots from the Tomatis process of filtration and gating of sound to create "active listening" and strengthen the middle-ear function. In addition to the Tomatis Method, Doman has used sound stimulation treatments and programs such as Sound Therapy for the Walkman, Auditory Integration Training, Auditory Enhancement Training, Samonas Sound Therapy, Fast For-Word, and The Listening Program.

Now Bob's son, Alexander Doman, is the third generation of neurodevelopmental specialists. Having worked extensively with sound programs at NACD, he says: "The Tomatis approach concentrated on retraining the voice through the ear and stimulating the brain with high-frequency sounds. The Joudry program [Sound Therapy for the Walkman] put some of the most important gains within the reach of many more people. Dr. Guy Berard's Auditory Integration Training emphasized how peaks in the audiograms (hypersensitivity to certain frequencies) created psychological problems. There was value in each approach, especially Dr. Tomatis's work. Yet none of the approaches provided all of the answers."

Although no existing sound programs were altogether suitable for their neurodevelopmental work, the Domans extrapolated what seemed appropriate for NACD families. Each intervention had value. Each method offered another piece of the auditory puzzle. Bob and Alex understood that restoration of auditory tonal processing was integral to auditory sequential issues. Therefore, their primary goal with clients using sound stimulation was normalizing auditory perception.

Says Alex: "We tracked thousands of children for many years during and following various sound therapy programs. We were seeing the benefits diminish after a few months to a year or more with a good majority of the kids, no matter what program they were doing. We saw the need for *booster programs*. For some of our clients, we also started people doing a shorter series, as few as two or three sessions.

"All of these deviations from the prescribed system reflected a shift of view on our part. We began to see that therapeutic auditory stimulation was an ongoing process. As soon as you leave a listening session, you're exposed to leaf blowers, traffic, loud thumping bass music, and countless other buzzes, hums, and whooshes. Many factors work to undo the benefits of the sound therapy. When kids are not so well organized, neurologically, they're especially susceptible. The therapeutic improvements involve laying down new neurological pathways, which need to be reinforced. With practice, they get easier to reinforce, but it's unrealistic to believe that reinforcement will never be necessary again."

Alex Doman continues, "So we knew we needed an ongoing program. The only cost-effective way was to make it home based. We saw that a home-based approach was by far most practical and accessible for the majority of our clients."[6] (For more on Alex Doman's work, see appendix E, "The Birth of a Sound Therapy.")

With this in mind, Robert and Alex Doman assembled a team of experts in psychiatry, psychoacoustics, music, and speech pathology. Combining their knowledge of neurodevelopment, their clients' reactions to other sound therapies, and this new team, the Domans created their own Tomatis-oriented program—The Listening Program. This eight-week, at-home program is designed to balance auditory perception. Treatment consists of fifteen minutes to half an hour per day spent listening to specially filtered and gated classical music and nature soundtracks. I am proud to have been part of the team that created The Listening Program. I coproduced this ground-breaking series with Richard Lawrence and The Arcangelos Chamber Ensemble.

In summary, sound stimulation programs such as the Tomatis Method, The Listening Program, and others retrain the auditory system to take in a fuller spectrum of sound. An open ear can assimilate more of the nutrients of sound—thereby facilitating stimulation of the brain and nervous system. This wider input also serves, according to Robert Doman Jr., "to remediate tonal misperception and distortions in hearing that have resulted from a variety of physical and environmental causes."[7]

PART TWO

Sound
Awareness

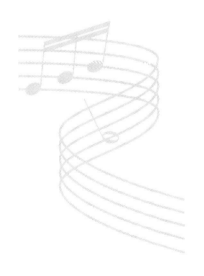

7 A New Awareness of Sound

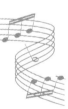

The prenatal research of Alfred Tomatis shows the hearing mechanism of the unborn child to be functional and alert five months prior to birth. The constant swoosh of blood flow, thumping of heartbeats, the high-frequency sound of the mother's ever-present voice, and the father's lower voice make up the soundscape of the womb. The sound levels inside the uterus actually get as high as 95 dB with every heartbeat. This is like being on the dance floor of a loud rock club on a Saturday night! As another point of comparison, a regular conversation between two people registers at 40 dB.[1]

So much for the notion of fetal tranquility. The fact is that very early on, we learn to tolerate noise. Fortunately, we have the neural facility to adapt, filter, isolate, and even ignore sound. A colleague who works with autistic children tells me that these kids often do not have a functional auditory filtering mechanism; consequently, many are so sound-sensitive that they painfully hear the electricity in the walls.

We are not equipped with earlids, so we take in every sound

around us. We may not be consciously aware of it, but the brain is analyzing every sound that vibrates against the eardrum. Our reptilian brain, the locus of an ever-present survival instinct, uses sound to assess safety. Our auditory system is always in a state of alertness. This does not mean that we are consciously listening to all the sounds we hear but, rather, that the auditory mechanism is perpetually processing. Imagine a computer that is on twenty-four hours a day, tuned with highly sensitive sound perception software to analyze the slightest disturbance of silence. This is the level of attention our auditory system maintains throughout our lives.

The creation of well-thought-out sonic environments is uncommon in our culture. Very few people consider the cerebral energy that is expended sorting out "garbage" sonic information. You may have noticed the effect of walking into a store or dining in a restaurant where sound is omnipresent. It may work positively; you comment on how nice the place is and go on with your task. Conversely, if the sound space rubs you the wrong way, you might decide to shop elsewhere or end up eating your meal feeling distracted and imposed upon.* If your primary response to a particular sound environment is irritation, the natural instinct is to remove yourself or the offending stimulus. In our noisy culture, however, we often cannot remove ourselves from sound irritants—be they in the home, office, restaurant, or shopping mall. The result is that we begin to shut down our internal hearing mechanism as a means of coping. This defense mechanism works when we need an escape or less input on the physical as well as the psychological level.†

---

* An encouraging sign of emerging sound awareness is evident in my local newspaper, the *San Francisco Chronicle*. In its restaurant section, a rating system now includes sound ambience in addition to price and overall quality. The sound rankings include "pleasantly quiet" (under 65 dB), "can talk easily" (65–70), "talking normally gets difficult" (70–75), "can talk only in raised voices" (75–80), and "too noisy for normal conversation" (80-plus).

† A case in point: I was riding on a bus in upstate New York when an elderly couple boarded. While the bus was in motion, the woman insisted on approaching the bus driver and asking him questions. She had a loud, high-pitched voice and an obnoxious manner. The driver asked her to sit down, referring to the CAUTION signs about interfering with the driver when the bus was in motion. This scenario was repeated another few times within the first hour, until the driver pulled the bus over and publicly rebuked the woman. Between each visit to the driver, she talked incessantly at her husband. I noticed that there was very little dialogue between the two. When we finally reached their destination, and as they walked by, I noticed that the man had large hearing aids on both ears. The question arises: *Did she talk this way because he was hard of hearing, or was he nearly deaf to avoid the sound of her voice?*

"Calling noise a nuisance is like calling smog an inconvenience," states William H. Stewart, a former U.S. Surgeon General, who suggests that "noise must be considered a hazard to the health of people everywhere."[2]

A new awareness of sound allows us to function fully in our society, noisy or not. The goal in life is to be an open, self-expressive, and healthy human being. We are equipped with the ability to *recycle* energy, be it food, light, or sound. These elements contain frequencies that can either energize or de-energize us.

If we become overloaded with sound, our systems begin to close down. The long-term effect is barely noticeable. Our ever-adaptive mind and body come to accept the shutting-down state as normal. Over a period of time, however, we begin to notice that we don't hear as well as we used to, we might be easily fatigued, or our focus seems scattered. A volume dial has somehow been turned down and we didn't even notice. Then one day we wondered how it had grown so quiet around us.

STRESS-INDUCED AUDITORY DYSFUNCTION

Auditory dysfunction is a very broad topic. Throughout part 1 of *The Power of Sound*, I explored the nature of sound and hearing. I also looked at the role of sound and listening through the filter of Tomatis, Doman, and others. When we put together the many pieces of auditory function, we see that the system has a greater importance than is commonly ascribed to it.

Popular perception of outer- and inner-ear function has centered on the interpretation of sound and the maintenance of balance. However, we now see greater ramifications when the auditory mechanism is not in full working order. If indeed sound is a vital stimulant for the nervous system, then the ear is the portal and the auditory system the delivery mechanism. Just as arteries and veins are vascular highways through which blood carries information, the auditory system is a fiber-optic network for the dissemination of sound impulse and energy.

In the following chapter, "Sonic Safety," I examine how noise damages the ear in two ways: acoustic trauma and noise-induced hearing loss. Be it a sudden shotgun blast or long-term exposure to high levels of noise, our auditory function can be affected—and often greatly diminished.

Noise, however, is not the only post-birth threat to normal auditory function. Childhood ear infections and illnesses, middle-ear fluid, and allergies can also contribute to diminished function. The work of Tomatis and Doman focuses on the remediation of auditory tonal processing.

The Tomatis concepts consider auditory function from a psychological viewpoint as well as physiologically. He speaks of the two muscles of the middle ear becoming flaccid when we shut out or shut down sounds we can't tolerate. As I explored Tomatis's thoughts about the impact of psychology on the ear, I began to wonder if additional layers of complexity could be laid down by stress and trauma. Two things tipped me off to this—personal experience and passing references within broader articles.

After a few years of extreme, compacted emotional stress—loss of community, loss of employment, premature birth of a child, tax audits, broken marriage—I began to notice aspects of my personality beginning to change. Mentally I was slowing down in my thought processing. I was not quite so sharp. I began mixing up letters when I typed at the computer—something that had never happened before. Also, I seemed to be having difficulty not taking everyday occurrences personally; as time went by, I was becoming emotionally overreactive. I felt like I was suffering from post-traumatic stress syndrome even though I didn't know what the actual symptoms of that disorder are. I felt like I had been through a war, and my nervous system was showing the effect.

While researching *The Power of Sound* I found an article titled "The Emerging Field of Sound Training," by Tomatis practitioners Billie Thompson and Susan Andrews. In their comprehensive eight-page piece, two sentences were of particular interest: "Poor listening can begin at any age and for any number of reasons. It might result from a health problem, an accident, a major lifestyle disruption, or from stress."[3] Because this was not the focus of their article (published in 1999), Thompson and Andrews left the coverage of stress and quickly moved on to other sound training topics.

Shortly thereafter I read an article by Robert Doman Jr., written in 1982, titled "Dominance and Emotionality." Once again I came across a solitary, one-sentence reference to stress and the auditory system: "Abnormal neurodevelopment may be caused by psychological, physiological, or environmental problems in childhood; deviations of a normal auditory development may also occur later in life due to stress or trauma."[4]

Given a sensitivity to this topic, my attention was rapt. Yet very few people were talking about it; the two references were all I could find. What is happening to auditory function due to stress and trauma? When we experience loss—be it family, job, money, or health—how does that manifest in auditory function, and what is the broader impact?

AUDITORY CROSS DOMINANCE— A POINT OF INQUIRY

One aspect of stress-induced auditory dysfunction that I find to be quite interesting revolves around laterality and auditory cross dominance, two topics that make my professional therapeutic associates cringe. "What is laterality? Nothing is simpler and nothing is more obscure," notes Dr. Tomatis. He concludes, "By laterality we mean the fact of being right-handed or left-handed."[5] *Lateral preference* is defined as "the predominant use of one side of the body over the other."[6]

In addition to right- or left-handedness, the concept of laterality includes feet, eyes, and ears. In most normal neurodevelopment, you are either right or left dominant. This means that if I am right-handed, I should ostensibly "lead" with my right foot, right eye, and right ear. Conversely, if I were left-handed, the same elements would line up on the left.

I have learned that the field of laterality is fraught with exceptions and disagreements. As a composer and producer, it is definitely not appropriate for me to state facts or offer opinions about a difficult aspect of human anatomy in which I have no training.* Still, once I was buoyed by a few brief professional references to the effects of stress and audition, I engaged in an inquiry into the effects of laterality and auditory cross dominance.

---

* For those interested in further exploration of the field of laterality, ample resources can be found on the Internet. Enter the word *laterality* on a major search engine. I recommend www.alltheweb.com.

Auditory cross dominance refers to a process whereby a right-handed person, with right-sided dominance, has a left-leading ear (or vice versa if left-handed). I have been told emphatically that there are no firm data on this phenomenon—only clinical observation. I have also been told of numerous gray areas concerning cross dominance, the least of which is the difficulty of scientific verification. Nonetheless, as I travel and teach internationally, I have the occasion to speak with various healthcare practitioners who work with the auditory system. When I informally broach the topic of auditory cross dominance, I am, without exception, met with nodding heads. It is from this context that I humbly introduce the following discussion.

Robert J. Doman Jr. comes from a lineage of medical and psychological mavericks, so it is no surprise that he dares walk into the zone of laterality and cross dominance. The following excerpt from his article titled "Dominance and Emotionality" was, as I noted above, one of the tip-offs for me that something was going on around the issue of stress and hearing . . . something worthy of further scientific exploration.[7]

The final stage in developing neurological organization—neurological efficiency is the establishment of cortical hemispheric dominance. Cortical hemisphere dominance refers to the establishment of a controlling hemisphere of the brain, separation of, or specialization of neurological function. This separation of function is possible when dominance has been achieved.

Dominance, that factor which permits cortical specialization, exists at such time when the individual has a dominant hand, eye, ear, and foot which are all on the same side. Specifically, the right handed individual need also be right eyed, eared, and footed, the left handed individual left eyed, eared, and footed.

Much has been written in the last few years relative to the specific functions of the dominant and subdominant hemispheres, the dominant hemisphere being that which is on the opposite side of the dominant hand, eye, ear, and foot. The person with right sided dominance has a dominant left hemisphere, the person with left sided dominance, a dominant right hemisphere.

One very significant function relative to learning which has not been mentioned in most of the literature is emotionality. As is music (it is not difficult to see the correlation between music and emotionality), emotionality is a subdominant hemisphere function.

Emotionality in the neurologically organized individual is controlled, it being subdominant. One of the problems associated with neurological disorganization is the lack of later dominance, lack of separation, and specifically relative to emotionality, lack of control of emotionality. In the disorganized individual, subdominant tends to control dominant, as opposed to the appropriate dominant control or balance. This lack of control is significant for all individuals with neurological disorganization.

Disorganized adults often (mental institutions are full of people who cannot) learn to cope, by creating conscious controls of emotionality. They develop screens between themselves and others, and often appear to be non-emotional because they have learned that they can either fight off emotion, or become virtually engulfed by their emotionality. These individuals are forced to live their lives limiting emotionality and protecting themselves.

We have learned to accept our inefficiencies, spending our lives with the pressures of attempting to cope with our problems, when solutions are available. Thousand of hours are spent in academic remediation, counseling, analysis, and thousands of dollars on medications to help us cope with neurological inefficiencies which are easily eliminated if we address and treat the cause.

An understanding of the relationship between neurological disorganization, dominance, and emotionality can dramatically improve many aspects of our lives, as well as those of our children.

Doman's observations come after working with thousands of children and adults. As a journalist, I pose these questions:

- Is there an effect of stress or trauma on the auditory system?
- What are the psychological issues that manifest themselves in the ear?
- How do they manifest?

- What is the effect of auditory cross dominance?
- What scientific basis is there for this?
- What causes mixed laterality and what are the solutions?
- What are the symptoms and how are they usually treated?
- Why is stress-related auditory dysfunction rarely spoken about?
- Could auditory cross dominance contribute to a country full of adults on Prozac and children on Ritalin?

For answers, I turned to three professionals who work with sound as a core medium of treatment. Interviews with Billie Thompson, Ph.D., Ron Minson, M.D., and Robert J. Doman Jr. can be found in appendix B and should be regarded as a continuation of this inquiry.

Within the larger context of audition, the subset issue of stress and auditory perception is microscopic. It appears that little attention has been paid to this important link. Yet every Tomatis practitioner will confirm that the psychological component of auditory function is significant. So will most occupational and speech and language therapists. For most of us, the *physiological* health of our hearing is never addressed until we notice that something is changing. Who among us has even considered the impact of our *psychological* state on our auditory system? This is a new way of thinking about sound, hearing, and human functionality.

In the future, our culture will understand sound as fuel and the ear as a portal for charging the nervous system. We will give our ears timely attention. We will tend to our auditory health just as we do our hearts, our eyes, and our teeth. In order for this shift in awareness to take place, we must understand that proper auditory function is not simply about passive hearing or balance. It is about the ability to engage in "active listening." This facilitates the loop of language → education → communication → social interaction. There is no aspect of normal living—home, family, employment—that is not dependent on these skills.

Sound is a nutrient for the nervous system. The goal is to learn how to use sound with the same awareness we would apply to food or drink. Moving from the psychological to the physiological impact of sound, let's take a look at the major body pulse systems. Understanding these systems, we can apply the principles of resonance and entrainment in our daily lives to support health and well-being.

THE MAJOR BODY PULSES

The heart, breath, and brain constitute the major pulse systems in the body. The beating of the heart not only lends itself to poetic interpretation but is also responsible for propelling vital blood throughout the physical mechanism. Without the proper intake and exhalation of air in the lungs, we would quickly perish. Finally, the electrochemical balance and tempos of our neurotransmitters allow our brains to monitor millions of events every second and coordinate a multitude of biologic systems.[8] Clearly, the proper functioning of these three systems is necessary for health. The mechanisms of the heart, breath, and brain are ideal subjects for the study of rhythmic entrainment: These systems are so conspicuously rhythmic that they are the perfect organs for resonant attention.

THE HEART

One of the largest structures of the body, the heart and its arterial system move the blood throughout the entire human body. The pulsing of the heart is produced by the alternating contraction (systole) and relaxation (diastole) of the heart muscle.

The heart begins its life-giving task shortly after conception and continues until the moment that we die. According to master drummer and sound researcher Reinhard Flatischler, our mother's heartbeat "is the first rhythmic expression to shape our consciousness." We gestate for nine months within this elemental pulsation, and forever after "there exists a pulsation within ourselves which embodies a specific tempo which relates to all other pulsations."[9]

So the pulse rate that we inherit from our mother, and her mother, and genetic generations before, becomes our major rhythm filter. Our levels of comfort, flexibility, and rigidity are tied to how close or far we are willing to venture from this major pacesetter.

The normal relaxed heart will beat between sixty and eighty times per minute. The continuous rhythm of the heart may run as low as fifty beats per minute (bpm) among athletes or go as high as two hundred bpm or more during illness or fever.[10] According to Flatischler, both the sympathetic and the parasympathetic nervous systems are in control of the rhythm of the heartbeat. "One stimulates, the other inhibits," he says. "The heartbeat is thus imbedded in the forces at work in our nervous system. But the final origin of this rhythmic power still remains a mystery."[11]

The source for the beating of the heart comes from a tiny valve located in the back of the massive heart muscle; this valve provides the electrical charge that makes the heart beat. As Flatischler notes, no one knows where the electrical charge comes from.

The heartbeat has had a strong influence on the tempo of music. Prior to the invention of the metronome, musical tempi were determined by the human pulse.[12] The difference between a slower adagio and a frenetic beat in music depends on how far it departs on one side or the other from the human heartbeat. Push up the tempo and you have military music; slow it down and you fall asleep.

Reinhard Flatischler spends his life traveling the world studying rhythm. Crossing the boundaries of all cultures, he has found that the body and its rhythms play a central role in music. Thus we find "a knowledge of the inner pulse in the music of all cultures." The melody of the heartbeat is imitated by drummers globally, from the Native American medicine men to the Japanese *taiko*. Highly complex eastern Indian rhythms are based on the heartbeat, using three tempo ranges that are multiples of the normal heart rate. In African, Latin American, and Asian music the pulse rate is clearly perceptible. Flatischler points out that Western classical music is no exception; music characterized by *tactus inter valor* (a fixed tempo of fifty to eighty beats per minute) was found in European music from the mid–fifteenth century until the end of the sixteenth century.[13] This tempo, corresponding to a slow to normal heartbeat, was the pulse underlying Bach's music.

THE BREATH

Normal breathing varies between twelve and twenty cycles per minute (cpm), which is three to five seconds per cycle. This changes in tempo with exercise and relaxation. Breathing can be slowed down during relaxation or sleep to cycles lasting six to eight seconds.[14] There is a reason that we feel so good at the seashore: The rhythm of the breaking waves often produces a relaxing cycle of eight seconds to which our breath rate entrains. This rate corresponds to the speed of our breath in deep relaxation. It is an excellent example of elemental entrainment.

Inhalation and exhalation are most often thought of as the sum total of the breathing process, but the rhythm of breathing is threefold. Many believe that the true point of power lies in the moment of stillness between breaths, an awareness of which we can cultivate. The moment of stillness is that instant that begins to expand—as though by itself—when we detach ourselves from activity and enter deeper levels of consciousness, as in sleep or meditation. As we allow ourselves to go deeper into this breathing process, we will find that the "letting-be" cycle of stillness becomes as long as the phases of inhalation and exhalation. At this point, we are breathing in a triple cycle rather than a dual.[15]

The dual cycle (inhale, exhale) is most easily observed after a fast run. The triple cycle (inhale, exhale, let be) is most easily observed watching someone in deep sleep. Flatischler believes that the dual cycle is associated with an active, extroverted attitude, while the triple cycle is a bodily expression of introversion. He believes that "duple-time and triple-time—two elementary phenomena in the music of every culture—are rooted in our physiology."[16]

The corresponding use of rhythm to affect human physiology lies in the relationship to duple and triple time. Flatischler believes that "rhythms that have three subdividing pulses in each interval make the listener more introverted and bring him or her toward an inner stillness, whereas the intervals containing the movement of 2 or 4 subdividing pulses will direct the listener toward outer movement and greater extroversion."[17]

THE BRAIN

The electrochemical activity of the brain produces electromagnetic waveforms known as brainwaves. These waveforms can be objectively measured with sensitive equipment such as an electroencephalograph (EEG). As long as you are alive, these continuous electrical waves circulate throughout your brain. As with cessation of the heartbeat, the lack of brainwave activity is a sign of death.

Research into brain-wave states began in the 1920s and has continued to evolve through the use of biofeedback instruments. Researchers have divided the range of brainwave activity into four categories. Each state can be associated with different mental characteristics, and each has its own recognizable cycle. Therefore, knowing which brainwave state is most conducive to an activity—be it peak output (high beta) or fully relaxation (theta)—allows for optimal accomplishment of that activity.

The four major brainwave states are:

1. *Beta waves* (14 to 35 Hz). These are found in the normal, waking state of consciousness. You are alert, with a focus on the everyday activities of the world. Beta is also present during states of anxiety, tension, fear, and alarm.
2. *Alpha waves* (8 to14 Hz). These accompany states of relaxed wakefulness, such as daydreaming and meditation. They are blocked by sensory awareness, conceptual thinking, and strong emotions. Alpha waves generally appear in the occipital region of the brain (the visual cortex) when the eyes are closed.
3. *Theta waves* (4 to 8 Hz). These are found in near-unconscious states, very deep meditation, and as you drift into or out of sleep. This rhythm has been connected to states of reverie and hypnogogic states that produce dreamlike imagery. It is difficult to maintain this state without training in the disciplines of meditation.
4. *Delta waves* (0.5 to 4 Hz). Found in the deepest part of the sleep cycle and in unconsciousness, these are the longest and slowest waves.

At any given time, the brain is not functioning in just one level of brainwave activity; it is the combination of these brainwave states that determines the focus of our activities. According to Anna Wise, an internationally respected brainwave feedback expert, "Each state that you experience entails a symphony of brainwaves, with each frequency playing its own characteristic part. Out of these symphonies come the art of Picasso, the dance of Martha Graham, the architecture of Frank Lloyd Wright, and the theories of Einstein."[18] The interrelationship of brain wave frequencies is what contributes to our various states of mental and subconscious awareness.

Brainwaves work in partnership with the heart rate and the breath rate, and all three body pulses are susceptible to the powerful effects of rhythmic entrainment.

$\mathcal{D}$

Even within our bodies, the natural heart rate, respiration, and brainwave cycles all entrain with each other. If we slow down our breath, the heart rate and brainwaves will follow; if we slow our brainwaves, heart rate and respiration will follow. The three pulses form a large rythmic loop, with each pulse system completely interdependent on the rhythms of the other two.

Listening to music through headphones causes entrainment to take place in the brain first, with the heart and lungs following. In an aerobics class, due to the rhythmic movement, the heart most likely is first affected, with the lungs and brain following suit. Likewise, the breath may become the lead entrainment pulse during yoga-style breathing exercises or while listening to Gregorian chant.*

CONCLUSION

What do I do with this information? you may be asking. If you are a musician or music producer, you will take these rhythms into account when you produce application-specific soundtracks. Knowledge of body rhythms helps you identify the specific sonic neurotechnologies that will help you coax the body to the tempo most conducive to an activity.

---

* Gregorian chant affects us in two ways. Each line is as long as a full breath. After a few minutes, listeners start to slow down their breath rates to match those of the singers. Natural entrainment at work! Another effect of Gregorian chant is the "charging" effect of the tenor voices. Dr. Tomatis recommends the use of chant instead of two cups of coffee. It has the perfect ingredients to create the body relaxed–mind alert combination identified as ideal for accelerated learning. For further information on the accelerated learning concept, I recommend *Suggestology and Outlines of Suggestopedy,* by Dr. Georgi Lozanov. A full citation is listed in the bibliography.

If you are a layperson looking to use music and sound with greater awareness, this information can reintroduce you to rhythms that have been going on in your body since the day you were born—or even before! Your body knows all about these rhythms; it doesn't even think about them but just autonomically controls them. In this chapter I have proposed that *you start thinking about this unconscious process.* By making it conscious, knowing which body rhythms are most conducive to a certain activity, you have an edge. You are learning how to use your body with your conscious mind. It's okay to leave the body on autopilot, but it's even more efficient to use your conscious mind with the rest of your body. This is the meaning of developing human potential. Human beings using music, sound, and other forms of frequency to sleep deeper, digest easier, think faster, concentrate longer, and heal. This is evolution.

Why do we need to do these things? would be the logical next question. If we lived in a serene and natural environment, we wouldn't. Our minds would be fresh, unstressed, and vital; our bodies would be well rested, healthy, and strong. Given that we reside in a new century of digital overload, though, the more natural and noninvasive tools we can use, the better.

If we combine an understanding of the vibrational nature of sound with the impact of resonance and entrainment, a picture should emerge of rhythmic beings using external sound to tune their internal rhythms.

Body tuning is not an exact process at this point; there are too many complex things taking place in the body. To imply that listening to music at eighty beats per minute will cause all systems to immediately meter out at 80 bpm would be making a false claim. Remember, the rhythms of the body are not entraining to outside stimuli only, but constantly to the body's internal rhythms as well. With entrainment, we are looking to operate within natural ranges. The body's pulses, like a little puppy, will follow a friendly rhythm. This is a natural process. And because sound is a subtle energy tool, we need to be even more aware of its impact.

Tomatis practitioner Ron Minson, M.D., agrees with the U.S. Surgeon General quoted at the beginning of this chapter. "When we see smog in the air, we become aware of what we are breathing," says Minson. "If people could see noise pollution as they see air pollution, they would never put up with it!" Given that sound is invisible, a strong awareness of the overall effects of sound pollution will serve us in both the short and the long run.

In the following two chapters I will examine sonic safety, explore current research, and make recommendations of positive ways to use music and sound in our lives.

8 Sonic Safety

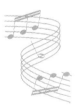In tandem with the visual experience of the world, the soundscape is a constant stimulus. Yet disproportionate to its influence, sound ranks as an environmental element to which we pay minimal attention. A growing number of researchers and theorists, however, are making sound—and responsibility for the soundscape—an environmental issue, looking deeply at its power both to disturb and to heal.

Beginning in 1972, government consideration and control of environmental noise was handled by the Environmental Protection Agency's Office of Noise Abatement and Control. This department was closed in 1982, though, and responsibility for noise control was returned to state and local governments.

City residents have long complained about noise: New Yorkers ranked it the number one problem in 1900 and still do so a hundred years later. Even the suburbs offer little escape. They've become an open-air stage for the din of leaf blowers, lawn mowers, garbage trucks, construction equipment, motorcycles, airplanes, and boom cars, those vehicles with more loudspeakers than square feet.

Environmental noise pollution, which began with the Industrial Revolution, is now a nearly ubiquitous problem. Almost no place is free from excessive noise, with exposure occurring not only on the streets and at work but also at home and even in the hospital.

SECONDHAND NOISE

The word *noise* is derived from the Latin *nausea*, meaning "seasickness." *Noise* generally refers to any loud, unmusical, or disagreeable sound. A potential problem arises here, though, as all three adjectives contain a subjective element. What is loud depends on the current state of your audiological health and your personal taste. If you have sustained hearing damage, sounds may register on you as either too soft or too loud—but not on someone with normal hearing. What is unmusical and disagreeable is a matter of taste in music; one person's noise is another's delight.

Here is the current state of American auditory health:

- More than thirty million Americans suffer from hearing loss.
- Exposure to excessive noise, not aging, accounts for 35 percent of hearing loss.
- One university study found that 61 percent of college freshmen exhibit some hearing loss.[1]
- The National Institute on Deafness reports that these losses begin as early as the preteen years and can result in sensory deafness, a permanent hearing loss.

DAMAGING NOISE

Noise damages ears in two ways. First, *acoustic trauma* occurs when an extremely loud sound strikes in an instant. One blast from a high-powered rifle can rip apart the ears' inner tissues, irreparably damaging your hearing. The scars that permanently dampen hearing remain. Second, *noise-induced hearing loss* (NIHL) develops insidiously over a period of decades. The most consistent finding in noise-induced hearing loss is injury to or degeneration of the 15,400 hair cells found in the cochlea. Repeated or extended exposure to dangerous noise levels attacks these delicate sensory cells, or cilia, whose job it is to transport airborne vibrations from the inner ear to the brain. The cilia are incapable of regeneration. By the time you get the signal that something is wrong—a ringing in the ears or a muffling of sounds—some of your cells may have died.[2]

Many things are not yet understood about the auditory mechanism. It is not known, for example, whether abrupt or inflated intensities of sound waves entering the cochlea cause direct mechanical disruption of the sensory nerves, or if a toxic biochemical reaction to the offending sound waves is the cause of damage to the cilia hair cells.

What *is* known, however, is that loud sounds cause constriction of blood vessels in the cochlea. This may result in damaging changes in the inner ear because of a lack of proper blood supply. This injury can be temporary—lasting minutes, hours, or days after the exposure to the noise—or it can be permanent. The loudness of the noise, how many times you were exposed to it, and how susceptible you are to it are the primary factors that contribute to a temporary or permanent hearing loss.[3]

If you have your ears checked by an audiologist, he will tell you that NIHL often begins at twenty-five to thirty years of age. Common symptoms are decreased ability to block out adjacent sounds and hypersensitivity to noise. When hair cells are damaged, sound perception may become jagged instead of smooth; sudden jumps in volume result from gaps in the cochlea's cilia.

My audiologist recently told me that the long-term effects of NIHL are analogous to skating on thin ice. From the surface it all looks the same, but underneath it may be thin; press too hard and you may fall through. With NIHL, an accumulation of cilia-cell damage can manifest over time or in an instant. A sudden very loud sound or a series of loud sound events can cause you to "fall through" into the zone of hearing impairment. Based on the cumulative loss of hair cells, hearing damage can take many forms, including tinnitus (ringing in the ears or noise sensed in the head), hyper- or hyposensitivity to sound volume, and diminution of hearing in specific ranges.

Who is most at risk for NIHL? The obvious recipients are those exposed on a consistent, long-term basis to occupational noise—firefighters, police officers, military personnel, construction and factory workers, musicians, aviation workers, farmers, and truck drivers, to name a few.

But outside the workplace some twenty million Americans are exposed on a regular basis to harmful levels of noise. Airplanes, recreational vehicles, lawn-care equipment, woodworking tools, some household appliances, chain saws, and live or recorded high-volume music are all nonoccupational sources of hazardous noise, and such noise is increasing in our environment every day. Experts have noted a corresponding leap in hearing loss at young ages. The unexpected culprit: headphones and portable cassette or CD players.

At the Los Angeles–based House Ear Institute, doctors and hearing specialists have studied since 1950 the effects of noise-induced hearing loss. "One important feature of NIHL," they say, "is that it is preventable in all but certain cases of accidental exposure. Legislation and regulations have been enacted that spell out guidelines for protecting workers from hazardous noise levels in the workplace and consumers from hazardous noise during leisure time pursuits."[4]

Laws and rules aside, there is no rehabilitation or twelve-step program for a noise-ravaged ear. All you can do is minimize further damaging exposure and hope that your rock 'n' roll days (or the equivalent thereof) were actually fewer than you now remember. While marked improvements are currently being made in digital hearing aids, they are expensive, and results cannot compare with the original equipment. Best solution: Practice safe sonics!

HEALTHY SOUND AWARENESS

Whether or not you have hearing loss, it's never too late to begin using ear protection and practicing hearing conservation. Much as we perceive temperature—one person may be hot while another is comfortable—each individual hears sound a little differently. As a consequence, susceptibility to noise and hearing loss varies widely.[5]

Previous hearing loss does not guard against additional auditory damage. While you may not be aware of it—because of your already diminished perception of harmful levels of sound—further erosion of the organ of Corti can still take place. It is never too late to begin to practice sound awareness.

As I have noted before, sounds are measured in decibels (dB), and each 10 dB increase represents a tenfold increase in sound energy. Thus 90 dB is ten times noisier than 80 dB. Indeed, the exponential nature of decibels is appropriately similar to the Richter scale for earth tremors.

Table 8.1 shows the decibel levels of common noise environments.

TABLE 8.1

Decibel Levels of Common Noises

NOISE	DECIBELS
Watch ticking	20
Whisper	30
Average conversation	40
Leaves rustling	40
Quiet neighborhood street	50
Dishwasher, microwave, blower on furnace	60
Alarm clock buzzer	70
City traffic	70
Noisy restaurant	70
Garbage disposal, vacuum cleaner	80
Busy city sidewalk	80
DANGER ZONE	
Battery-powered siren on toy ambulance	90
Lawn mower	90
Screaming child	90
Subway platform	100
Power drill, chain saw	100
Blow dryer	100
Snowmobile	100
Automobile horn	110
Snowblower	110
Noisy video arcade	110
Rock concert	100–130
Boom cars (when turned up)	125–138
Jet engine at 100 feet	130
Gunshot	140
Jackhammer	180

The standard sonic health formula is based on the proportion of amplitude and length of exposure. How loud and for how long are the factors determining whether hearing damage takes place?

In human adults, 80 dB is the maximum sound intensity that will not produce sensorineural loss regardless of duration.[6] In other words, no matter how long you listen to something at 80 dB, you do not have to worry about ear damage. Above 85 dB, you start playing with auditory fire. Cilia cell damage worsens with length of exposure and higher dB levels. With every 10 dB increase in sound, a quantum jump in effect takes place.

The following standard of noise-level safety is based on decibels and time-exposure levels determined in 1971 by the U.S. Department of Labor, Occupational Safety and Health Administration. In 1984, on further research, 90 dB for eight hours was changed to 85 dB. Therefore, use table 8.2 as an indicator. It was created for the workplace, and the duration per day may be higher than what is truly healthy for your ears.

TABLE 8.2
Permissible Noise Exposures[7]

SOUND LEVEL (IN DECIBELS)	DURATION PER DAY (IN HOURS)
90	8
92	6
95	4
97	3
100	2
102	1.5
105	1
110	0.5
115	0.25 or less

SAFE SONICS

So how do we live in our noisy culture without becoming sound paranoiacs? The goal is to protect our wonderful hearing mechanisms so we can enjoy the beautiful sounds of our planet; it would be a tragedy to lose the ability to perceive the sounds of a flute, our children's laughter, a loved one's voice, and nature. Serious hearing loss does not necessarily substitute silence for other sounds; often they are replaced with tinnitus, or ringing or buzzing sounds in the head. Hearing damage is not something to take lightly. It will affect you for the rest of your life. Here are some precautionary measures.

- *Limit your exposure to sounds over 85 dB.* If you must be around sounds over this level, minimize the amount of time around each exposure, and wear ear protection.
- *With headphones, observe the following:* Keep the volume down;* limit yourself to one hour at a time and let your ears rest. Be extremely careful using headphones when you are exercising or at work (see chapter 9).
- *Give your ears a rest.* Alternate quiet and noisy activities. Don't go directly to a rock club after a loud sports event; wait a few hours before going out in a snowmobile if you work at a noisy job site.

HEARING-PROTECTION DEVICES: EARPLUGS AND EARMUFFS

If you have to shout to be heard, your sonic environment is too loud. Based on intensity and length of exposure, consider adding earplugs or earmuffs to your repertoire of health aids.

Earplugs are available easily and cheaply at any hardware or drugstore. Don't let your kids go to a rock concert without them. (Some organizations routinely pass out earplugs at rock concerts. One such exemplary group is Hearing Education and Awareness for Rockers, or HEAR. See "Soundwork Resources.") Earplugs are made of foam, silicone, or wax, with noise-reduction levels ranging from 20 to 30 dB. Cotton in your ears is a nice concept, but it won't effectively diminish excessive sound waves.

---

* Most portable stereos can amplify music to as loud as 110 to 130 dB. Over time, many people prefer listening levels that rank within the harmful range. If you listen with headphones to a portable tape or CD player with a ten-digit volume wheel set at 4 or higher, you may be contributing to hearing loss.

Earmuffs can be found in sporting goods stores. They tend to last longer than earplugs, may afford better protection, and may be more comfortable, depending on the weather. The term *earmuffs* (as in *ear mufflers*) does not refer here to the kind used for warmth; rather, these are special ear protectors specifically designed for protection from loud sound.

Your personal and professional requirements will determine which combination of earplugs and earmuffs can afford you the proper protection. For maximum effectiveness, muffs and plugs must be correctly worn, maintained, and replaced as needed.

Noise-intensive activities that can contribute to NIHL and for which you should take appropriate measures by wearing earplugs or earmuffs and limiting time per exposure include very loud TVs and stereos, leaf blowers, lawn mowers, snowblowers, and power tools in the home; among children's toys, watch out for certain battery-operated cars, sirens on toy ambulances, some musical night lights, and toy vacuum cleaners.

Snowmobiles, jet skis, motorcycles, amd model airplanes (if flown indoors), as well as real and toy firearms, are recreational items that can lead to NIHL.

CONCLUSION

Because our ears don't actually bleed after a blast of fireworks or a rock concert, we don't comprehend the self-induced damage. But the cells are hurting inside the inner ear. As mentioned previously, more than thirty million Americans suffer from hearing loss. "About 75 percent of hearing loss in the typical American is caused not by the aging process alone," says William Clark, a senior scientist at the Central Institute for the Deaf in St. Louis, "but by what you've done to your ears throughout your lifetime."[8]

While the concept of hearing-protection devices is novel in a nonindustrial setting, it is time to consider using them. Given the increasing noise of Western society and research clearly delineating irreversible noise-induced hearing loss, we would be foolish not to take appropriate measures.

As with secondhand tobacco exposure and increased exposure to ultraviolet light owing to our diminished ozone layer, sound pollution now requires us to take appropriate measures to safeguard an important organ of perception and pleasure. Even if you do not need the earplugs, conscientious sound awareness will go a long way toward preserving your aural well-being.

9 Music and Sound in Your Life

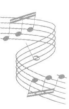 To this point, I have examined the physics of sound and the mechanics of hearing. I have looked at the effect on the body of tone (resonance) and rhythm (entrainment). The elegant theories of Tomatis and the discoveries of Doman have shed light on the physio- and psychological effects of sound stimulation. Finally, understanding body pulses and looking at sonic safety issues have brought me to practical suggestions that embrace all of the above topics.

In this chapter I look at personal applications of psycho-acoustic principles. From "Music for Babies" to "Music in the Hospital," selected research into the effects of music and sound will be combined with suggestions on how you can use sound in a positive and effective manner.

Be aware of the power of sound; use it consciously. As with any substance, there can be positive and negative applications. *Think of music and sound as thinking people's drugs.* They can enhance, arouse, or depress. Like food, water, wine, sex, and pharmaceuticals, it all comes down to frequency and dosage. The question becomes: *How often and how much?* Applied to the effectiveness of auditory stimulation as well as nervous system balance, the answer is always individual. This is the nature of sound: subtle, powerful, personal.

A comprehensive list of musical resources is given in the "Sound Remedies Catalog" 📖 (see page 285). These recommended selections are offered as a starting place. I believe that given the differences among individual nervous systems, what works well for one may have a different effect on another. Therefore, applying the principles of resonance and entrainment to each individual circumstance is the preferred method of effective sonic prescription. *Think of music and sound as self-help for the nervous system.* Compile your own lists based on personal preference and the intention of the application.

MUSIC FOR BABIES

In 1998 a few states in America actually legislated applications of classical music for infants and young children. In Georgia, every newborn leaves the hospital with a classical CD or cassette—a gift from the state! Florida now requires all its state-funded childcare facilities to play classical music every day. What was the genesis of this idea?

Scientists who have studied infant brain development say that infants can develop sensitivity to music as young as four months of age.[1] However, according to Dr. Tomatis, sound processing is not a new function at all for the newborn. He believes the unborn child has been hearing for four and a half months prior to birth.[2] Therefore, once the baby is born and the outer and middle ear switches from liquid to air induction, the baby's auditory mechanism is 100 percent functional.

On birth, a baby's brain is a mass of neurons. The potential for learning physical and mental skills turns into reality as neuronal pathways connect with different sections of the brain. The first few years will determine the child's ability to learn for the rest of his or her life—for during these early years, nerve cells form and connect at an astonishing rate.[3]

The latest research shows that music is actually perceived in many areas of the brain. According to a 1998 study from the University of Texas, music experts determined that rhythm is tracked by the cerebellum, melody perceived by the temporal lobes, and interpretation of musical notation accomplished in areas on the right side of the brain that correspond to areas on the left that process language.[4]

The circuitry for spatial reasoning and mathematics lies in or near the brain's cortex. The function of musical perception takes place in part in the same area. When a baby hears music, it stimulates this part of the brain, resulting in an increase in the newborn's neuronal development. Theoretically, this should lead to better brain functioning in math and spatial reasoning—increased neuronal circuitry is a collateral result of the perception of music. Additionally, language and music are both forms of communication that rely on highly organized variations in pitch, accent, rhythm, and timbre. While these are discrete cognitive systems, both language and music are rich in harmonics, the overtones of a sound that give it resonance and distinction. In language, sounds are combined into patterns—words. Music does the same patterning with melodic phrases.[5]

In an experiment by Sandra Trehub, a developmental psychologist at the University of Toronto, and reported in *Discover* magazine, repeated intervals were played to six-month-olds, with the intervals raised or lowered occasionally to determine if the infants could decipher the difference in the pattern. They could, especially when the test intervals were perfect fifths or fourths. Clearly, there is an interrelationship between music and language.

It is assumed that by exposing babies to complex musical structures, their brains will by necessity develop neuronal connections. The chemical interaction of neuronal connections is a natural response for the interpretation of incoming data. In this instance the data happen to be in sonic form. The fact that math, language, and spatial reasoning skills benefit from neuronal development spurred by musical input is perhaps a happenstance of cerebral neighborhoods. In other words, brain functions that border or share the musical perceptual areas (that part of the brain's real estate, so to speak) may prosper by association.

MUSIC IN THE CARE OF THE NEWBORN

By the time the unborn child is six months in utero, he or she not only hears music but also responds, interacts, differentiates, and even has preferences.[6] Researchers have found that a fetus will jump in rhythm to the beat of an orchestra drum. The unconscious memory of the maternal heartbeat in utero appears to be the reason that a baby is comforted by being held against someone's chest or is lulled to sleep by the steady ticking of a clock. Regardless of culture or caregiver, babies are instinctually held with their heads near the heart. The mother's heartbeat has been the sound that dominated the unborn child's world.

Other voices and familiar sounds add harmony to the progressive composition of the uterine symphony. From the sixteenth week, the unborn child is capable of hearing. He or she has much to listen to, because the pregnant abdomen and uterus are very noisy places. As you can imagine, the ongoing blood flow through the placenta is a nonstop river of sound. Studies of the newborn's auditory capacity suggest that infants prefer high-pitched voices to low pitches. This makes sense; Mama's voice—in the high frequency range—was an ongoing prebirth phenomenon. According to psychiatrist and Tomatis practitioner Ron Minson, "It's well known that there is a higher incidence of learning disabilities in adopted children than in the general population." In Tomatis circles it is widely held that a baby taken from its natural sonic environment—away from its natural mother—will tend to "close down" instead of the normal reflex of "reaching out." These terms are metaphorical because Tomatis is referring not to an actual physical reaction but to a psychological one that quickly translates into physiological ear and brain manifestations. For further information on this subject, contact a Tomatis practitioner (see "Soundwork Resources").

In selecting sounds and music for the newborn, consider the type of music that the mother has been listening to pre-birth, along with the baby's response to the music. Familiar pieces will assist the infant in feeling secure in an enormously new environment. Much like a child or adult, a newborn seeks familiarity. That which we recognize makes us feel safe.

SOUND AWARENESS FOR BABIES

Words, math, spatial perception, and music are all intertwined in the brain. You might expect that if you could stimulate one capacity, the others would prosper. Following that line of thinking, why not surround the baby with numeric equations? By stimulating the mathematical part of the brain, wouldn't that also increase the neurons connected with musical processing? Probably not.

The cerebral triggering that occurs through the ears is different from what occurs through the eyes. Physiology textbook authors readily admit that knowledge of the brain's auditory perception—while advanced—is incomplete. Let it suffice to say that sound and the ear play a role in the development of the nervous system very different from that of the eyes, nose, and mouth.

Classical music for babies? Absolutely. They will learn beauty and form. They will be mesmerized by the sounds; gentle harmonies will soothe them. Perfection exists within complex classical music as well as in the simplicity of a single melodic line.

But which music? you may ask. Using your understanding of entrainment, determine what you would like to accomplish. If you wish to help your baby sleep, use adagio and lento (slow) movements. If you wish to calm an uncomfortable baby, use simple music—pieces with light densities of orchestration, such as acoustic guitar solos and harp and flute duets. It will be easier on the nervous system of a tired parent and child if the sound source is uncomplicated and takes less energy to process. To distract or entertain a little one, pick what you like. Remember, always keep it soft and gentle. Loud, sudden sounds will scare a baby. This is never the goal with music, and it will defeat your purposes in using music to enhance and support.

Best of all . . . sing to your child. Regardless of the magnificence of the classical repertoire, the mother's sweet, loving voice is the ultimate analgesic for a baby. The only thing that comes close is the father's voice, especially if he has been vocally present during the pregnancy. According to Dr. Tomatis, the more a newborn hears the mother's voice, the more he or she will reach out for reconnection. This is the best thing for a developing baby.

Recommended Selections: 📖 See "Sound Remedies Catalog."

MUSIC FOR TEENAGERS

The amazing transitional time between childhood and adulthood seems to fall loosely into the category of adolescent years—twelve to nineteen. During these teen years, raging hormones cause the body to change as sexuality emerges. A driver's license allows heretofore unknown freedom. Social interaction intensifies. Preparation for college causes academic pressures to increase. Choices abound: *What do you like? Who is in charge and why? What do you want to do with your life? When are you going to leave home?* These are big questions that go to the root of security, groundedness, and self-esteem. The soul searching of this time can cause anxiety and produce stress. Finding ways to deal with the quantum changes looming ahead is a well-worn rite of passage. Music and teenagers is a match made in heaven . . . or some might say hell! Let's find out why.

"Music has strong effects on behavior and can do so by communicating moods and emotions." As sound researcher N. M. Weinberger notes, numerous studies attest to music's powerful influence on mood and emotion.[7] According to a renowned pioneer in psychiatric aspects of music, Dr. Peter Ostwald of the University of California, San Francisco, music is "a form of social behavior . . . a symbolic emotional experience."[8] Moreover, music may provide a form of nonverbal communication whose meaning is ineffable—it cannot be captured in words. Perhaps music exists because of the need for expression of emotions that "can only crudely be measured or described in words."[9]

"Therefore," Weinberger concludes, "music can rapidly and powerfully set moods and do so in a way not as easily attained by other means. (Even if adequate to the task, the written word cannot do so as quickly and, when used, often must convey a particular setting, content and visual imagery that itself interferes with or shifts thoughts.)"[10]

Given our understanding of the power of music and its evocation of mood and emotion, there is another piece to add to the puzzle—that of guided imagery. How do words and music together influence us?

There has been much research on this topic. However, one recent study makes a concise statement: Music and guided imagery actually alter hormonal output. In a 1996 study titled "The Effect of Selected Classical Music and Spontaneous Imagery on Plasma B-Endorphin," researchers explored the effect of music and verbal imagery. What they were looking to determine was if silence, music alone, or music with guided verbal imagery could cause a decline in the secretion of a stress hormone. A significant decline in the hormone was found in the group of volunteers that used music and imagery combined. No other group demonstrated any significant changes.[11]

What is guided imagery? Simplistically, I would define it as a psychological tool that intentionally uses language to paint conscious and subconscious images for a specific therapeutic effect. This methodology can be used for relaxation, for self-induced healing, or in a psychotherapeutic context. When words are used in conjunction with music that complements the imagery, a very powerful match of verbal and nonverbal cues is sent to the brain. Quite often the creation of a trance state facilitates a deeper induction of the guided imagery. And what can create trance? Rhythm and entrainment.[12]

If we understand the effect of music to elicit emotion and mood and the ability of words to stimulate and label feelings, a picture emerges of the powerful combination of words, rhythm, and music. Add to the mix a vulnerable teenage psyche and we have a recipe for considerable influence. Let's look at seven recent reports and studies and see what these different perspectives add up to.

RECENT RESEARCH

"Adolescents and Their Music." In a 1989 issue of the *Journal of the American Medical Association,* Dr. Elizabeth Brown reported: "During adolescence, teenagers are expected to develop standards of behavior and reconcile them with their perceptions of adult standards. In this context, music, a powerful medium in the lives of adolescents, offers conflicting values. The explicit sexual and violent lyrics of some forms of music clash with the themes of abstinence and rational behavior promoted by adult society. Identification with rock music, particularly those styles that are rejected by adults, functions to separate adolescents from adult society. Some forms of rock music extend well beyond respectability in fulfilling this definitional role. Total immersion into a rock subculture, such as heavy metal, may be both a portrait of adolescent alienation and an unflattering reflection of an adolescent's perception of the moral and ethical duplicity of adult society. Physicians should be aware of the role of music in the lives of adolescents and use music preferences as clues to the emotional and mental health of adolescents."[13]

"Adolescents' Interest in and Views of Destructive Themes in Rock Music." In this 1987 University of Florida study, the goal was to determine musical preferences and views on homicide, satanism, and suicide (HSS). In all, 694 middle and high school students were given questionnaires of structured and open-ended questions. Nine percent of the middle school students, 17 percent of the rural, and 24 percent of the urban high school students were HSS rock fans. Three quarters of these fans were male, and nearly all were white.

Of the remaining non-HSS fans, a large proportion shared the concern of adult citizens and professional groups about destructive lyrics in rock music and their effects.[14]

"Adolescent Suicide: Music Preference as an Indicator of Vulnerability." Researched in 1992, this study from Australia investigated possible relationships between adolescents' music preferences and aspects of their psychological health and lifestyle. Of the girls, 74 percent preferred pop music; 71 percent of the boys preferred rock and heavy metal. Significant associations with suicidal thoughts, acts of deliberate self-harm, depression, delinquency, drug taking, and family dysfunction appeared to exist with those respondents who preferred rock or heavy metal. This was especially true of the 26 percent of the girls who expressed a preference for rock or heavy metal.

Feeling sadder after listening to the rock or heavy metal appeared to distinguish the most disturbed group. Researchers postulate that these students—11 percent of the poll group—are the most vulnerable to acting out the lyrics or themes from the music.[15]

"Differential Gender Affects of Exposure to Rap Music on African Americans." Thirty African-American males and thirty African-American females, ages eleven through sixteen, from an inner-city youth club in Wilmington, North Carolina, were recruited for this 1995 study. They were shown nonviolent rap videos that contained images of women in sexually subordinate roles. They also read a vignette that involved teen dating violence perpetrated by a male. Some parts of the group did not see the videos.

Responses showed a significant correlation to gender. Acceptance of the use of violence did not vary for the young men after watching the videos. Conversely, female subjects who were exposed to the videos showed greater acceptance of the violence than did females who were not exposed.

Prior studies have shown that exposure to violent rap music did, in fact, tend to lead to a higher degree of acceptance of the use of violence, including violence against women.[16]

"The Influence of Misogynous Rap Music on Sexual Aggression Against Women." This study focused solely on the effects of misogynous rap music on men. Conducted in 1995 at Ohio's Kent State University, the purpose of this research was to determine the effect of cognitive distortions concerning women on sexually aggressive behavior in the laboratory. *Misogyny* is defined as "hatred of women." The misogynous rap music used in this study contained frequent references to both sex and violence. These songs often referred to women as "bitches" and "hos" and suggested that women enjoy coercive sex. The rap songs used for the neutral listening contained no references to sex or violence and were primarily concerned with the problems of social injustice facing African Americans in America.

Twenty-seven men listened to misogynous rap music and twenty-seven men listened to neutral rap music. Participants then viewed neutral and sexual/violent film vignettes and chose one to show to a female confederate. Among the participants in the misogynous music group, 30 percent showed the assaultive vignette and 70 percent showed the neutral. Among the men who listened to the neutral rap music, only 7 percent showed the sexual/violent video; 93 percent showed the neutral vignette.

These findings suggest that misogynous music facilitates sexually aggressive behavior and support the relationship between cognitive distortions and sexual aggression.[17]

"The Relationship between Heavy Metal and Rap Music and Adolescent Turmoil: Real or Artifact?" Adolescents and their parents were surveyed to investigate the association between heavy metal and rap music and adolescent psychosocial turmoil. Adolescents who preferred heavy metal and rap music were compared with those who preferred other types of music. Results indicated that adolescents who preferred heavy metal and rap music had a higher incidence of below-average school grades, school behavioral problems, sexual activity, drug and alcohol use, and arrests.

Researchers in this 1994 study noted, however, that the majority of heavy metal and rap listeners are male: "What we may be seeing are merely behaviors associated with being an adolescent male."[18]

"The Immediate Effects of Homicidal, Suicidal, and Nonviolent Heavy Metal and Rap Songs on the Moods of College Students." This 1995 study from Appalachian State University examined the impact of homicidal, suicidal, and nonviolent heavy metal and rap songs on the moods of male undergraduates. There were no effects of song content or music type on suicidal ideation, anxiety, or self-esteem. Also, researchers found that male adolescents reported feeling a release of negative emotions—in a positive, nondestructive way—when listening to heavy metal music.[19]

SOUND AWARENESS FOR TEENS

If you survey the titles of these research studies, you might think that I purposefully looked for the most damning and negative reports I could find. Not so. In my extensive literature reviews of medical and psychology journals (where most recent research is reported), these papers were the sum total of what I discovered. Combing through the popular press (major magazines and daily newspapers), these were the articles I found: "Sonic Boomers: Turning Up the Volume"; "Is Rock Music Rotting Our Kids' Minds?"; "Rock Doesn't Rot Anybody's Mind . . . But Heavy Metal Just Might"; "Midlife Music"; "Decibel Disciples: Young-at-Heart Head Bangers and Their Heavy Metal Way of Life"; and "Does Rap Music Need a Warning Label?"

With the exception of "Midlife Music," all the articles questioned the negative effects of rock, heavy metal, and rap music. "Rock music has been decried as a scourge of society since it was first introduced to the American public by Bill Haley and The Comets in 1955," states Mary Ballard, a psychology professor and specialist on the impact of the media on adolescents and children. This may be because the foundation of rock 'n' roll was built on defiance, rebellion, and the expression of youthful angst. Ballard continues: "Two subgenres of rock, heavy metal and rap, may best exemplify both the insurgency and the disenfranchisement experienced by many adolescents. At the same time, heavy metal and rap music often embody the worst fears of the parents of this generation's youth, that is, sex, drugs, and violence. Thus these two types of rock music have become the center of a controversy that has reached from the sermons of small town churches to hearings on Capitol Hill."[20]

Sex, drugs, and violence . . . In the 1960s the famous lifestyle slogan was Sex, Drugs, and Rock 'n' Roll. However, many things have changed since then. AIDS, crack cocaine, and handguns have tarnished the battle cry of the counterculture. Things are very different for our children from when we grew up in the heady days of the original Woodstock. The 1990s began a different chapter, with music continuing to play a unique role— but the stakes are higher now.

Since rock 'n' roll emerged almost fifty years ago, it has become the auditory anthem of individuating teenagers. One of the things that has changed, however, is the ubiquity of music among today's teens. Due to new technologies such as portable players and lightweight headphones, music is now a constant companion. In the *Journal of the American Medical Association*'s report "Adolescents and Their Music," Dr. Elizabeth Brown noted that between the seventh and twelfth grades, the average teenager listens to 10,500 hours of rock music, just slightly less than the entire number of hours spent in the classroom from kindergarten through high school.[21]

This statistic is staggering. I have a six-year-old daughter. What did I just present her for the holidays? A portable CD player and a dozen very carefully chosen CDs. I was not intentionally enrolling her in the music "habit." I wanted to introduce her to the joy of music, for her to discover different styles. I want her to know music as a good friend—a place she can go when there are too many words. I selected show tunes, silly tunes, and Irish, Gregorian, and Jewish holiday music. I included world-beat albums for children and musical dramatizations of Mozart, Vivaldi, and Handel. I'd rather she listen to music than sit mindlessly in front of a TV.

Yet many parents, researchers, and lawmakers draw correlations between escalating violence and graphically sexual or violent rock lyrics. They point out that children with headsets live in an unmonitored world of repetitive suggestion. Many believe that at least TV is a public forum that can be experienced as a family and discussed and processed as such.

Aren't the adolescents who spend 10,500 hours listening to music practicing the art of choice? Aren't free will, preference, and judgment important parts of honing adult skills? This book has spent a great deal of time advocating the concept of the intentional use of music and sound. Does anyone force children to listen to something they don't like, or do they gravitate to the music that resonates emotionally or physically for them?

If teenagers have feelings of frustration, rage, and despair, they will find music that addresses those issues. Perhaps this is why the major consumers of heavy metal music are teenage males. What are the issues on a teenage girl's mind? Love, tenderness, "doing it"! Who buys the millions of albums of clean-cut, cute eighteen-year-old male sex symbols? The fourteen-year-old girls. What are the themes of this music? Best friends, love, tenderness, and the like. Recall who did all the screaming at the early Elvis or Beatles concerts.

Seguing to the year 2000, let's examine the effect of heavy metal and rap music from a psychoacoustic vantage point. The primary musical elements of rap consist of fairly slow rhythms on a drum machine (extremely periodic) and lots of up-front bass. This is sonic Valium! The rhythm slows the nervous system. The preponderance of bass does not energize the nervous system; rather, it is discharging. Add the lyrics, rapped in a periodic cadence. This style of speaking, along with the rock-steady percussion, facilitates trance. Recall that at the beginning of this section on teens, I spoke about the power of music and guided imagery. Rap music is an extraordinary sonic tool. It contains all the elements of a therapeutic device. The question, however, is whether its guided imagery is positive or if it embraces and imparts negative values. Some is positive and some is not. Rap stars booked on murder charges are not exactly the kind of role model that any parent wants. Yet isn't this situation—one that has overtaken and crossed all racial boundaries—a reflection of our culture? Or is it defining our culture?

Heavy metal follows in many of the same footsteps as rap, with lots of bass but faster rhythms. Where rap seeks to keep it slow and low, heavy metal music accomplishes the same blowout of the nervous system through overload—lots of distortion turned up very loud. The themes of head-banger music tend to be on the negative side. Not much political or social awareness here. Yet who is forcing a fan to listen? What is it about this music that attracts the white teenage male? Aside from the fact that his parents cannot stand it, it makes him feel good. Those bass tones hit right in the gonads. Few young men are constantly sexually active, but they are hormonally active. Perhaps they are attracted to this music because it actually settles them down . . . in the same way that rap grew out of the inner city—young black men "chilling out," keeping from exploding from the frustration of watching their brothers and friends die on the streets or end up in jail.

What attracts one kid to death metal and another to Christian rock? For some, identification with a particular musical style indicates resistance to authority and provides an outlet for personal troubles or conflicts with parents or school. For others, music provides relaxation and entertainment, soothes emotions, and creates a groove to dance and clap to. Ultimately, music will not turn a good kid bad. But it can influence a troubled kid and reinforce a negative direction.

Rock is an extraordinary American art form. In any of its varied approximations, rock music is not the problem. If anything, rock—or any other form of music—is an indicator of resonance. We are attracted to that which is most familiar. If a teenager is drawn to lyrics about suicide or Satan, this is a wake-up call.

The music is the messenger. Don't shoot the messenger! Instead, welcome the opportunity to make genuine, authentic, patient pathways into your children's minds and emotions. Listen to what they are saying by what they are listening to. These are the keys, and they are in your hands.

MUSIC FOR SENIORS

The research that I have come across on music and seniors tends to focus on the use of music for remediation of depression, anxiety, Alzheimer's and Parkinson's diseases, and dementia—in other words, using music for healing. This is valuable information, but in the second section—"Sound Awareness and Seniors"—I will address the use of music and sound as enhancement tools for elders who are active and vital in their lives.

MUSIC AND HEALING: RECENT RESEARCH

"Soothing Sounds: Even Raucous Tunes May Be Relaxing." Research indicates that depressed seniors can benefit from listening to music. However, it is recommended that the music selected first match the mood of the listener, then lead to slower and more relaxing pieces as the session continues.[22]

"Effects of Music Therapy Strategy on Depressed Older Adults." Music has been used as a form of therapy for older adults in residential and adult daycare centers. Studies have documented the effects of music on the quality of life, expression of feelings, involvement with the environment, awareness and responsiveness, positive associations, and socialization in these settings.

In this research study, however, music was explored in the home with senior adults who had a history of depression or acute anxiety. Home-based music therapy is seen as an alternative to pharmaceutical drugs that might have side effects or interfere with existing prescriptions, as a palliative coping strategy for the relief of pain and anxiety, and as a therapeutic support for the homebound or those who cannot afford psychotherapy.

This study showed that depression, distress, self-esteem, and mood greatly improved when a daily regimen of listening to music with therapeutic support was instituted. Another study group commenced a daily self-administered music therapy practice. A third group, the control group, had no music or therapeutic support. Both of the groups that heard thirty to sixty minutes of music a day saw much improvement in symptoms. Therapeutic support had the greatest result. However, the group with music and no therapist showed impressive positive results when compared to the control group with no music. Follow-up testing after nine months showed that self-administered music listening sessions when symptoms arose produced the same positive effects as did daily use of music. In other words, there was a learned response.[23]

"Music Therapy: Doctors Explore the Healing Potential of Rhythm and Song." "Music therapists are a unique breed of musician-counselors, with specialized training in the use of rhythm and melody to improve psychological and emotional well-being. They work with individuals and groups in psychiatric hospitals, nursing homes, rehabilitation centers, community mental health centers, residencies for the developmentally disabled, and correctional facilities."[24]

Researchers are finding that drumming and music can improve motor coordination in people with Parkinson's disease and evoke long-forgotten memories in Alzheimer's patients.

According to neurologist Oliver Sacks, author of *Awakenings*, "Music can be a crucially important aspect of therapy. Often people who can no longer use or understand language and cannot achieve conceptual thought can respond to music. I've seen patients who couldn't take a single step but could dance, and patients who could not utter a single syllable but could sing."

According to music therapist Louise Lynch, director of musical activities at an adult daycare center, "Music is very often the only thing that older demented adults will respond to." Alicia Ann Clare, director of music therapy at the University of Kansas in Lawrence, states: "Music gives them a window of time to come out of the confusion. Rhythm provides structure and security. It's anxiety-reducing." Lynch observes that "the rhythm helps organize them in time and space."

Sacks speaks about the effects of music and rhythm after the sound has stopped. "One of the striking things about music," he says, "is that people not only join in but they often stay organized for a time afterwards." According to Sacks, nobody knows quite why music has the effect on Alzheimer's patients that it does. The measure of lucidity may come from music's power to stimulate memories. Memory, he says, is the key to a sense of self.

"We are historical, generational creatures," he notes, "and without memory we lose our identities. Music is one of the most powerful ways of calling out the identity. You have to find the right music, the music that calls the person by evoking certain memories."

In the field of Parkinson's disease, research into the effects of rhythm therapies in improving the ability of patients to walk has been very promising. Some have walked 50 percent faster at the end of studies than when they began. Given that Parkinson's is a degenerative disease, Dr. Michael Thaut, director of these studies, asks, "Can we stem the long-term decline of these Parkinson's patients? That's the burning question." His studies continue.

SOUND AWARENESS AND SENIORS

The category "seniors," which by various estimates will soon include the front end of the enormous bubble of baby boomers *and* their parents, is becoming a very large segment of the American population. Therefore, this is the ideal group of people to practice proactive auditory restoration.

Auditory restoration refers to the process of tuning up the auditory mechanism so that it takes in as full a spectrum of sound frequencies as possible. Based on the belief that sound is energy and the ear is a primary portal to the brain and nervous system, the logic is that the more sonic fuel we can take in, the better. What inhibits this flow? The ability to perceive sound through the outer, middle, or inner ear. Other than physiological damage or deformity to the outer ear that would affect the flow of sound, I am essentially speaking about the middle and inner ear.

As I discussed in chapter 7, "A New Awareness of Sound," psychologically induced (stress-induced) hearing dysfunction is a middle-ear issue. Through the process of auditory retraining and sound stimulation, a sub-functioning middle ear can be retuned, its flaccid muscles retonified. This allows the middle-ear mechanism to transfer a fuller spectrum of sounds to the inner ear. The net effect: enhanced energy, alertness, and increased active listening.

Beyond physical health, a primary concern of seniors is maintaining a sharp and focused mind. Given that inner-ear processing diminishes with age, another concern is being able to hear.

Sound stimulation addresses both these issues. Although inner-ear hearing loss cannot be restored, tonified middle-ear function allows us to use what we've got left more fully.

Where can you partake of sound stimulation and auditory retraining? There is a new generation of soundwork products and practitioners specializing in auditory retraining. Most use derivations of the Tomatis Method. In-clinic and at-home programs are now available. (See "Sound work Resources" for a listing of sound stimulation products and practitioner networks.)

MUSIC AND EARLY EDUCATION

It seems that barely a week goes by without the appearance of another research study about the effects of music on education. The following headlines say it all: "Music Training May Boost Memory"; "Music May

Help Neurological Therapy"; "Beautiful Music Improves Brain Power"; "Musical Links for Scientists and Mathematicians of Tomorrow"; "Improved Maze Learning through Early Music Exposure in Rats."

On the brink of a new century, there is little doubt that legitimate scientific research can verify the power of music. Rather, the only questions are, *To what degree?* and *How soon?* and *When will music, as an educational aid, be implemented on a mass level?* As research accelerates, there is mounting evidence that music and young children are a very good match.

RECENT RESEARCH

"Early Music Training Alters Brain Anatomy." A research team from Germany discovered that the corpus callosum—the central bundle of nerve fibers connecting the two hemispheres of the brain—was significantly larger in musicians who had studied at an early age than in nonmusicians. Nerves that control motor function on both sides of the body pass through the corpus callosum. The researchers believe that musical training in early life lays down either additional "wiring" or better-insulated wiring, resulting in better communication between the two hemispheres.[25]

"Music Has Long-Term Effect on Abstract Reasoning Skills." An inner-city daycare center was the locale where thirty-three three-year-olds were tested. Nineteen children were provided with weekly piano lessons and daily group singing sessions. Fourteen children did not receive any musical training at all. After eight months, the musical group showed great improvement in working with puzzles—a standard test for mathematical reasoning skills. In a larger follow-up study, researchers found that children who participated in voice and piano studies increased their spatial-temporal IQs by a 46 percent mean. Those children who received no musical training improved by 6 percent. Spatial IQ is important to higher brain functions such as mathematics.[26]

"Music and Math." Using first-graders, a Rhode Island control group was given the district's standard music and art training. The experimental group was given *more intensive* instruction in music and art. At the beginning of the test, the experimental group rated below the control group. After seven months, the experimental group had pulled even with the control group in reading, and considerably bypassed it in mathematics.[27]

"Music Training Boosts Memory." In Hong Kong, psychologists found that word memory increased by 16 percent in adults who had learned a musical instrument as a child. The study involved thirty college students with a minimum of six years of musical training prior to age twelve and thirty students with no prior musical instruction. The musically trained were found to be better at recalling words read to them from a list. Interestingly enough, they were no better at recalling and drawing simple designs from memory. The researchers note that the left planum temporale region of the brain, behind the left ear, is larger in musicians. This is the part of the brain that also handles verbal memory.[28]

"Improved Maze Learning through Early Music Exposure in Rats." Rats were exposed in utero and sixty days after birth to either complex music (Mozart's Sonata K. 448), minimalist music (Philip Glass), white noise, or silence. By day three, the rats exposed to the Mozart completed the maze more rapidly and with fewer errors than did the rats assigned to the other groups. The difference increased in magnitude through day five. This suggests that repeated exposure to complex music induces improved spatial-temporal learning in rats; similar results have been found in humans. These tests suggest a similar neurophysical mechanism for the effects of music on rats and humans.[29]

SOUND AWARENESS AND EARLY EDUCATION

Music is a more potent instrument than any other for education.

—**Plato (347 B.C.E.)**

Increased communication between cerebral hemispheres, 46 percent spatial-temporal IQ improvement in three-year-olds, improved math skills in first-graders, better word retention by adults who studied music as children, maze-racing rats that accelerate to Mozart: comical? Yes. Serious? Yes. How did Plato know that music is a more potent instrument than any other for education? He probably observed that students who played music excelled in other areas as well. He didn't run clinical trials and get written up in psychology journals. He simply noted what was in front of him.

What clinicians are finding, in test after test, is that young brains benefit with the simple application of this fun activity. What could be better for education? Yet in the era of budget-cutting in public education in America, the arts have been the first thing to go.

What can you do with your children?

1. *Sing with your children.* This is a great way for them to learn a sense of rhythm, practice phonics, make up rhymes, and have fun with you. Locate local music-for-children events. Bookstores often host weekend morning children's musical events.
2. *Introduce them to musical instruments.* Have instruments—even a little drum or tambourine—available for them to play with. My six-year-old daughter pounds on the piano (she can play "Do, a Deer," from *The Sound of Music*) and sings with a tiny guitar that she cannot functionally play but loves to play with. Fun is the goal at this age.
3. *Buy your child a cassette player.* There are *wonderful* children's books on tape available in record stores (they are orchestrated). Additionally, clever and sweet musical recordings abound, produced specifically for youngsters. It is far better for the development of your children's minds to be listening to music or a musical story than to be sitting in front of a TV. Just as when you read them a story, when children listen to music their imagination is busy making up a visual story. This practice is lost when they sit passively in front of a TV, with all of the images provided.
4. *Have music playing in your house.* The more your young children hear different kinds of music, the more interest they will focus in that direction. Engage with them about what you are hearing. For instance, you might point out which instrument is playing, then relate this to a visual representation in person or in a picture.
5. *Make instruction available.* If your children show an interest in wanting to learn more about music, inquire about teachers who specialize

in nonpressured, gentle instruction. Some children are started in disciplined and rigorous music study at five years old. In this instance, parents are motivated to give their children a head start as professional musicians. There are pros and cons to such early immersion. My suggestion is that early music training should be entered into only if the child enjoys and gravitates to music. This is a motivation different from creating a child prodigy. Music should never be a forced endeavor; the purpose is to enhance the learning process and to have fun. If it grows into something more serious, this is the child's natural inclination and you can support it. Forcing a child into music, however, can create lifelong avoidance. A time-tested and lovely introduction to music for children is the Orff Method. (See "Soundwork Resources.")

6. *Be a music education activist!* Reprint the information about this research from this book or download research from the Internet (keywords: "music and learning" or "music and education") and bring it to your local school administration. This steady flow of favorable research and a public show of support will help to reinstitute music into the public school curriculum.

Here is an inspiring example of community-based music in education: I was recently staying in a hotel in Phoenix, Arizona. As I sat in the Jacuzzi one quiet afternoon, the pool area was suddenly invaded by two hundred enthusiastic high school students. They were from Hellgate High School in Missoula, Montana, and had just arrived to march in the New Year's parade the following day. As I queried my exuberant hot-tub mates, an inspiring story began to unfold.

They came from a school with a student body of thirteen hundred—of whom six hundred were involved in at least one of many music programs, including choir, orchestra, and jazz bands. When I spoke with their highly respected music director, John Combes, I found that Missoula is a city with a long tradition of artists, a community that consistently values the arts in its schools. All children begin choir in grade three. By grade five they can continue with an instrument if they desire. Most of the students in the marching band had begun playing together in the fifth grade and continued throughout their public education. In fact, the fifth-grade music instructor, John Schuberg, works hand in hand with the high school music director, who in turn works closely with the local college music department, which is headed by Schuberg's wife.*

I then spoke with a few of the parent chaperons and was told that the band room is where their kids can be found during lunch and after school, and that the teaching faculty fully supports the program. If there is a mandatory marching rehearsal at the same time as a wrestling practice, the coach sends the students to the marching rehearsal. This level of community backing is inspiring and effective. The social context of music here is a healthy umbrella—with all kinds of residual benefits—for these teenagers to grow up under.

Recommended selections: 📖 See "Sound Remedies Catalog."

MUSIC FOR FOCUS, CONCENTRATION, AND LEARNING

This is an area I have spent a great deal of time investigating. As a writer—with dozens of magazine articles under my belt—I am very familiar with the all-night writing sessions required to meet the 10 AM FedEx pickup deadline. I don't drink coffee or use drugs. Sharp focus starts to lag after midnight. What to do?

I started experimenting with different audio products that claimed increased concentration as a benefit. To my delight, I found a few albums that were extremely effective in helping me hold concentration and maintain productive energy. After I had personally benefited from sound as a productivity enhancer, my vision of the power of music and sound expanded. My investigations into music as a healing art accelerated into an analysis of music for learning and productivity.

Our modern-day use of music to enhance learning is nothing new. In 1970, *Psychic Discoveries Behind the Iron Curtain* devoted a few pages to

* This is the same community that hosts the Chalice of Repose Project. See "Soundwork Resources."

the work of the Bulgarian psychiatrist Georgi Lozanov. He had developed a process he called Suggestology, a conglomeration of techniques—with music as an integral part—designed to create smarter students. The government of the Soviet Union fully supported his work, thinking that if it could not beat America in the arms race, it would overwhelm us by creating more intelligent people. Lozanov's work came to be widely researched and enthusiastically accepted in the West as the basis for accelerated learning. His work is clearly documented in *Superlearning* and *Superlearning 2000* (again, see the bibliography for more information).

The bottom line of Lozanov's work is the concept *body relaxed–mind alert*. His premise is that there is an ideal psycho- and physiological state in which the brain is most receptive to new information. Creating the right level of relaxation in the body and alertness in the mind is the challenge. Music is a key to this.

One of the pleasures of being involved in the unfolding field of psychoacoustics is that both the public and the media already love music. They do not have to be convinced that there are things to be gained from the listening process beyond pure enjoyment. Music is universally adored; that it has meaning beyond entertainment is widely reported and positively received.

In November 1998, at a meeting of the Society for Neuroscience in Los Angeles, multiple clinical studies about music were enthusiastically reported by the press. Studies have revealed direct evidence that music stimulates specific regions of the brain responsible for memory, motor control, timing, and language. For the first time researchers also have located specific areas of mental activity linked to emotional responses to music. Canadian researchers have discovered that music activates different parts of the brain involved in emotion, depending on whether it is pleasant or dissonant.[30] The brain interprets written musical notes and scores in a special area on the brain's right side. This region corresponds to an area on the opposite side of the brain known to process written words and letters. In studying the brains of expert musicians, researchers uncovered a link between music and language.[31]

In a study of classically trained musicians, researchers discovered that male musicians have significantly larger brains than do men without extensive musical training. Researchers believe that the brain grows in response to musical training the way a muscle responds to exercise. The area of the brain called the cerebellum, which contains about 70 percent of the brain's neurons, was about 5 percent larger in male musicians. The cerebellum grows as a result of the constant practice of the virtuoso motor skills needed to play an instrument. (As an interesting sidenote, researchers found no such brain increase in female musicians, but said they may not have studied enough women to be certain.)[32]

Repeatedly, studies are showing that music engages the brain at almost every level. Even allowing for cultural differences in musical taste, researchers found evidence of music's power to affect neural activity no matter where they looked in the brain, from primitive regions found in all animals to the more evolved regions thought to be distinctly human. Harmony, melody, and rhythm each initiate distinct patterns of brain activity involving both the right and left sides of the brain. Melody affects both sides equally; harmony and rhythm seem to activate the left side of the brain more strongly than the right.[33]

In 1993 researchers at the University of California at Irvine found that college students who listened to Mozart's Piano Sonata K. 448 for ten minutes prior to taking a spatial IQ test scored eight points higher than those who did not. The concept is that listening to music might somehow enhance the brain's ability to perform abstract operations immediately thereafter. This phenomenon, known as the Mozart effect, has received a great deal of media attention due to the highly publicized, popular book of the same name by Don Campbell (see the bibliography). However, the university research team actually suspects that listening to *any* complex musical piece can produce similar results.[34] It is continuing its study, and has found that attempting to replicate it has produced mixed results. The team's report, published in 1998, states that "more work is needed before practical applications can be derived."[35]

The bottom line is that our ability to measure the quantitative impact of music—from Mozart or from any other composer—on the brain is gaining in sophistication. This allows us to specifically understand why we perceive Mozart differently from Beethoven, where in the brain these perceptions take place, and how we can consciously use this information to enhance our lives.

Sound Awareness and Music for Focus and Learning

As clinical studies evolve and rapidly build on one another, they confirm Plato's observation: "Music is a more potent instrument than any other for education." He knew this twenty-three hundred years ago! Unfortunately, while this truth is not disputed, it *is* ignored. Apparently, we are still trying to figure out why music is so potent.

As I've noted, Dr. Georgi Lozanov believes that in the body relaxed–mind alert state, concentration, memory, and imagination are heightened. To induce this state, Lozanov used mostly the adagio movements from the baroque repertoire. Most of these pieces were sixty beats per minute, corresponding to a relaxed heart rate. In the following few pages, I will demonstrate my own thought process as I used Lozanov's concept as well as those of resonance and entrainment to build a sound library that facilitates intensive concentration and clarity of thought. The main question to consider is: *What music will relax my body while stimulating my mind?*

For my writing, I have created a workspace that is as conducive as possible to maximized productivity. It is well lighted and secluded; my phones are turned off and there is nobody around. Still, a great studio does not guarantee that my brain is working optimally! Thus, I rely on music and sound for energy, focus, and inspiration—but they must not interfere or distract. If they become obtrusive, then soundwork is counterproductive.

I love bossa nova, jazz, and world music, for instance. However, they are not *appropriate for me* when I write. They are great when I am doing other office or creative tasks that do not require intensive focus. In those instances, I am looking for energy, stimulation, and ear candy. The sweetness of this music is similar—*for me*—to a great chocolate-chip cookie: It gives me a rush. Other people prefer sour to sweet. Everybody is different, in food and in choice of sounds.

Here are *my* sound tools for enhanced concentration:

- *Entrainment at work.* The goal is music between fifty and seventy beats per minute. Slower will put you to sleep; faster will make you want to get up and move. (There are times when you will want to do both of these things in the learning process. Pick your times.) Fifty to seventy bpm corresponds to the ideal relaxed heart rate.

- *Resonance at work.* Higher-frequency sounds—those in an upper range, such as high violins, woodwinds, and voices—*charge* the nervous system. An abundance of lower frequencies can *discharge* the system.

- *Gregorian chant.* Dr. Alfred Tomatis alludes to Gregorian chant as the equivalent of two cups of European-strength coffee, and I wholeheartedly agree. High tenor and soprano voices are stimulating (resonance); slow and long vocal phrases slow my breath (entrainment). A perfect sonic alchemy of body relaxed–mind alert. I play chants very softly in the background with my CD player on repeat. I can use this soundscape for hours at a time and not even know it is there. Nonetheless, I really miss it when it is not.

- *Baroque and other classical music.* I find this to be a sticky wicket: Some classical music works wonderfully for me, but much does not work at all. Remember, when this music was written, it was not intended as a productivity tool but instead for the Church, the royal court, or entertainment. Consequently, all kinds of wonderful musical events take place within a given movement that may not be conducive to concentration. If melody, complexity of harmony, or density of arrangement takes your attention, the music will fail as a productivity tool. Indeed, some believe that classical music cannot be used at all because of its *distraction challenge.* These extraordinary pieces of music were not created to be sonic wallpaper that doesn't disturb. They are living testaments to the continuum of human struggle, emotional landscape, and sacred devotion portrayed by the most gifted composers in the Western world. *So what to do about this challenge?*

  1. *Find compilations* sequenced from classical recording archives. In the best of these compilations producers have found existing pieces whose tempo ranges between fifty and seventy beats per minute and that feature a lot of high-frequency orchestration (high strings). The string section is the dominant force of any symphonic work, but it is not just lots of violins that do the trick.

Effective works offer a balance of orchestration among the varied instrument families, melodic and harmonic structures, and tonal ranges.

My personal experience with compilations of prerecorded classical music is a lack of consistency. A case in point: Think of a beautifully soft and sweet movement from Mahler. Then, three minutes into the movement, the composer goes harmonically ballistic for no apparent reason. This lasts about a minute and creates a lot of tension, leading to a great release on return to the serenity that I was enjoying. It is a great compositional tactic to keep us from falling asleep—but not effective as a soundwork application. Still, compilation producers will use such a piece because without its one-minute harmonic side trip, it is perfect.

2. *Applied Music & Sound recordings.* I am a founder of this company and have coproduced multiple albums for the Sound Health Series in response to the distraction challenge of classical music soundwork applications. *What is different about these compilations?* My coproducer, Richard Lawrence, and I select pieces based on specific psychoacoustic criteria. We then rearrange the music as necessary to create soundtracks that relax the body, stimulate the mind, and do not intrude. Then The Arcangelos Chamber Ensemble rerecords these baroque and classical masterworks. Since our first release in 1996, the Sound Health Series has been adopted by entire school districts, children's learning disability centers, and Tomatis and assorted other clinics throughout North America and Europe. Additionally, parents of children with homework and people faced with the need for clarity and focus in their own work use Sound Health recordings on a regular basis.

We have made it easy for the nervous system to get the benefits of music for learning and focus. Among many psychoacoustic refinements, consistent pulses in the music make entrainment a gentle and effective process. We have also simplified melodic structures where necessary, either by complete omission of a phrase or by deleting the lead melodic line, allowing the subtle inner harmonic voices to become dominant.

To grasp what I mean, imagine yourself at a live performance of the symphony. You see all the players on stage working away diligently in precise harmony and interaction. However, your brain focuses on the main melody, and the other 75 to 95 percent of the orchestra recedes to the background. The Sound Health Series brings out many of the parts being played by the background players. The extraordinary beauty of the lead lines is generally supported with simplified harmonic structures by these players. For the purposes of the mental immersion sound application, isn't this exactly what you are looking for: simplified sonic support? By occasionally deleting the main melody, we are tapping into the original bedrock of the composition—which has been there all the time, but obscured by the fanciful lead lines and featured instrumentalists.

The enclosed 💿 CD, *Music for The Power of Sound,* has many examples of these techniques. The Bach Allegro Assai (track 12) amply shows the process of simplified melodic structures.

3. *Music with light density.* Musical density affects the central nervous system. An easy way of thinking about this is in comparison with a computer. The more information it has to process, the more it needs faster microchips. Do you have a computer with a speed of 300 MHz or a 400 MHz processor? Computing is all about the *amount* of information and the *speed* at which it can be handled. This is no different from the human brain. How much information can your brain absorb quickly?

Music that features thick arrangements (complex density) requires more processing attention and speed. With this image in mind, consider how you want to spend, or allocate, your brain's processing mechanism. In my own case, for instance, when I am in an intensive mental immersion time, the less complexity, the better. Too much complexity in the music distracts me; it "borrows" some of my attention to analyze the incoming auditory signals. A four-part counterpoint (four separate melody lines tensing and releasing with each other) with full symphonic background requires a lot more processing than does a single or double instrumental line. I also avoid music with lyrics in my native tongue; I don't want to hear other words or thoughts while I am organizing my own.

I use music that is light and spacious: solo acoustic guitar, solo flute, solo piano, duos or trios. These ensembles, by virtue of the small number of instruments, tend to be simpler and thus demand less processing! The sounds still charge the system, entrainment can take place, and the simplicity lends unobtrusive beauty. Nature recordings, too, with or without music, can be lovely. However, be aware that a lot of tacky combinations have come onto the market. I have listed some of my favorites in "Sound Remedies Catalog."

4. *Music or sound with binaural beat frequencies.* Binaural beat frequencies (BBFs) are a means of achieving whole-brain synchronization. This is a good thing when concentrating! If you are not opposed to using a set of comfortable headphones, you will find certain recordings that embed these specific frequencies into their musical tracks to be very effective. (For more information on BBFs, see chapter 12.)

MUSIC IN THE CLASSROOM

All of the preceding discussion applies to the use of sound in the classroom. If I were a teacher, chalkboard and music system both would be obligatory.

The effectiveness of music in the classroom is well documented. The core concepts of Lozanov and accelerated learning have been wonderfully honed and are worth further exploration if you are a teacher and want to incorporate sound on a rigorous level. Three books I recommend are *Rhythms of Learning: Creative Tools for Developing Lifelong Skills,* by Chris Brewer and Don Campbell; *The Mozart Effect for Children,* by Don Campbell; and *Learn with the Classics,* by Ole Andersen, Marcy Marsh, and Dr. Arthur Harvey. (See the bibliography for complete information.)

Recommended musical selections: 📖 See "Sound Remedies Catalog."

MUSIC FOR FITNESS AND ATHLETICS

Much attention is paid to the use of music as an adjunct to fitness and athletics. There was no TV network coverage of the first Olympiad, but it would be a safe bet that the musicians were there. Where better to use the power punch of entrainment to motivate a stronger workout or training session? Still, note that of the following research excerpts, two speak of the dangers inherent in certain commonplace usages of music in the fitness arena.

RECENT RESEARCH

"Wired for a Workout." Research indicates that listening to music while exercising enables people to work out longer before feeling exhausted. Men increased their time by 30 percent, women by 25 percent, before exhaustion set in. Most listened to rock 'n' roll. Researchers believe there is nothing magic about rock music; the important thing is to pick music that is enjoyable. The researchers did not discover new music-muscle connections but, rather, came to the conclusion that this effect is most likely due to the music's ability to distract.[36]

"Rhythmic Golf Training." Waltzes, cha-chas, mambos, and other music are all part of an innovative program called Rhythmic Golf Training taught in Deerfield, Illinois. Created by a golf pro and a ballroom dancer/golf enthusiast, this program teaches students a pre-shot routine, set to rhythm, much like a dance step that enables them to move with the beat. It is based on the concept that music allows the mind to become focused and relaxed. The creators often have their students hit the ball with their eyes closed while listening to music. They believe that closing off one sense heightens others—instead of just seeing the rhythm of movement, you learn to hear and feel it, too.[37]

"Music Can Help Learn a Sport Faster." By concentrating on a rhythm, sports specialists say, you accelerate the process of mastering a sport and help your body discover the best biomechanical way to move. Your body, when you listen to music, moves with greater efficiency and synchronization.

This causes less muscle contraction. Consequently, your joints are more stable and the risk of injury decreases.[38]

"Music and Hormones." A rehabilitation specialist in Eugene, Oregon, uses music to help people recovering from injuries. He says, "Musical rhythms tap into our more primitive brain centers and act to override some of the conscious centers that control pain and fatigue."[39]

"Specific Tempos for Injury Recovery." By using music at specific tempos—120 beats per minute—pacing for recovery-oriented exercise is facilitated. Specific tempos help exercisers maintain a workout rate that will produce a desired target heart rate.[40]

THE RISK OF MUSIC IN A FITNESS ENVIRONMENT: RECENT RESEARCH

"Feel the Burn, Don't Hear It." Legislation has been filed in Massachusetts requiring health clubs to post warnings about the dangers of exposure to loud music and to provide earplugs if the volume exceeds 90 dB, which is about as loud as a lawn mower. A survey that monitored ninety health clubs nationwide found noise levels in 60 percent of these clubs to exceed 110 dB, or the equivalent of a chain saw. Thirty minutes of ongoing exposure is enough to risk lifelong hearing damage, says the author of the study, an audiologist.[41]

"Headphones and Working Out." Fitness experts say you double your risk of permanent hearing loss when you work out with headphones. The reason for this is that aerobic activities—such as brisk walking and running—force the body to divert blood from the ears and direct it to the legs, arms, and heart. This abnormal blood flow makes the hair cells in the cochlea more vulnerable to loud music.[42]

SOUND AWARENESS FOR FITNESS AND ATHLETICS

As is common in the world of sports and fitness training: *Use it or lose it*. Given the two most important studies I've seen, the phrase can be adapted to fitness and music: *Use it but don't abuse it!*

Audiologists say that the legislation in Massachusetts has called attention to a widespread, hidden health menace. Combine the effects of music at 110 dB—which after thirty minutes is enough to cause permanent hearing damage—with the new research about how the body diverts blood from the ears to the legs, arms, and heart during brisk walking, running, or working out, and we're talking high impact!

What a terrible dichotomy. We devote valuable time to fitness programs intended to improve health. But in more than half of all aerobic studios, the sound is loud enough to damage our ears. Those of us who prefer a long jog over a country back road with beautiful music in the headphones may be irreversibly damaging our ears.

I used to ski while listening to Steely Dan's rock music or Mozart's allegro movements. It was one of the most exhilarating activities I have ever experienced. I loved it because it helped me to "dance" with the mountain, and I skied better than ever. I had so much adrenaline from the increased rhythmic push that even my last run of the day, with my tired legs, was a nonstopper all the way to the bottom of the mountain. For fifteen minutes I was youthfully invincible!

Talk to me about the ringing in my ears fifteen years later. Yes, it could have been all that loud rock music I played as a teen and in my twenties. Could have been the skiing. It doesn't matter now. The ear does not regenerate damaged cells. Once they're gone, they're gone.

Take this as a word of advice and pass it on to those you love. *Exercise and music are a great pair—quietly.* This may seem like it defeats our purpose—after all, we want the extra push from the sonics. But read the stats. Our ears and brains are not getting along with the way we have incorporated music into our fitness routines. Aerobics teachers will have to become better motivators and not depend on the latest high-volume hip-hop to keep tired students pushing. Who would have thought that headphones and exercise were an unlikely hazard? But it is, unfortunately, true. This information needs to be common knowledge.

If you choose to use music, be cognizant of its volume. Given current research, headphones are probably not a good idea unless you play the music very softly. If you want the energy or adrenaline bump from entrainment, speakers seem to be a safer bet.

Pick music that falls into the desired beats per minute (bpm) range corresponding to your fitness activity.

TABLE 9.1

Preferred Beats per Minute for Various Fitness Activities[43]

ACTIVITY	PREFERRED BEATS PER MINUTE
Aerobic dance	126–192
Stationary bike—heart patient (50 bpm)	100
Stationary bike—average to high fitness level (80 bpm)	160
Jogging (10-minute mile)	150
Running (8-minute mile)	166
Running (6-minute mile)	180
Rehab. walking (30-minute mile)	90–100
Health walking (20-minute mile)	120
Fitness walking (15-minute mile)	140
Race walking (12-minute mile)	160
Race walking (10-minute mile)	180
Rowing machine (25 strokes per minute)	200
Ski simulator	100–140
Stair stepper	80–120
Swimming (crawl, 60 strokes per minute)	120

Note that these numbers are determined by a statistical average. Tempos will vary according to your fitness level and age.

MUSIC IN THE WORKPLACE

Does music enhance the work environment? What happens when the volume of industrial noise is always way up? What about music after work? There are some interesting results from recent studies.

RECENT RESEARCH

"Music via Headphone Boosts Job Performance." University of Illinois researchers found in a study of 256 office workers that listening to music of the individual's choice soothed frayed nerves, drowned out distracting office chatter, boosted mood, and significantly enhanced office performance. Also among the positive effects: greater satisfaction with the employer and reduced interest in switching jobs.

Job performance in simple clerical work was increased by 14 percent; in more-complex jobs, by 7 percent. Those who didn't do well wearing headphones were people who had to talk on the phone a great deal and those with more complex jobs that required greater attention.[44]

"Hearing Protection Device Use among Industrial Workers." Research in North America has shown that the percentage of workers exposed daily to harmful noise (over 85 db) varies between 30 and 60 percent across industries. In certain industries, it may reach as much as 95 percent. Yet the percentage of workers who take measures to protect their hearing is surprisingly low, despite regulations requiring their use.

With noise exposure—as with chronic exposure to other environmental hazards—the negative health outcome is gradual; the timing of possible damage is uncertain; and no visible, immediate damage is apparent from any one exposure *Hearing loss becomes manifest only after several years of noise exposure.* In the short run, then, no one is able to perceive either the benefits of using hearing protection devices or the damage incurred from nonuse.[45]

"Heart and Blood Disease Greater in Noisy Industries." Studies indicate a greater prevalence of cardiac and peripheral vascular disease and hypoglycemia in workers in very noisy industries than in those employed in less noisy industries.[46]

"Using Music to Forget a Hard Day's Work." For some executives, making music is just about as sweet as making money. Be it opera or rock, cabaret or country, music represents for them the ultimate escape from the rigors of corporate life. For some it is the realization of a lifelong aspiration even as they make their careers in the very different world of business. Lawyers, CEOs, psychologists, and stockbrokers use their previous musical training as an adjunct to their professional careers for stress reduction and personal revitalization and creativity.[47]

> **Rules of Thumb**
>
> • If you are in an office, use music wisely. It can be of great assistance.
>
> • If your workplace features loud industrial noise, use ear protection.
>
> • You will not know that you have lost your hearing until it is irretrievably gone.

SOUND AWARENESS FOR MUSIC IN THE WORKPLACE

Music and the office are a natural match. The challenge is personal preference and control. If you can have your own sound system, either with headphones or without, you have the best opportunity to use music and sound to enhance your work life. If you work at a computer with a CD-ROM drive, you can play any regular CD and hear it directly through the computer (if it is equipped with speakers) or through headphones plugged into your computer.

Sound and rhythm create mental and emotional environments. What is most conducive to your task? Do you need help concentrating or simply staying awake? Do you want to be energized or sedated? Is there a big meeting coming up? Are you uptight about a presentation you have to give? The intentional use of music in the office is a perfect soundwork application.

- *For enhanced concentration and mental immersion,* revisit "Music for Focus, Concentration, and Learning" (page 121) to refresh yourself on all the information you need to use music to increase concentration. If your office work is conducive to uninterrupted headphone usage, take advantage of the binaural beat frequency selections I've listed in "Sound Remedies Catalog." And classical or other music in the range of fifty to seventy beats per minute will be your best bet.
- *Staying awake, increased energy.* This is the best time for up-tempo, fun music. Pull out the jazz, country, reggae, pop, or classical allegro movements. Turn up the volume a bit. Be considerate of those around you; they may not need the sonic hit you are looking for. If you wear headphones, remember that high volumes close to the brain might give you two things: the energy endorphin rush you are looking for and dead auditory brain cells.

- *Music in industrial settings.* If there is ongoing noise in your work-place, be careful. Rather than using music turned up higher than the noise, you will be auditorily better off if you wear earplugs. You want to guard your delicate and precious hearing mechanism. Replacing one sound with another, louder sound may bring you temporary psychological relief, but it will also cause hearing damage.

Headphones

Headphones come in many varieties and prices. Earbuds—small, comfortable transducers that fit right into the ear canal—allow you to listen at *very low levels* and do not block out external noise. They also do not require over-the-head binding; their small wires follow your jawline, proceeding from under your chin to the connector on your sound system. (Because they lack headgear, earbuds are good for bedtime listening.) You can listen to your soundtracks and be in a conversation with an associate at the same time. The opposite of this is the closed-ear system, whereby the entire ear is covered by the headphone. This will block out external noise to a degree determined by the quality of the headphone.

Earbuds can be purchased for as little as $10. Closed-ear head-phones range anywhere from $25 to $250. As a point of reference: My professional closed-ear headphones, used in studio mixing and mastering, cost $150. For normal use, a good closed-ear set shouldn't cost more than $60.

In the long run, however, a set of $100 headphones will be much better for your ears than a less expensive model. With higher-quality headphones, you do not need to turn up the volume to achieve a full spectrum of sound. You can listen quite quietly. With cheaper head-phones, you need higher amplitude to achieve a full bass and treble response. Consequently, you often listen at a volume not conducive to auditory health.

Finally, I recently spoke with an office manager who is an avid head-phone user. She was concerned that, when she used headphones in areas of high ambient noise levels, she had to turn up the volume higher than was probably best in order to hear. She wanted to know what to do.

If your ears are ringing when you take off your headphones, you are listening at too high a volume and may be causing hearing damage. A rule of thumb is that if you can't hear someone talking to you while you listen, the volume is too high. Also, be aware of listening with headphones for too long. Your ears may habituate to the sound, and your inclination will be to turn up the volume—especially if you are trying to shut out surrounding noise. After an hour, let your ears rest for fifteen minutes or more. Headphones are a major source of noise-induced hearing loss. Be very careful with them.

An emerging field of study centers on the masking of sound, referred to as noise cancellation. The concept is that by finding sounds of equal frequency, you can essentially create a sonic block, or neutralization, of the offending noise. This has to do with different methods of phase and interference with the offending sound waves. If you have a particular noise problem and an employer willing to look into what can bring relief, I encourage you to take advantage of the Internet using the keyword "noise cancellation."

Remember also that if the attractor for disease is compromised immune function, sound pollution contributes greatly. Interestingly enough, long-standing bad odor, bright lights, and continuous bad tastes are not tolerated. Sound seems to be the only sensory input that we are surrounded with but have little control over. Bear this in mind as you enthusiastically bring music into your workplace. Everyone brings his or her own lunch to meet his or her own dietary requirements; use sound in a similar fashion. Think: *Nutrient Sound.*

MUSIC IN THE HOME

RECENT RESEARCH

"The Housing Environment and Women's Health." This 1978 Canadian study examined three indicators of the quality of the home environment affecting the mental and physical health of married women with children: perceived space and privacy problems; structural deficiencies in the dwelling; and the nonstructural deficiencies of noise, cold, and pests. The good news in this study was that while noise, cold, and pests "adversely influence health, they are not a major cause of poor health." Although researchers have been concerned about the medical consequence of excessive noise, their conclusion was that the "trauma of noise may bring to the surface a scarcely submerged tension and result in an emotional outburst."[48]

In other words, noise, cold, and rats are not as lethal as dioxin or asbestos. This is reassuring!

"Human Response to Environmental Noise." It is estimated that noise levels in the United States increased more than 11 percent between 1986 and 1996. It is predicted that these levels will continue to grow at least as rapidly as the general population, and that noise from air traffic will increase at an even more rapid rate.

Prolonged exposure to environmental noise has been related to impaired scholastic performance and learning ability, higher blood pressure, and lowered tolerance of frustration. Researchers have identified nonauditory health effects of noise as indirect, cumulative, and stress related. They caution that studies of noise's effects on nonauditory function are inconclusive at this point.

There is, however, a growing body of research indicating that noise effects are psychologically mediated. It has been noted that individual differences in response to noise are striking. On average, more than 50 percent of variations in reactions to noise can be accounted for by psychological factors. Several investigations suggest that physiological effects and health complaints are closely related more to subjective reactions to noise than to noise itself.

Adverse reactions to noise arise predominantly from two factors: the perceived inability to control your exposure and the appraisal of an event as threatening important personal needs or goals. The appraisal of noise as a noxious quality of the environment, while often subjectively based, may still trigger stress-related effects. These can include blood pressure increases, increased catecholamine secretion, and inhibited immune system functioning.

Researchers add, "A person's home is a different context for evaluating control over noise than it is for evaluating control over other ambient stressors such as air pollution. The home can be an escape from exposure to air pollutants. In contrast, noise impacts that penetrate the interior of the home represent an inescapable violation of the safety presumed of a primary setting."

The study concludes with the following: "Noise may not be etiologically related to any given disease but may enhance susceptibility to disease in general and, thus, may cause a wide variety of physiological and psychiatric symptoms."[49]

SOUND AWARENESS AND THE HOME

We know that uncontrolled amplitudes of extremely low or high frequencies can cause physiological reactions. From the research just discussed, we understand that under normal circumstances, there is no such thing as "noise disease" per se. However, stress, which is a psychological perception, is known to weaken the immune system. If noise causes stress, weakened health may be an indirect consequence. It is an interesting note that the penetration of noise into the home represents an "inescapable violation of safety." This statement points to the auditory dilemma of the day: the control of our auditory environment.

From research, we understand that some people are more sound sensitive than others. This can originate either from auditory damage whereby we can no longer block or filter out extraneous sound very well or from an inherited and normal sound sensitivity. Either way, our homes are our last bastion of sonic defense—the place where it is hoped that we have some control over the environment. This control is the opposite of what we experience when we are out and about in town.

I used to live in New York City, and there is no better place to test the adaptability of the auditory function. I never knew what sounds—sirens, screeching car tires, a cappella singing, foreign language bantering, crying babies, laughing friends, boom boxes galore—I would encounter and therefore process next. A sound feast! Remember, the initial purpose of hearing is survival. In New York, your ears have quite a workout. Our homes are the place of release where *we* choose what sounds, or silence, we will enjoy or tolerate.

In your abode, why put yourself in a position where you must *tolerate* the soundscape? If you share the space with others, inform them of the effect of sound and the importance of having a place of sonic control. The sound environment of where I live is the most important thing about it to me—more important than the visual.

Not everyone is auditorily aware. Therefore, politely set your sonic boundaries with relatives and roommates. Determine your needs for music and silence and politely make your arrangements. Remember, everyone has different requirements. Don't be a sonic dictator, but don't be a sound victim either.

MUSIC IN THE CAR

I have found no research on this topic, but common sense goes a long way. Two levels of awareness can be addressed with music: staying alert and staying calm. There is a big difference between music used on a long, unobstructed highway journey and music used in rush-hour traffic.

HIGHWAY DRIVING

When we are traveling long distances, the role of music is to keep us alert. Long journeys mean we are behind the wheel for extended, often monotonous periods of time. Putting entrainment to work, this is the time to use up-tempo music. Pick out your favorite jazz, rock 'n' roll, or big-band selections. Alternate these with classical music. The goal is to keep your brain from habituating, so keep the music and the tempos varied. Entertainment also helps keep the mind active. Books-on-tape and instructional audio programs are thus excellent for long drives.

RUSH-HOUR AND CITY DRIVING

"Road rage" reflects the level of stress felt when maneuvering in too small a space with too many cars. This is the time to use music that will keep you both alert and relaxed. Whereas faster tempos are recommended for road trips, in the city—where patience is a necessity—mid-tempos (sixty to ninety beats per minute) are suggested. As with enhanced learning, where body relaxed–mind alert is the preferred state, city driving demands a similar state. Classical music (adagio alternating with allegro movements) and light jazz both have medium tempos and often feature high-frequency instruments. As you know, the higher-frequency sounds tend to energize the nervous system. This aids in maintaining alertness. Consequently, music with high strings, flutes, and saxophones is a good choice. As always, it comes down to taste. By applying the principles of resonance and entrainment, you can determine which music is uplifting to the neurological system and which actually has the opposite effect. Talk radio is also good for maintaining alertness because it is keeping the mind engaged. Still, the goal is to stay calm and cool, and music can have a big influence on this.

MUSIC IN THE HOSPITAL

RECENT RESEARCH

"Music to Operate By." This study found that surgeons are likely to do a better job at the operating table if background music is playing. They also have lower blood pressure and pulse rates and perform better at nonsurgical mental exercises while listening to music. The quickest, most accurate performances with the least physical stress come while the surgeons are listening to music of their choice. And they perform better with less stress when listening to music chosen by the experimenter than with no music at all.[50]

"Relaxation Therapy Works." With a $1,500 budget, some cassette players, headphones, and special cassettes were purchased by a children's hospital in Palo Alto, California. Special attention was paid to compiling a sound library with wide appeal. Three categories were included:

- *Therapeutic music.* Soothing background music and natural sound effects help decrease stress and encourage relaxation (all ages).
- *Disease- and symptom-specific guided imagery.* With or without music, a narrator helps patients target disease, insomnia, and anxiety, then eliminate them with images (ages five-plus).

- *Stories.* These are designed to provide distraction from pain and help children control stress (ages two through twelve).

The patients who found the tapes especially helpful were those with ulcers, bronchospasm, rheumatoid arthritis, asthma, depression, and insomnia. Because there is a psychological component to most illness, all patients can benefit from relaxation and imagery.[51]

"Music and Pattern Change in Chronic Pain." Music was investigated for its use in altering the perception of chronic pain among women with rheumatoid arthritis. Researchers found that sedative music—characterized by a regular rhythm, predictable dynamics, harmonic consonance, and recognizable vocal and instrumental timbre—created a relaxation response that included decreases in heart and respiratory rates, muscle relaxation, sleep, decreased oxygen consumption, lower metabolic rates, and a reduction in circulating corticosteroids. In addition, activated psycho- and physiological responses included endorphin release, autogenic conditioning, and distraction. For critically ill intensive-care patients, significant reductions in blood pressure, anxiety, depression, and pain perception took place following the introduction of music into the environment. Likewise, reductions in nausea and vomiting followed music therapy among cancer patients undergoing chemotherapy.

There were conflicting results regarding the effects of various types of music on anxiety. Researchers suggested that personal preference regarding the type of music used, rather than arbitrary labeling of type (sedative or stimulative), is a significant factor. Reports also pointed to a significant decrease in heart rate and an improvement in mood among cardiac patients in response to classical music.

In relationship to pain reduction, researchers found that the pain perception threshold increased while patients listened to music for a period of time following the sonic intervention. It appears that patients are able to move beyond their pain during the time of listening. It was posited that humor, imagery, sound frequency, breathing, and touch are the essential dimensions of pain transformation.[52]

"Music and Birthing." Researchers determined in this study that if music was used as part of the woman's preparation for birth, music therapy was beneficial also during labor. Music, along with a positive mental attitude, helped the woman relax, so she required less medication. This in turn led to a better outcome for the baby, because there was no respiratory depression caused by transplacental transfer of drugs.

During normal deliveries and cesarean sections (under epidural anesthesia) music has a role to play as a distraction, altering pain perception, decreasing anxiety, and being part of the celebration of birth.[53]

"Music Therapy in the Care of the Premature Newborn." Neonates, like adults in critical-care settings, react adversely to the stressful environment of modern intensive-care units. This is reflected in heart rate variations, decreased oxygen saturation levels, wide fluctuations in blood pressure, and increased levels of agitation. Additional negative reactions may include increased myocardial oxygen consumption, cardiac arrhythmias, and reduction in peripheral and renal perfusion.

High levels of ambient light, along with loud noises and sleep interruption, are now being recognized as potential stressors of the preterm infant. Exposure to noise levels above 80 dB has been identified as one cause of hearing loss in young children. Sound levels in a neonatal ICU have been measured as averaging between 70 and 80 dB, with effects intensified rather than diminished by the incubator.

Researchers studied the effects of taped intrauterine sounds on seventeen agitated, intubated premature infants. The sounds were combined with synthesized vocal singing. The studies concluded that oxygen saturation and behavioral state improved significantly during the playing of the taped sounds.

What types of music should be played for the preterm infant? Care must be taken with the neonate to ensure that any music therapy given is indeed therapeutic and not just for the comfort of the ICU staff. Music is made up of several components including rhythm, tone, pitch, dynamics, melody, and harmony. High pitch creates tension; low pitch promotes relaxation. Rhythms of more than ninety beats per minute can also cause tension, while a slower rhythm can cause suspense or fear. A tempo of sixty beats per minute can be soothing. Dynamically, the measured intrauterine noise level is said to be 80 to 95 dB. To achieve the desired decibel level with the neonate, researchers suggest music be played at a volume of 80 dB, at a distance of three inches from the baby's ear.

Music in the environment of a developing infant has been shown to improve oxygenation and may also enhance brain development.[54]

"The Impact of Music on Newborn Colic and Circumcision Pain." Parents were instructed to follow three courses of action with colicky babies. The first was to continue whatever they usually did to try to soothe the babies. In the second, mothers chose a selection of music and played it for half an hour, regardless of whether the babies were crying or calm. In the third, mothers put on the music half a minute after the babies stopped crying and gave them plenty of loving attention; if the crying started again, they switched off the music, attended to the baby's needs, and gave them no other attention until the crying stopped.

The first and second courses of action had no effect, but after six to seven weeks the third had reduced excessive crying by about 75 percent.

Neither tapes of intrauterine sounds nor music could offset the effects of circumcision pain.[55]

"Hospital Noise—Level and Potential Health Hazards." Except for noise-induced hearing loss, there is no known noise-induced disease. However, human beings can react to noise psychologically (with fear, annoyance, anger, agitation, or pleasure), and any of these reactions can then alter the physiological state.

In addition, noise produces recognized physiological changes in the endocrine, cardiovascular, and auditory systems, as well as affecting sleep. A well-established effect of noise on the human cardiovascular system is vasoconstriction. Most of these changes do not cease on repeated exposure to noise.

Simply put: Just because we are exposed to lots of irritating noises doesn't mean our systems adapt to them. We don't get used to them—if they irritate, they just keep on irritating!

If these physiological changes become extreme, noise becomes a health hazard. Researchers have found that noise levels in incubators, recovery rooms, and acute-care units are of sufficient intensity to interfere with sleep and possibly to damage hearing in patients receiving certain antibiotics. The pituitary-adrenal axis has an extremely low threshold for stimulation by noise—as low as 68 db. The average noise levels in the recovery room, acute-care unit, and incubator exceed this intensity.[56]

SOUND AWARENESS AND THE HOSPITAL

Here are some of the conclusions we can draw from the above research:

For surgery. Surgeons are likely to do a better job at the operating table with background music. If the music is of their preference, it is all the more effective. Therefore, in a pre-op conference with your doctor, find out what kind of music he or she likes. If it corresponds with your personal taste, you've got a good match. If it doesn't, decide who needs the music more—you or the surgeon. I suggest you put yourself first in this department and let the surgeons worry about their own stress. That's their job. Your job is to absorb the positive effects of your surgery and heal as quickly as you can.

Music will accomplish the same thing, in different degrees, for you and your operating team. It reduces the stress hormones and keeps everybody relaxed. The surgical team will operate more efficiently; you will recover and heal more quickly.

One of the many facets of surgery is the use of anesthesia. You need this pharmaceutical intervention for pain reduction and numbing purposes. Anesthesia is a good thing; it is also better to have less than more. The sooner your physical system can resume full custody of your bodily functions, the better it is for your recovery. Music can help you do this. Whether you are awake or asleep during surgery, you will benefit from music being played.

What music does is blunt the stress hormones, including norepinephrine, epinephrine, and growth hormones.[57] When these hormones increase, blood pressure and bleeding during surgery also increase. To keep stress and blood pressure down, more anesthesia is used. The more anesthesia, the longer the period of time when your body is not fully producing natural healing agents—which increases the possibility of complications. Better to use the music of your preference to stay relaxed during surgery and reduce the amount of anesthesia. The music's effects will continue in the recovery room, even after it stops playing. Music will also help you recover and get you home faster.

For extended hospital stays. A hospital is an institutional setting designed to facilitate various activities and situations. Unfortunately, hospitals' sonic environmental design—that is, their noise levels—are not the most beneficial for rest and recovery. Patient satisfaction studies have shown that environmental factors can significantly affect clinical results.[58]

Within an institutional setting, how can you create a sonic environment conducive to healing and recovery for yourself or for those you love? Interrupted sleep patterns, hospital employee noise, procedures for other patients, and the incessant sounds of commercial TV do not lend themselves to ideal sonic healing space. The noise and distractions are often an impediment to efficient recovery. Yet the hospital must function, and noise is a part of everyday activity.

The answer to this is actually simple: earplugs, headphones with portable cassette or CD player, and appropriate recordings. There are several goals:

- To create as much of a chance for uninterrupted sleep as possible
- To establish relaxation and reduce anxiety
- To provide positive entertainment
- To use sonic tools for self-directed healing (meditation and self-hypnosis, for example)

By establishing auditory insulation from the institutional setting, you lay the groundwork for faster recovery. What you are essentially doing is applying the principles of sound awareness. If you cannot control the environment around you, control it within your ears. This can be done.

Earplugs are a wonderful way to mask noise. They come in all shapes, sizes, and prices. When you want to sleep, meditate, or tune out of the environment, use the plugs; they are the equivalent of eyelids, and they can help give you a sense of control over your personal environment even in a situation that may feel overwhelmingly out of control. Take back your personal sound space. Establish auditory boundaries.

Headphones are an integral part of auditory boundaries, too. Use earplugs when you want quiet; use headphones when you want auditory stimulation or sedation. The more you can use sound, the less you are dependent on medication.

Sound Equipment in the Hospital

Your body is in flux when you are hospitalized. You are likely to be under the influence of pharmaceutical drugs that may have side effects. For example, certain antibiotics can create a lower threshold for noise stimulation—as low as 68 db. Therefore, a simple rule of thumb about headphone usage is to *keep the volume low*. You do not need loud sound to mask existing noise levels. (If your roommates play the TV too loud, politely ask them or a nurse to turn it down or to use a headphone system themselves.) Just as we instinctively recognize the need for personal space in the physical realm, hold on to the image of auditory boundaries. This is a state of mind assisted by the earplugs and headphones. Volume is not the factor for establishing your own sound zone, though.

Headphones, like earplugs, also come in all shapes and sizes. See page 135 for some useful information on headphone types.

You will also need a portable cassette or CD player, which can easily be plugged into the wall. This way you don't have to worry about battery replacement. A portable cassette player can be had for under $30; portable CD players run $50 and up. Those in the $100 range are usually more reliable.

For a total of $100 to $200, then, you can purchase a sound system: earplugs, headphones, and portable sound music player. This is a very small price to pay for a great deal of comfort. Many hospitals have portable equipment and a tape library. Request this, or ask for a visit from a hospital music therapist, who can directly assist you in this process.

Sound library for the hospital stay. In the hospital you want music and sound recordings that help you sleep, keep you relaxed, distract or entertain you, and assist in self-directed healing. The most important thing to remember is that sonic space is your private space. *Listen to whatever helps you feel better.* If you like big-band music, use it! Opera, country, zydeco? It is your choice, and no one even knows what you are listening to. This is a completely private zone. Do what you like!

Over the last twenty years, numerous series of recordings have been created by notable medical and psychological authorities for self-directed healing. They contain many psychoacoustic techniques to assist that process. Music and guided imagery make a great mix: Research has shown that their combination reduces specific stress-producing hormones, including Plasma B-Endorphin and ACTH.[59]

Other recordings contain specific psychoacoustic techniques with a strong emphasis on resonance and entrainment. In some cases, binaural beat frequencies are employed (see chapter 12). I recommend this technology in a hospital setting; it may amplify the effectiveness of soundtracks. If you have any kind of a condition that may contraindicate the use of this psychoacoustic application, especially anything having to do with seizures, consult your doctor first.

See "Sound Remedies Catalog" to get started or to trigger your imagination. As you will see, almost all of the recordings listed there were created specifically for therapeutic applications.

PROGRESSIVE SOUND HEALTH FOR THE HOSPITAL ENVIRONMENT

A Reno-based company, Healing Healthcare Systems, recognizes the need for sonic environments that support the process of healing and recovery in the hospital setting. It has created—with the utmost attention to practical requirements and marvelous aesthetics—video and sound programs used within hospitals on a systemwide basis. This work is so exemplary of conscious therapeutic applications of music and sound that I have included more information in "Soundwork Resources."

PART THREE

A Guide to Soundwork Techniques and Applications

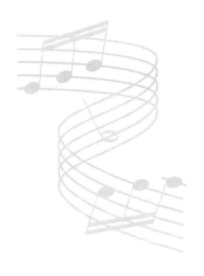

A Matter of Distinctions

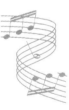

In part 1, I explored the nature of sound and hearing. Part 2 suggested personal applications of a new sound awareness. Now let's turn our attention to the professional applications of soundwork techniques, the therapeutic uses of sound, and sonic neurotechnologies. Psychoacoustics is the overarching theme under which I will explore these topics.

As I have discussed, psychoacoustics is the study of the perception of sound. How we perceive sound can be broken down into how we listen, what our psychological responses are, and what the physiological effects of music and sound are on the human nervous system.

In this context *applied psychoacoustics* refers to the practical application of music and sound. The subject of *The Power of Sound*, in its entirety, is applied psychoacoustics. The level of specificity here in part 3, however, will be appreciated by professionals who wish to integrate soundwork into their healthcare practices, musicians who want to focus their craft on psychoacoustically designed programs, and educators who want to fully understand the components of applied music and sound. Understanding the inner mechanics of psychoacoustic programs will be of value to all readers.

To start, a few subtle yet important delineations are appropriate. Let's compare sound therapy and music therapy, healing and curing, and tone and music.

SOUND THERAPY AND MUSIC THERAPY

Over the past few decades, new forms of auditory-based therapeutic practices have been gaining momentum. In this book I refer to the use of sound as an agent of change as *soundwork*. Joining the ancient global wisdom of indigenous healers with the high-technology precision of the Western world, individuals are now able to use sound as a vibrational tool of transformation—and know what and why.

According to N. M. Weinberger, a sound researcher and archivist of music research at the University of California at Irvine, research into the neurological reactions and effects of music has grown tremendously in the last ten years. The major reason for this is recent development of imaging technologies to scan the activity of the human brain.[1]

Some call this newly burgeoning field sound therapy. I prefer to use the term *soundwork* because the term *therapy* generically implies healing or fixing. The use of sound to effect change goes far beyond fixing. Controlled vibrational interaction can also be transformational and of great value in enhancing what already works in our lives. Therefore, *soundwork* applies to the intentional use of music and sound for either therapeutic or life-enhancement purposes.

In the last fifty years, music therapists have combined the use of music with psychological and physiological applications in hospitals and in private practice. The success of music therapy has rendered it a legitimate modality within the domain of Western medicine. The up-and-coming field of soundwork, however, presents a radically different approach based on the powerful interaction between the vibrational frequencies within sound and the body and mind.

While music therapy and sound therapy seem quite similar because they both use sound to create change, they are actually very different approaches. Music therapy is psychologically oriented, using familiar music to enhance relaxation, comfort, and enjoyment. (For more on music therapy, see appendix F.) Sound therapy, on the other hand, uses the principles of resonance, entrainment, and vibration to effect changes in tissues and organs; it is thus neurologically oriented.

I must point out that soundwork does not preclude music therapy. Psychological reactions will take place whenever music is present. Likewise, music therapists cause vibrational interactions to take place when they play a familiar melody to trigger memory. I make the distinction because although soundwork and music therapy often use the same material, the primary approach and intention may be different.

HEALING AND CURING

The goal of soundwork is the enhancement of human function through the use of music and sound. This broad approach includes enhancement of what works as well as healing of what could be better. In the context of soundwork, I define *healing* as the process of regaining balance. *Balance* is, in turn, the continuing development of equanimity. In balance, right action seems to occur: The body's innate wisdom compensates and adjusts. Healing looks beyond the symptom to the root of the distress; it addresses the gestalt of the mind, heart, spirit, and body. Healing is different from curing: Sometimes we find healing but not a cure. We may find balance and ease yet still suffer—even die. There can be healing in dying, contrary to the view in Western medicine that sees death as failure.

However, to label a modality as *healing* may undermine its effectiveness and prevent us from understanding it. This is especially true when dealing with subtle energy or vibrational formats. The effect of music and sound is influenced by mood, fatigue, brainwaves, heart rate, and temperature. What works for me may not work for you. What works today may cause a different reaction tomorrow. There are no guarantees. To find the most effective individual prescription of sound is the challenge. Therefore, I recommend great caution and modesty in labeling intentionally created music and sound programs.

Says Weinberger, "The secrets of nature don't reveal themselves easily. . . . Understanding the relationship between music and human mental processes and behavior requires a commitment of resources, time, and the dedication of skilled investigators."[2]

TONE AND MUSIC

When soundwork is focused therapeutically, there is a marked difference between the use of music, with its rhythmic and harmonic complexity, and the use of single tones or extremely simple tonal patterns. Dr. Randall McClellan has discovered that the therapeutic uses of music are characterized by two distinct approaches: Songs made up of rhythm and melody have traditionally been used for general healing purposes, whereas specific tones and mantras have been used for their vibrational properties to treat specific parts of the body. The significance of these approaches is that they "represent two distinctive but equally valid philosophies and methods." A song, "which for the sake of convenience may be referred to as *music healing,* begins the healing process through its influence on the emotions and mind first and the physical body second." A tone or mantra, on the other hand, "which may be referred to as *sound healing,* treats the body through resonance first and affects the emotions and mind second."[3]

Songs use the mind and emotions as a doorway in. Again, this psychological approach is the basis of music therapy. Tones or sound therapy goes straight for the physiological impact, directly resonating the body.

In the future, sound healing (through tones) may be considered prescriptive and comparable to highly specific pharmaceutical drugs, while music healing may be perceived as an over-the-counter remedy, effective and generalized. In time, we may find *sound* healing most effective in alleviating chronic physical conditions, and *music* healing part of the regimen of well-body maintenance. People may come to incorporate a daily sound bath into their schedules, recognizing sound health as just as necessary for overall wellness as daily food and exercise.

11 The Building Blocks of Therapeutic Sound

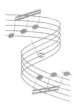 There are many tools in the musician's toolbox. Against the backdrop of tonal centers, counterpoint, and rhythm, a player understands the use of different scales. In the West a scale is an arrangement of notes in a specific order of whole and half steps. Trained musicians know where tone rows make sense and when a pentatonic blues scale is creatively congruent. With rhythm, a musician understands that a time signature of 4/4 (four quarter notes to a measure) will not work for a waltz (3/4), and that syncopated polyrhythms are great for jazz but not so good for lullabies. Timbre, harmony, rhythm . . . these are some of the building blocks of music.

Adding psychoacoustics to the musical canvas requires understanding resonance and entrainment. These elements are essentially the scales of psychoacoustic composition; the knowledge of resonance then informs the tones and rhythms that we play. Once a musician moves into the realm of application-specific composition, many rules change. Some of the building blocks of music take on another dimension when applied in this manner. For example, in a psychoacoustic context, the timbre—or the color of a sound—is looked on as tone. This triggers a thought process about how and what this tone resonates. Rhythm implies entrainment. Now the beat is related to the desired rate of internal pulses. And harmony is not so much about consonance and dissonance as it is about sonic density and the effect of data, complex or simple, on the nervous system. In this chapter I will look at musical components from a different slant—a psychoacoustic vantage point.

In her highly regarded book *Sounding the Inner Landscape: Music as Medicine* (see the bibliography), Kay Gardner identifies the following therapeutic elements of music:

Drone. A drone is a long, uninterrupted sound, or set of sounds, underneath the music. The musical term *ostinato*, or pedal point, refers to an accompaniment figure that is repeated.[1] In Western music a drone might consist of a bass line of a few low tones. Melody lines are then played against the drone by other instruments. Drones are quite common in Indian music. An open-stringed instrument such as a tamboura or vina will play a repeating chord consisting of three or four notes. A sitar will then play a melody over the drone. Bagpipes also have non-changing low tones that accompany higher melodic tones. Drone tones are usually long and low. Like a bed of sound, drones provide an emotional sense of security. As single tones, drones may be a vehicle for resonating specific parts of the body.

Repetition. When a musical phrase is repeated, the listener becomes comfortable. Repetition creates a hypnotic or relaxing effect in which the listener is moved into a receptive state. Repetition with rhythm or simple melodic phrases can create a trance state.

Rhythm. The effect of rhythm springs from the natural reaction of pulses in the body: heartbeat, breath cycle, brainwaves. Rhythm may accelerate or slow these pulses through the vehicle of entrainment.

Harmony. The emotional content of music is contained in its harmony. With the use of inner harmonic phrases, dissonance resolves to consonance and tension is released. Complex harmony challenges the listener emotionally; simple harmony is used for meditation, centering, and visualization.

Melody. This is the primary element that we hear in a composition. It is a succession of single notes. The power of melody is its ability to take away the listener from physical awareness. In guided visualization, melody allows visual fantasies to take shape. Beginning with Pythagoras, melody has been prescribed as anesthesia because of its power to soothe.[2]

Instrumental colors. In Western music the study of instrumental color is known as orchestration. The timbre of each instrument is determined by the uniqueness of its harmonic content. This is what makes a violin, a trombone, and an oboe sound so distinct. Each instrument resonates the listener in a specific area of the body.

Form. The structure underneath all the other elements is the form. Form is the organization of a composition. For example, a sonata form consists of three main sections: exposition, development, and recapitulation. (In lay terms, a sonata form is like a well-organized speech: You are told what you will hear, you hear the themes with embellishment, and you are reminded of what you just heard.) The form of a pop song is usually verse, verse, chorus, verse, chorus, chorus, bridge, modulated verse, chorus infinitum. Different styles of music have their own forms. Be it a fugue or a morning raga, the form provides a sense of stability.

Intent. Perhaps the most important element in therapeutic music is the intention of the musical team. Is the music offered with pure intent? Is it possible that music is a carrier wave for the vibration of those playing and composing? If the choice of harmonies, colors, and intervals is a reflection of the psycho- and physiological tonus of the person creating the music, couldn't this information be transmitted in sound like an electrical impulse through a fiber-optic cable? I believe that this is the case. I don't know it from research: It is my intuitive and anecdotal truth. Consider the following . . .

If I write a piece of music to salve a breaking heart and I'm good at my compositional job, this music will resonate with other people who share a memory of that occurrence. As fellow humans, perhaps we recognize the intervals between the tones, or the tensions and releases. Maybe we see—or, in this case, hear—ourselves in others.

When we listen to music, our psychological defenses usually are down. We are open and vulnerable on the emotional and psychic levels. If we "see" sound as a sonic snapshot of another's psyche, don't we then bathe ourselves in another?

This is all very subtle and subjective. I can refute these hypotheses with other examples. Some of Beethoven's most beautiful works were written while he was in pain, but you don't hear it in the music. Other compositions have been written by hateful racists, yet you wouldn't know it unless someone told you. Or would you? Is it a matter of sensitivity? Where is the line of believability on this issue?

Music is a powerful energy transmission, yet its power lies in its subtlety. We may not *consciously* be aware of the intention of those behind our music, but our higher consciousness—the inherent wisdom that knows how to grow a human out of two cells—reads the information encoded inside the sound wave.

If a musician is angry or scared when making a recording, this emotion can be subtly recognized in the phrasing or dynamics. This may not be discernible to our normal ear, but it is interpreted and recognized as fear or anger in some part of some auditory center of the brain. Or if a composer such as Brahms consciously prayed for divine intervention before he put pen to paper, and prepared himself to write down the music he "heard," we will recognize those sounds because we have the ability to "hear" on that level as well. I believe that in our gross physical bodies, auditory sensitivity is pretty dense. Perhaps recognition of intentionality takes place in the unused gray matter.

The iso principle. *Iso* means "equal." Applied to therapeutic music, the iso principle consists of initially matching the mood of the music to that of the listener and then slowly changing that mood, tempo, or timbre in the direction you want to bring the listener. Essentially, it is a gentle coaxing of listeners from their existing body and mind-set, by means of something familiar, to another space conducive to the sound application.

A composer must always consider the audience. This is true for a film composer as well as a pop songwriter. In a psychoacoustic context, the end listener is especially important. If you are writing for a bedridden cancer patient, the tempos, orchestration, structure, and conclusion you choose will be different from those you would incorporate into a soundtrack for healthy people unwinding from a hectic day.

After the audience question is answered, the next issue concerns rhythmic destination. This is where the iso principle applies. Let's assume that your listeners are at the end of their days. Chances are they are in a low beta brainwave state (12 to 15 Hz), because they have been mentally active all day and are starting to slow down. By first rhythmically matching their existing brainwave and heartbeat states, then gradually slowing down the pace, you have met them at their own tempo. Through the process of entrainment, they will essentially follow you as you gradually slow the tempo. If you created a tempo *too* different from their existing rate, they would most likely not be able to relate sonically; they'd simply tune you out. Your efforts become ineffective at this point. The idea is to bring about gradual change.

Harmonics. The harmonics of sound may be the most important part of actual sound waves. I have not been able to locate verifiable scientific research into the effects of harmonics. However, the effects of harmonic resonance on the electrical fields of the body have been referred to in numerous anecdotal explorations of sound.[3] The natural acoustical harmonic frequencies duplicate ratios found throughout nature, the human body, classic art, and architecture. Let's take a look.

Simply put, harmonics are a series of tones that vibrate above a fundamental note. Known as *overtones* or *partials*, these softer tones are pure, clear sounds. Harmonics exist in our voices and in all instruments and are responsible for the unique sounds of each.[4] Even if you cannot hear the harmonics, they are there.

If I play a low C on a piano and hold down the key, you will hear a series of other tones begin to sound. They will not be as loud as the fundamental note (the struck C note), but you will hear other strings on the piano begin to resonate and sound. Many of these sounds will be octaves of the original C note. Other tones will be intervals of a fifth or a third. Within the overtone series triggered by any single note, almost every other note is sounding, although you cannot consciously hear them all—especially not the higher overtones. But you can hear the first few harmonics.

One of the most interesting things about harmonics is the frequency ratio between the successive notes in any harmonic series. Each note in the harmonic series is a geometric multiple of the fundamental. The first overtone is vibrating twice as fast as the fundamental at a ratio of 2:1. The second overtone is vibrating three times as fast as the fundamental (3:1). This continues up the series—for instance, the eighth overtone is vibrating nine times as fast (9:1), and so on. Each of the different speed frequencies corresponds to a different note.

This is how harmonics relate to therapeutics—through the concept of wholeness. Sound researcher Jonathan Goldman states: "In the 1920s Hans Kayser, a German scientist, developed a theory of world harmonics based on the Lambdoma.* Kayser found that the principles of harmonious structure in nature and the fundamentals of harmonics were essentially the same . . . that the whole number ratios of musical harmonics corresponds to an underlying framework existing in chemistry, physics, crystallography, astronomy, architecture, spectroanalysis, botany, and the study of other natural sciences."[5]

Herein lies the interrelationship of music with the rest of the world and beyond. The harmonic ratios found between certain intervals (the distance in pitch between two notes) corresponds to ratios found in DNA, in the proportion of many (but not all) leaves, flowers, fruit, shells, and some animals. The Golden Section is a specific geometric proportion. The use of this formula can be seen in Egyptian pyramids (thirteenth century B.C.E.), in the Parthenon at Athens (fifth century B.C.E.), as well as in other ancient buildings in Athens and Rome.[6]

According to Goldman, "The Golden Section often involves proportions which relate to the ratios found in the major sixth (3:5) and minor sixth (5:8). The proportions of the body adhere to these ratios."[7]

---

* The Lambdoma, also known as the Pythagorean Table, is an ancient musical mathematical theory that relates music to ratios. It is credited to Pythagoras.

Gardner poses the question, "Why be concerned with divine proportion in music? If music with healing intent is to be written with both aesthetics *and* function in mind, it is reasonable to use a form, or musical direction, that defines natural growth, expansion, beauty, proportion, and balance in nature." She continues: "Wouldn't a piece of music in a form that relates to listeners at the biological level (from molecular structure to brain functioning) as well as the perceptual level (as in visual appreciation and aesthetics) be most effective as a way to define the direction of listening, bringing the listener into balance with the basic and universal patterns of life itself? Music written using the divine proportion is bound to be of value in the field of healing music precisely because of its directional relationship to life cycles and to the forms of universal consciousness."[8]

Gardner speaks of using the proportions of the Golden Section as a compositional device. Goldman refers to the interrelationship of the ratios found in the harmonic overtone series with math, physics, and the natural sciences. They all tie in! Says Goldman: "The universe is harmonically related."[9]

It is because of the interrelatedness of harmonics (and their ratios) and so many other natural structures that harmonics are important. If we bathe the body in natural healthy sound frequencies, it can only have a beneficial effect.

SYNTHESIS AND HARMONICS

Unfortunately, electronic, digitized music loses its precious partials—the overtones of sound. It is for this reason that I moved into 100 percent acoustic soundtracks. However, a note to musicians: I suggest you pause before throwing synthesizers and samplers out the window. There are times when you may need sounds that cannot be duplicated by live players. A case in point: While producing an album that required musical accompaniment for theta and delta zones—the slowest, most unobtrusive soundtrack conceivable—I wrote a piece for a full string section. It required very long single tones, some as long as three minutes before a change. At the conclusion, one of the players came into the recording booth. I thought she was going to hit me with her viola. She was so angry that she asked if I was trying to injure her.

Apparently, the combination of being late in a session when the players were already tired and the rigor of holding these extremely long tones caused her to be concerned about her own muscular damage. This was a very real complaint and possibility, and a lesson I will not forget. For the psychoacoustic effect necessary for my goal, I was asking players to do something not natural to their instruments. It was at that point that I remembered digital keyboards and samplers. No concern about muscular damage here. Although I could not get the same harmonics that I would with a real string section, the desired effect superseded the aesthetic sound. My rule of thumb in relationship to electronic and acoustic sounds: I use electronics only if they are creatively congruent or therapeutically relevant. I suggest you use acoustics whenever possible.

CONCLUSION

There are many things to consider when it comes to application-specific soundtracks. Drone, repetition, rhythm, harmony, melody, timbre, form, intent, the iso principle, harmonics, acoustics, synthesis . . . these are the basic building blocks of music regardless of the intent. But when the intent is music that informs and supports positive outcomes in human function, a different sensibility moves in.

I remember when I was a songwriter. I would have an inspiration, go into the studio, and sit at the piano, looking to find the musical phrase that fit with a snappy lyric. I knew the formula for pop music radio formats: three minutes and forty-five seconds with lots of sing-along choruses and a modulated bridge between final verses. All I needed was the key to the lock; once I found it, inspiration was complemented by craftsmanship and the process evolved. Depending on the time of day and the graces of the creative muse, a new song would emerge in the coming hours or days.

With psychoacoustics, it is the same thing. The creative impulse still needs to take place. And there are formulas. The major difference is that there is an additional layer of consideration. Just as a musician considers the relationship of tone, rhythm, and harmony, so a psychoacoustician thinks about the relationship of resonance, entrainment, and density. Just as a jazz player uses the extensions (ninths, elevenths, and thirteenths) beyond the major triad, a psychoacoustician considers the heart rate, breath, and brainwaves.

In many cases application-specific music can be simpler than music designed for entertainment. Simplicity is most often the order of the day. The complexity comes in the interrelationship of sound and body. Psychoacoustically, we play two instruments—that of tone and that of body.

Sonic Neurotechnologies

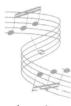The brain has been called the final frontier of the human body.[1] While organ transplants become commonplace and genetic engineering develops at quantum pace, the gray matter that occupies central headquarters is our least understood anatomical territory.

The complexity and speed of processing in the brain is staggering. Consider the following: The human brain must process millions of stimuli per second for at least 4.5 hours a day to remain conscious and not fall asleep.[2] There are 100 billion neurons in the brain's frontal lobes alone. And it is common knowledge that only a small percentage of the brain mass is consciously used. Consequently, it's not surprising that higher brain efficiency is a state many seek. What may raise eyebrows, however, is the way in which this increased access, and/or repair, is being pursued—through the ear and the medium of sound.

Two diverse approaches to the processing of sound frequencies hold great interest.

Filtration/gating techniques have been honed in Tomatis clinics worldwide. By gradually gating and filtering out the lower 8000 Hz of music, and then adding the frequencies back in, a retraining of the auditory processing system occurs. The effects of filtration and gating are felt on a psychological, neurodevelopmental, and physical level. Another approach to sound processing is the field of *binaural beat* frequencies. By listening through stereo headphones to slightly detuned tones (i.e., sound frequencies that differ by a prescribed number of Hz), sonic brainwave entrainment takes place. Facilitating a specific range of brainwave states may assist in arenas such as pain reduction, enhance creativity, or accelerated learning.

Representing two distinct approaches to therapeutic sound, filtration/gating and binaural beat frequencies currently define the growing field of "sonic neurotechnologies." I have coined this phrase to describe the arena of soundwork that depends on the precise mechanical manipulation of soundwaves to bring about desired changes in the psyche and physical body. As you will see in the following discussion, these two technologies—used in different settings—have roots in neurology, physiology, and psychology.

SOUND STIMULATION/FILTRATION AND GATING

In the broadest definition, sound stimulation can be defined as the excitement of the nervous system by auditory information. Sound stimulation auditory retraining narrows the focus. In this context, a precise application of electronically processed sound, through headphones, can have the effect of retraining the auditory mechanism to take in a wider spectrum of sound frequencies. An ear that cannot process tone properly is a problem of great magnitude. As discussed in previous chapters, sufficient auditory tonal processing is a prerequisite to normal auditory sequential processing.

A definitions refresher will be helpful at this point. According to neurodevelopmental specialist Robert J. Doman Jr.:

- Auditory tonal processing (ATP) may be defined as the ability to differentiate between the tones utilized in language.

- Auditory sequential processing (ASP) is the ability to link pieces of auditory information together.

Auditory *tonal* processing is a basis for more complex levels of auditory sequential processing. ASP is the ability to receive, hold, process, and utilize auditory information using our short-term memory. As the foundation for short-term memory, ASP is one of the building blocks of thinking.

Sequential processing functions are fundamental to speech, language, learning, and other perceptual skills. The ability to interpret sound efficiently provides the neurological foundation for these sequential functions. Per Doman, "many people who have experienced auditory processing deficits have seen their sequential functions return and/or improve when proper tonal processing is restored."[3]

The primary sound application used in the remediation of impaired tonal processing was created by Alfred Tomatis. Further discussions cannot take place without absolute acknowledgment of his pioneering research (see chapter 5). The current field of sound stimulation auditory retraining evolves from Tomatis's discoveries of the powerful effect of filtration and gating of sound.

In the context of auditory retraining, let's define these terms:

- *Filtration* means the removal of specific frequencies from an existing sound recording, be that the music of Mozart or a recording of a voice. Through the use of sound processing equipment, it is possible to isolate and mute certain frequency bandwidths. With filtration, any part of the low, mid, or high end of a recording can be withdrawn and reintroduced at will. On a visual level, imagine erasing the bottom part of a picture and then eventually drawing it back in. This is filtration.
- *Gating* refers to the creation of a random sonic event. This is accomplished by electronically processing a soundtrack so it unexpectedly jumps between the high and low frequencies.[4] While not always pretty to listen to, the net effect of this sound treatment is an extensive exercising of the muscles of the middle ear. The combined process of filtration and gating creates a powerful auditory workout.[5]

And for good reason! The middle ear mechanism must work very hard to translate the complexity of the "treated" incoming sound.

HISTORY OF FILTRATION/GATING (F/G)

The process of F/G is traced to the brilliant work of Tomatis. One of his great contributions to science was to redefine the role of the ear to the human body. In addition to hearing and balance, his research proved that sound also stimulates the nervous system. Therefore, if our ears do not function properly, a major source of energy is underexploited.

According to Tomatis, high frequency sounds are the most beneficial for "charging" the nervous system. This is one of the reasons why he began to filter out the lowest 8000 Hz of sound in his sound therapy method. Subsequently he discovered that it was not enough to bathe the ear in high frequencies if the internal auditory mechanism was not properly tuned. Extensive gating techniques were created to tone the two tiny muscles of the middle ear so that a full spectrum of sound could be transmitted to the inner ear and the brain could perceive a full spectrum of sound.[6]

Tomatis accomplished the F/G of soundtracks, mostly of Mozart's music and Gregorian chant, with the creation of a device called the "Electronic Ear." This complex series of sound-processing gates, filters, and equalizers can be adjusted for individual sound "prescriptions." The Tomatis Method, in its entirety, is comprised of three interlocking elements: sound stimulation, audio-vocal activities, and therapeutic consultation. The Electronic Ear plays a central role in the sound stimulation and vocal activities.

As is common with the creation of a successful methodology, other practitioners experiment, combine, and mold the original into new approximations. This has been the case with the F/G techniques of Tomatis. While the foundations of the Tomatis Method were laid in the 1940s and still evolve, derivations of his filtration/gating process began surfacing in the 1980s.[7] The common focus has been on reeducating middle ear auditory pathways. This has been accomplished through the electronic modification of music and sound.

One of the earliest extensions of F/G outside of the Tomatis Method was a series of tapes made by Canadian Patricia Joudry. She recognized the power of the Tomatis Method after gaining great benefit from the therapy. However, because there were few clinics in North America, she felt it was better for those who could not logistically arrange a clinical program to have some portable version of the method. Her series is known as Sound Therapy for the Walkman, with a book of the same title.

Another method, known as Auditory Integration Training (AIT), was created by Tomatis's patient cum student and colleague, Dr. Guy Berard. He created a machine called the Audiokinetron and applied his method of sound stimulation primarily to children with autistic spectrum disorders. From this work evolved another device, also modeled on the Electronic Ear—the Audio Tone Enhancer/Trainer. This sound processing machine was known as the BGC.

Billie Thompson, Ph.D., played a large role in introducing the Tomatis Method to America. Her Listening and Learning Center is located in Phoenix, and she keeps offices on both east and west coasts. Dr. Thompson has written or edited numerous articles and books on Tomatis and has witnessed the Tomatis progression. She observes, "The Society of Auditory Integration Training (SAIT) was organized for those providing AIT using the BGC and Berard machines, but the organization's activities declined following a 1996 incident in Florida that resulted in confiscation of equipment and the FDA's decision to stop importation of the Audiokinetron."[8]

At this point, emphasis on Electronic Ear–style devices that could process any soundtrack played through it shifted to the creation of CDs that were pre–filtered and gated. Medical and therapeutic claims evolved into auditory education and training.

What actually takes place with the filtration/gating of sound? For the answer to this question, I turned to Denver-based Tomatis practitioner, Ron Minson, M.D. After traditional medical and psychiatric practice, Minson was certified by Tomatis and reemerged as a highly qualified sound therapist. Applying ten years of clinical experience with filtration and gating at the Center for InnerChange, Minson has become a leading F/G designer for The Listening Program—a recent entry in the field of sound stimulation auditory training.[9] This at-home program is designed primarily for children and adults with learning disabilities and other auditory tonal difficulties and uses low-level F/G techniques appropriate to non-clinical application.[10]

Minson says: "Filtration and gating and are two of the sonic neurotechnologies central to the Tomatis Method and a core principal in The Listening Program. In the Tomatis Method, gating is achieved by using a low channel where the base tones are emphasized and the high tones are diminished and a high channel where the reverse occurs—namely the low tones are diminished while the high frequencies are accentuated. The purpose of gating was originally to exercise the muscles of the middle ear. But it was also found that this random, unexpected event promoted active listening.

"The exercising of the muscles of the middle ear in a scientific and precise manner is important in the reeducation of the ear, especially following ear infections, premature birth, allergies, or any event that may have delayed the development of listening and language. The proper functioning of the middle ear muscles is essential to protecting the ear from excessively loud sounds, for filtering out background noises, for focusing on foreground conversation, and also to facilitate the easy and fluid expression of language."

I queried Dr. Minson about what innovations have taken place in the technology of gating. "In TLP we have developed two different processes for gating," he says. "Firstly, gating is done manually rather than by a machine. This provides a more natural effect. Although the gating is generally in synch with the musical pulse, it is also accomplished in a somewhat random way. Additionally, there are a few totally random gates. Secondly, a unique gating technique superimposes a highly-filtered track with a less-filtered track. The highly-filtered track emphasizes the alerting high frequencies while also promoting active listening. Randomness further facilitates the production of new brain pathways. Research has shown that novel, unexpected events stimulate the formation of dendritic connections between brain cells."

Understanding that filtration is an interlocking technique with gating, I asked Dr. Minson to elaborate on his experience with this process. "The second sonic neurotechnology that Tomatis used was called filtration and consists of the gradual removal of low frequencies, arriving at filtered music where all sounds are essentially 6,000–8,000 Hz or above. This is the 'scratchy' sound with which Tomatis listeners are so familiar. The high frequencies invite a deeper and more precise listening, even to the point of enhancing inner listening, promoting the development of insight and intuition." According to Minson, the experience of listening to higher frequencies promotes increased awareness, creativity, higher consciousness, motivation, and energy.

"In our environment we are bombarded by noise-polluting, low frequency sounds of machines, autos, and more. They are low frequency, energy-depleting sounds that make one tired and irritable. To make matters worse, we are subjected to penetrating, very high frequency tones that are used as warnings, setting off our internal alarms, flooding our nervous system with adrenal hormones (adrenaline, norepinephrine, cortisol) that push us into a stressed fight/flight response. This includes the sirens, horns, fire alarms, and smoke detectors that pollute our environment to the point where we stop listening in order to survive. The perception of high frequency sounds needs to be retrained."

Through a gradual process of filtering out low frequencies the ear becomes aware of what to listen for and is trained to grasp and 'feel' the rich, high tones that nourish us. "I have observed in listeners a marked increase in mental and physical energy," says Dr. Minson. "With this increased energy and motivation there is a accompanying decrease in irritability and depressed mood. Clients often report that their dreams are more active, that they feel more creative and have the ability to realize their desires. While they appear more awake and energized, their thinking is definitely more clear."

In The Listening Program, the scratchy and often irritating sounds of filtered music originated in the Tomatis Method have been greatly reduced by improved studio techniques and recent innovations in software. "We have maintained the effectiveness of the filtration while increasing the aesthetics of the music and sound," says Minson. "This has been accomplished by a more gradual process of filtration and by slowly cross-fading a highly filtered track with an unfiltered track. These advanced engineering processes result in soundtracks that are much easier to listen to."

Dr. Minson provides the following filtration/gating summary:

Filtration—a removal of specific frequencies

The effect of higher frequencies:

- Energizing and alerting
- Enhances creativity
- Improves mood and sense of well-being
- Increases awareness and motivation
- Enhances communication
- Awakens the listening process

Gating—a random sonic event

The effect of gating:

- Promotes active listening
- Retrains muscles of the middle ear. The significance of these muscles:
  - Important in the process of conducting sound
  - Protect the ear from loud sounds
  - Amplify soft sounds
  - Provide accurate perception of sound[11]

A NEW GENERATION OF SOUND STIMULATION METHODOLOGIES

The efficacy of F/G has been proven more in empirical result than in independent scientific research. Over the last forty years, Tomatis's method of sonic stimulation has been tested on over a million clients worldwide.[12] However, research lags the growth rate of the field. Minson, Thompson, Madaule, and other North American sound stimulation practitioners are scientifically oriented, highly credentialed, and well-spoken. They will confidently share the wealth of results they have personally witnessed from sound stimulation auditory training. Yet the exact understanding as to why "scratchy" Mozart has worked miracles is not so easy to articulate.

According to Dr. Thompson, "The demand for more sound-based services in the United States is growing as individuals recognize that these methods offer a new solution for disabilities and deficits that have heretofore resisted change or been untreatable."[13] However, lack of funded research to prove efficacy has hindered the outreach of these clinically-proved therapeutic models. The biggest casualty of all is that many learning disabilities—not to mention numerous other tonal processing considerations—would become successfully addressed with the widespread distribution of F/G methodologies to school systems, prisons, and clinics. However, because of the web of government regulation, insurance considerations, and competing pharmaceutical interests, sound stimulation therapies will have to go through the onerous process of public acceptance.[14] The loss is to the numerous people who could be helped in the meantime. Thompson concludes, "While the FDA requires that clinical products be safe for the U.S. public, educational products do not fall under its control."[15]

The following two programs exemplify a new generation of sound stimulation methodologies. Both offer educational applications of F/G. These methods are currently available for use by trained therapists and educators.

The Listening Program (TLP) is a team effort of neurodevelopmental experts Robert and Alex Doman, Tomatis practitioner Ron Minson, speech pathologist Lori Riggs, psychoacoustic producer Richard Lawrence, and myself.[16] Combining innovative F/G techniques with newly recorded, psychoacoustically refined classical music, TLP represents an interdisciplinary approach to auditory retraining. TLP is an at-home program requiring CD player and headphones only. The eight-week program is listened to for half an hour daily. Approximate cost is $300. Two-day professional trainings are conducted in America and Europe. TLP is available to the public through specially trained therapeutic and educational professionals.[17]

Listening Fitness was created by Paul Madaule, a patient cum student of Tomatis. As founder/director of The Listening Centre in Toronto, Madaule is a leading Tomatis authority and author of When Listening Comes Alive.[18] Listening Fitness uses many of the elements of the Tomatis Method. However, it has been recast for therapeutic and educational professionals to use in their own practices.

The Listening Fitness Program consists of the Listening Fitness Trainer (LIFT), a portable, battery-run audio unit that uses a microprocessor to modify music from a Walkman or your own voice. LIFT is specially designed to play these sounds in a pulsating manner that exercises and develops listening. The LIFT comes with a headphone and microphone set for listening and vocal exercises. The cost of the equipment is about $1,000. Three and a half days are spent for initial training and certification. Over the following 6–12 months, students learn how to use the Listening Fitness Trainer within their professional practice or school and work under supervision with ten clients.[19]

SUMMARY

The filtration/gating discoveries of Tomatis fit like a hand in a glove with Doman's auditory tonal/sequential processing theories. Tomatis developed his F/G techniques to improve listening skills and tone the ear. He determined that in addition to listening and balance, the auditory function serves as a major integrator for the nervous system as well.

Doman, working exclusively in the field of neurodevelopment, was looking for a key to help unlock impaired sequential processing. For Doman, sound stimulation is one of those keys. Tomatis's F/G has provided a means by which auditory function can be improved.

BINAURAL BEAT FREQUENCIES (BBFS)

The term *binaural beat frequencies* describes a neuroacoustical phenomenon that takes place when the brain perceives one tone in one ear with a slightly detuned tone in the other. As a means of measuring the difference between these two tones, the brain creates a third "phantom" tone, unheard elsewhere. This is known as a binaural (two-ears) auditory beat.

Whereas filtration is the process of subtracting specific sonic frequencies from a soundtrack, creating the BBF effect is an additive process. De-tuned sine-wave tones are mixed into a soundtrack of music, nature, or white noise. Sometimes the two tones can be heard, other times they are sub-audio. This is a subjective decision on the part of the producer. For the greatest effect, headphones or stereo speakers placed in proximity to each ear are recommended.

The phenomenon known as binaural beats was discovered by the German researcher H. W. Dove in 1839. He found that binaural beating (an actual *wah-wah* effect similar to vibrato) took place when separate frequencies were introduced into each ear, for example, a tone of 100 Hz in the right ear and a tone of 108 Hz in the left. The brain strives to bridge the gap by creating a third tone that is the actual difference between the two; in this example, 8 Hz.

According to the biophysics authority Dr. Gerald Oster, the binaural beat exists only as a consequence of the interaction of auditory signals occurring within the brain.[20] The sound of the binaural beat will only be heard with the participation of both ears. If one ear is covered and only one tone is heard, the brain will use normal auditory measurement senses to determine tone, amplitude, timbre, etc. The phenomenon of BBFs is a consequence of measurement.

This natural process of sonic measurement takes place not only in humans but in other animals as well. Simply put, as a sound wave passes around the skull, each ear gets a different portion of the wave. When the wave length of a sound signal is longer than the diameter of the skull, the brain hears the inputs from the ears as out of phase with each other. Binaural beat expert F. Holmes Atwater states that "it is this innate ability of the brain to detect phase differences between the ears that enables the perception of binaural beats."[21]

BBFs can only be heard when the tones used to produce them are of low pitch.[22] Binaural beats are best perceived when the carrier frequency (the tone in each ear) is about 440 Hz.[23] Oster explains that above that frequency the "beats" become less distinct and above 1500 Hz they vanish altogether. On the lower end of the scale—below 90 Hz—the beats become confused with the tones used to produce them. In layman's terms, this means that when two slightly detuned notes in the range between the second F on the piano and the sixth G (third G above middle C) are sounded, the BBF effect will take place. Beyond these ranges, other auditory mechanisms measure the difference between two or more presenting tones.

The question arises: Can this process be harnessed for psychoacoustic applications? The answer is yes. Let's explore two major by-products of BBFs: whole-brain synchrony and sonic brainwave entrainment.

Whole-brain Synchrony

In order for the brain to decipher the difference between two tones, the superior olivar nuclei in the brainstem creates the electrical signal of measurement. The by-product of this response is known as whole-brain synchrony—a natural brain state that occurs occasionally, and momentarily, throughout the day. At these times of bilateral hemispheric synchronization, coherent brain power is at its height. According to speech-language pathologist Suzanne Evans Morris, "When there is synchronization in brain frequencies in the same area of both hemispheres, it is much easier for information transfer to occur on the two sides of the brain, probably as a result of the entrainment itself. This simply makes us more efficient and able to deal with information in an easier way."

However, this idyllic mind state—referred to at its maximal effect as the "AHA!" or "Eureka" state—is not accessible on command. But with the application of specific audio tones to each ear, access to this prime state of awareness is increased. Says Morris, "If we can increase and control the amount of time that we spend in a synchronized state we simply function more harmoniously."[24]

The cerebral hemispheres—commonly referred to as the right and left brain—are like two separate data-processing modules; they are each complex, cognitive systems that process information both independently and in parallel. Research indicates that when the two frontal lobes of the brain are synchronized, the power of the brain is significantly increased. By using certain frequencies, one can produce a coherent and unique brainwave state. [25] Binaural beat pioneer Robert Monroe called this state "hemispheric synchronization" or Hemi-Sync for short. [26]

Sonic Brainwave Entrainment

In addition to whole-brain synchronization, an entrainment effect can also take place. Once the third "difference" tone is created, brainwaves will speed up or slow down to match the speed of the binaural beats. BBFs become a method for sonic brainwave entrainment.

Sound researcher Michael Hutchison states, "When precisely controlled tones are combined in the brain, the olivary nucleus begins to become "entrained" or resonate sympathetically to this "phantom" binaural beat, like a crystal goblet vibrating in response to a pure tone. As the olivary nucleus becomes entrained, it sends signals upwards into the cerebral cortex that mix with the existing patterns of brainwave activity there to produce noticeable state changes."[27]

The electrochemical activity of the brain produces electromagnetic waveforms known as brainwaves. These waveforms can be objectively measured with sensitive equipment such as the electroencephalogram (EEG). As long as one is alive, continuous electrical waves circulate throughout the brain.

Beta, alpha, theta, and delta waves pulsate at particular frequencies that are measured, just like sound waves, in cycles per second (Hz or cps). Through the use of BBF recordings, we can change brainwave rates to states most efficient for a specific task. According to brainwave biofeedback expert Anna Wise, we are not only in beta, alpha, or theta at any given point. Throughout the brain, a complex matrix of brainwave states exists. However, the cortex has predominant brainwave states corresponding to certain activities. We are alert with the fast beta brainwaves, alpha waves make us daydreamy, theta waves are experienced when meditating or falling asleep, and delta is the deepest part of the sleep cycle. The cortex seems to be the primary recipient of the entraining effect of BBFs.[28]

Says Atwater: "Perceived as a fluctuating rhythm at the frequency of the difference between the two auditory inputs, binaural beats originate in the brainstem within the contralateral audio-processing regions called the superior olivary nuclei.[29] This auditory sensation is neurologically routed to the reticular formation[30] and simultaneously volume-conducted to the cortex where it can be objectively measured as a frequency-following response."[31]

Three original federal patents in the field of altering brain states through sound were issued to sound researcher Robert Monroe in 1975 for the use of binaural beats in altering consciousness. Leslie France, a former coordinator of The Monroe Institute's Professional Division, says, "When a listener's environment is dominated by sounds of certain frequencies, the listener tends to reproduce those frequencies within his/her own physiology."[32]

Sonic brainwave entrainment is perfectly suited to the binaural beat concept. As previously mentioned, if we put a 400 Hz tone in one ear and a 410 Hz tone in the other, the brain will hear 10 Hz (in addition to the 400 and 410 Hz tones). The reticular formation insures the brain will then come to meet this 10 Hz pace and lower (or raise) the brainwaves to match it. The brain's electrical pulse of 10 Hz corresponds to the alpha brainwave state. If we put a 400 Hz tone in one ear and a 415 Hz tone in the other, the brain will hear 15 Hz, corresponding to a beta state.[33]

In other words, sonic brainwave entrainment basically leads the brain, following externally created combinations and sequences of sound, into targeted arenas of consciousness—be it an alpha state or theta ramping down to delta. The binaural beats can be changed at will by changing the sound patterns. The Monroe Institute, located in Faber, Virginia, has demonstrated that methods to access different states can be learned from recordings that contain the sound frequencies that stimulate or facilitate BBFs and then recreated from memory.[34]

THE MONROE INSTITUTE

Current exploration of the field of binaural beat frequencies cannot take place without bringing the late Robert Monroe into the picture. His contributions to the field of sonic technologies—brought about through extensive research conducted by the institute he founded and funded—brought him great respect during his lifetime and continues to this day.[35]

In the mid-fifties, Bob Monroe was a successful radio/TV producer and multiple-station owner when he began to have spontaneous, often frightening extrasensory experiences that drastically altered his life.[36]

Monroe was surrounded by sub-audio radio and television frequencies many years prior to his unusual experiences. Additionally, he had been an in-house volunteer with experiments seeking a sonic solution for insomnia. Monroe subsequently linked his experiences with exposure to sound waves. In a desperate attempt to understand the effect of soundwaves on his psyche, Monroe initiated research focused on the effect of sound frequencies.

What began as the research and development division in his private radio-production business grew into the world-renowned Monroe Institute. Over the past four decades, Monroe subjected his investigations to vigorous scientific and anecdotal experimentation. He pioneered, or improved upon, basic technologies used by other sonic brain enhancement organizations.

The fundamental premise of The Monroe Institute is that "focused consciousness" contains the solutions to questions of human existence. "From its investigations into consciousness, The Monroe Institute seeks practical applications," reads the preface of the institute's brochure.[37]

Since the 1950s, the Institute has been identifying and evaluating the effects of different sound patterns, blending them into complex combinations which have proven effects on mental states. These sound patterns, barely audible to the human ear, become powerful, noninvasive tools for the exploration, development, and maximization of consciousness. Under the steady aegis of the Monroe family, the institute has created inner exploration tools (including Hemi-Sync, discussed above) from which anyone can benefit, using individual timetables and personal objectives. The fact that these tools are self-controlled contributes to the unique power of this technology.

Whether it be in sleep/dreams, accelerated learning and memory, physical or mental health, pain reduction, meditation, physical coordination, creative problem solving, or stress management, the applications of Monroe's sound tools are vast. Results are achieved by sustaining a focused, coherent brain/mind state. What is most amazing is that these effects are accomplished with an audio tape or CD player and headphones. Hemi-Sync frequencies are layered underneath music, nature, or white noise. Some soundtracks include guided imagery or vocal instructions.

BBFs were not invented by Monroe. Indications are that they were used thousands of years ago in Tibetan temples to facilitate prolonged meditation by the monks. In those days, detuned cymbals called *ting-shas* were used. However, there is no larger archive of current research to be found than at The Monroe Institute.[38]

Institute research is concentrated in three distinct areas: clinical and applied research done by members of the institute's professional division, basic technical research done by university or institutional laboratories, and applied research done at the laboratory at The Monroe Institute. A sampling of research efforts and anecdotal reports reporting beneficial brain-state changes associated with Hemi-Sync's binaural beats include: changes in arousal states, attentional focus, and levels of awareness leading to sensory integration, pain management, treatment of children with developmental disabilities, peak and other exceptional experiences, enhancement of hypnotizability, treatment of alcoholic depression, and positive effects on vigilance, performance, and mood.[39]

BBFs: Recent Research

To give an indication of the growing interest and varied applications of BBFs, I have selected the following four research projects. They were conducted in England and the United States using different binaural frequency formats.

Hemispheric-Synchronization During Anesthesia. In a 1999 study conducted in England, the possible pain-relieving effect of hemispheric-synchronized sounds, classical music, and blank tape were investigated in patients undergoing surgery under general anesthesia. The study was performed on 76 patients, aged 18 to 75 years.

The general anesthesia was standardized and consisted of four elements: propofol, nitrous oxide/oxygen, isoflurane, and fentanyl. The purpose of the fentanyl is to keep the intra-operative heart rate and arterial blood pressure within 20 percent of pre-op baseline values.

The results: Patients to whom hemispheric-synchronized sounds were played under general anesthesia required significantly less fentanyl compared with patients listening to classical music or blank tape. The mean values of fentanyl: hemispheric-sync sounds/28 micrograms, classical music/124 micrograms, and blank tape/126 micrograms.[40]

Binaural Auditory Beats Affect Vigilance, Performance, and Mood. In 1997 a joint study from the departments of Psychiatry and Behavioral Sciences at Duke University Medical Center and the Center for the Study of Complementary and Alternative Therapies, School of Nursing, at the University of Virginia was released.[41] This study was designed to investigate whether different patterns of binaural beat stimulation could produce changes in level of alertness manifested in behavior and mood. Twenty-nine people, with an average age of 32 years, participated in the research. Their task was the detection, during a thirty-minute continuous stream of information, of 180 duplicate letters on a computer screen. Instructions emphasized continuous monitoring, rapid response, and good performance. Mood assessment tests were administered before and after the tests to assess task-related changes in mood. Research participants listened through headphones to different binaural beat matrices during each of the three testing periods.

The authors concluded that "the results of the study provide evidence that presentation of simple binaural auditory beat stimuli during a 30-minute vigilance task can affect both the task performance and the changes in mood associated with the task." They found that binaural beats in the beta frequency range were associated with relative improvements in target detection and reduction in the number of false alarms compared to the binaural beats in the theta/delta range. Scores on their confusion/bewilderment scale rose significantly during the theta/delta frequency stimulation. Changes observed in this study suggest that the theta/delta binaural beats produced a subjective impairment in the ability to think clearly for a task requiring a narrow focus of attention. Results also suggest that the negative changes in mood produced by a monotonous task may have been partially ameliorated by the presentation of the beta-frequency binaural beats. Given that beta frequencies are present during active thinking processes, and theta/delta frequencies are most frequently found during sleep, this was not a surprise. Nonetheless, scientific research demands that this level of scrutiny be accomplished.

"The phenomenon of auditory beat stimulation and its psychophysiological consequences deserve further study" state the authors of the study. "Little is known about the mechanisms that may be involved in the transduction of simple auditory changes into changes of mood and performance demonstrated here. However, the results of this study demonstrate clearly that simple binaural-beat auditory stimulation can influence psychomotor and affective processes."[42]

Their recommendations: "There may be potential applications for the self-control of arousal, attention, and performance. There may be potential applications of these performance-enhancing signals in situations that demand high levels of continuous sustained attention and performance, such as commercial highway driving or air traffic control. Performance-enhancing stimulation may prove useful in other occupational tasks as well. Conversely, binaural-beat stimulation that decreases arousal may have applications in the treatment of insomnia or stress."[43]

A Study of Cognitive Substance Abuse Treatment with and without Auditory Guidance. This 1996 study was conducted at the Mount Edgecumbe Hospital in Sitka, Alaska. Twenty-eight Native Alaskan/American (NAA) men were being treated for alcoholism in a five-week in-hospital chemical dependency therapy and education program. In this study, auditory tapes containing binaural frequencies were utilized as part of the treatment program.

In the Results and Discussion section of the study, the authors state: "This small group study on the effects of cognitive/self-regulation therapy augmented with auditory guidance in treatment and six-month and projected one-year post treatment behavior assessments indicates the following: mean scores on four clinical scales (depression, hysteria, paranoia, and psychasthenia) clearly relevant to substance abuse were significantly reduced in comparison to cognitive/self-regulation therapy alone. The value of auditory guidance training appeared confirmed somewhat in reducing self-reported stress." The authors conclude that while "Only limited data was obtained on the 'success' of augmenting cognitive/self-regulation therapy with auditory guidance training, there were some indications that adding auditory guidance training may help reduce the monthly amount spent by NAAs failing to refrain from substance abuse, lengthen the period that NAAs remain abstinent, and increase the percentage of total abstinence for NAAs completing substance abuse programming."[44]

Music and Hemi-Sync in the Treatment of Children with Developmental Disabilities.[45] Dr. Suzanne Evans Morris works with developmentally disabled children. Her specialization is communication disorders in children with severe motor dysfunction. In this study, published in 1996, the role of music and music with Hemi-Sync was explored in the rehabilitation of 20 developmentally disabled children. The children ranged in age from 5 months to 8 years, with an average age of 2 years. Children had received diagnoses of cerebral palsy, mental retardation, autism, and uncontrolled seizure disorder. All children were referred to Morris because of severe feeding and pre-speech problems. Eighteen of the children were nonverbal and nonambulatory.

Music was included in the child's program as a way of creating an auditory environment to make learning easier. Music with a tempo of 60 beats per minute was selected to provide a quieting background and a regular rhythm and rate which was similar to the tempo of the heartbeat and walking rhythms. This style of music is generally thought of as "superlearning music," because it has been shown to increase the learning and retention rate of verbal materials. Sixty beats per minute takes on an added significance in Morris's circumstance. This rhythm also corresponds to the tempo of a baby's sucking rhythm.

Morris reports that the response to this "superlearning music" was very positive. "Most children became calmer and less distractible during the therapy sessions. Several showed a more normal response to touch and an increased ability to organize sensory information." While the improved reactions were noted during times of therapy, Morris reports, minimal carryover of the improved sensory organization took place when the children were out of the therapeutic environment. Because of the positive responses, albeit temporary, Morris began studying the addition of Hemi-Sync auditory tapes to see if there was a difference.

The frequency in which the Hemi-Sync material was used varied per child. Eighteen children (from the original twenty) continued to receive therapy, consisting of one to eight 45-minute therapy sessions per month. Hemi-Sync tapes were also provided to families of eleven of the children for use during play-learning sessions and for falling asleep. Tapes were used for one month to three years, with the majority of children using the tapes for four to six months.

Says Morris, "The child's nonverbal responses to therapy were carefully documented. Each change of expression, body movement, shift of attention, etc., was interpreted as a means of communicating like or dislike, comfort or discomfort with what was occurring at that moment. These nonverbal reactions became the clearest clues indicating whether a musical or Hemi-Sync background was acceptable to the child's system. Nonverbal responses were positive in 18 of the 20 children."[46]

The purpose of the observations was to obtain a clinical impression of the role which Hemi-Sync in a musical format could play in the feeding and pre-speech rehabilitation of the child. The study was explorative in nature and formal data was not collected. However, clinical records described activities, the child's response, and the type of auditory background which was used.

Dr. Morris found that children who continued to receive music with Hemi-Sync showed positive behavioral changes in therapy. As a contrast, these changes were not evident in sessions with no music or with no Hemi-Sync. While positive changes were also noted with the "super-learning music," the degree of change and permanence was more pronounced when Hemi-Sync was combined with the music. There were five behavioral areas that showed the greatest change with the addition of the binaural beat frequencies: disorganized sensory input, distractibility, motor coordination difficulties, fear of change in vulnerable areas, and benefit to others sharing the Hemi-Sync environment with the child.

The results of this informal study, says Morris, "Show that Hemi-Sync in a musical format can be an effective adjunct to a pre-speech and feeding rehabilitation program. It serves to enhance the effectiveness of a program which is appropriate to a child's needs. The fifteen children (75 percent of the group) who made gains in the program had not made similar gains when the program was implemented without the Hemi-Sync background. Significant changes occurred in thirteen of these children within the first two Hemi-Sync sessions."

Dr. Morris states that a point of reference for a child's skills and behavior without the Hemi-Sync music background must be established. Therefore, any changes with the addition of the Hemi-Sync can be more significantly interpreted. She found that the effectiveness of Hemi-Sync appeared to be cumulative; children responded more consistently to sessions with Hemi-Sync as their experience with the signals increased. She says, "As the child experienced a more balanced and organized way of dealing with the sensory input for learning it became easier to re-create this new organization when the Hemi-Sync signals were not present. It is significant that major permanent changes were seen in children who experienced Hemi-Sync less than three hours per month. Hemi-Sync contributes to long-term changes in the child's abilities and ways of organizing information."[47]

CONCLUSION

With the combined tools of sonic brainwave entrainment and resonance, soundwaves are able to modulate brainwaves through the use of binaural beats. Now, one can determine that an afternoon spent in mid-beta would benefit concentration, or that low alpha is best for deep stress reduction.

As the authors of the vigilance and performance studies noted, "Only the most recent studies include sufficient experimental controls and can be considered as scientific investigations. Even so, the value of potential applications of a technology for self-control of EEG patterns and states of consciousness argues for continued investigation of the binaural beat phenomenon and its psychophysiological effects.[48]

The versatility and potential for BBF technology is impressive. Beyond all claims, personal experience is the true arbiter. Over the last ten years, I've extensively partaken of this technology. Recordings that contain BBFs have been of great value in stress reduction and deep rest. My most regular use of BBFs is for increased concentration and focus.

Filtration and Gating techniques were originally created for physio/psychological interventions. However, pragmatic applications are emerging as well. Tomatis found that he could accelerate the learning of foreign languages by training the ear to hear language-specific frequency ranges. The "Japanese ear" is different from the "American ear." Hence the Japanese difficulty with the "r" sound. Per Tomatis, if you can't hear it, you can't say it.

Tomatis is now retired and no longer training professionals in his method. In North America there are about twenty-five people who had the honor of being trained by the master. As F/G techniques evolve, so does the exploration of combining with other therapeutic or educational modalities. Innovation is a natural progression as the originators pass their creative mantles.

Robert Monroe probably never met Alfred Tomatis. There is no mention in any of their combined publications. However, if they had met, it would have been a most interesting exploration. While their methods and motivations are completely different, they are tied together inextricably through their passionate use of sound. They shared the tools of resonance and entrainment. They have moved the field of soundwork immeasurably forward.

Sonic neurotechnologies must be used carefully and wisely. BBF and F/G soundtracks can be powerful tools. Consequently, proper consideration must always be afforded.

The therapeutic use of sound, like any new tool, requires discipline, education, and strict observance of ethical standards. There is currently no established licensure in the use of sonic neurotechnologies. Therefore the onus of responsibility for handling the changes that occur as a consequence of the application of these methods falls clearly on the practitioner. Sound is a marvelous adjunct to an existing profession. Therapists and educators will do well in performing due diligence and acquiring proper training.

13 Applied Psychoacoustics for Healthcare Practitioners

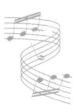

Soundwork is a natural complement to other treatment processes. Music and sound have a wide range of therapeutic applications. A case in point: Music can be a superficial balm, calming the nerves of anxious patients in a waiting or treatment room. In the surgical theater, however, music has a much stronger effect. In a recent U.K. study, specific music programs significantly reduced the quantity of anesthesia needed.[1] Music and sound can be a simple adjunct to or a central structure in the architecture of your practice.

Some of you are medical practitioners; others look at soundwork from a psychotherapeutic vantage point. Some readers work with modalities falling under the rubric of holistic healing. My goal in this chapter is to help you understand how soundwork can be added to your practice. You will find simple and elementary suggestions, universal in their application. Likewise, a review of highly sophisticated soundworking techniques will be presented. I also provide an overview of advanced techniques—each by itself worthy of a book. References and resources will be abundant. Consider me a guide, showing you where to explore sound techniques in the in-depth manner required by professional healthcare and educational practitioners.

Before proceeding, a disclaimer is apropos: I am neither a therapist nor a health professional. I am a musician, record producer, and sound researcher. The information I offer is based on my cocreative experiences as a psychoacoustic producer with healthcare providers of many stripes. I have developed programs with medical doctors, psychiatrists, neurodevelopmental specialists, and biofeedback experts. In the collaborative process and follow-up, I've had the privilege of observing how sound programs are employed in various practices. Consequently, the greatest service I can render to the educator or healthcare practitioner (HCP) comes from my knowledge of sound and how it is being used. I will not be providing sonic prescriptions but, rather, reasserting basic concepts for your consideration. Consider this chapter an overview of soundworking possibilities. Adapting this information to your specific health or education modalities is in your hands.

Recommended Reading

If you are just beginning your exploration into the therapeutic applications of sound, a good starting place is to look at how others are using sound. The following books are an excellent introduction to the various facets of sound and how other professionals use them. For complete information on each, see the bibliography.

The Book of Sound Therapy: Heal Yourself with Music and Voice, by Olivea Dewhurst-Maddock, 127 pages.

Music: Physician for Times to Come, by Don Campbell, 355 pages.

Sonic Alchemy: Conversations with Leading Sound Practitioners, by Joshua Leeds, 300 pages.

Rhythms of Learning, by Chris Brewer and Don Campbell, 317 pages.

WHAT CAN SOUNDWORK BRING
TO MY PRACTICE?

Depending on your practice—healthcare, psychotherapy, bodywork, education—sound can complement your work in any number of ways. The following five vignettes illustrate how chiropractor, psychotherapist, bodyworker, anesthesiologist, and psychiatrist integrated soundwork into their respective practices.

Jeffrey Thompson, a chiropractor, discovered that he could adjust subluxations painlessly and more effectively with sound than with his physical manipulations. He has since become one of the leading sound researchers in America. His work includes the development of sound products and sound tables and the invention of equipment used to decipher NASA sound recordings. Dr. Thompson is currently founder and director of the Center for NeuroAcoustic Research at the California Institute for Human Science. Psychoacoustics is part of the core curriculum he teaches to graduate psychology students. (See "Soundwork Resources.")

Molly Scott found soundwork so effective in her psychotherapy work that she developed a model known as Resonance Therapy. This use of music and sound has become the framework for her therapeutic practice and doctoral dissertation. Dr. Scott travels internationally teaching her innovative use of the voice in a psychotherapeutic context (see "Soundwork Resources").

Vickie Dodd has been an Aston Patterning bodyworker for twenty-plus years. Her successful use of sound has so permeated her practice that it is now equal to the physical modalities she uses. In her book *Tuning the Blues to Gold* she says, "Everything that has occurred in our lives is recorded in our bodies. These events are recorded in our tissue as memories that actually exude a Sound that can be engaged and integrated by our own voice. Sound is a truly powerful medium. Sound touches where hands and words cannot reach."[2] (See "Soundwork Resources.")

An anesthesiologist (and former saxophone player) in Atlanta loved music so much that he brought recordings into the operating room. He found that the music not only reduced the tension of the medical teams but also calmed the patients to such a degree that his use of anesthesia was remarkably diminished. Dr. Fred Schwartz then became instrumental in recording internal womb sounds that have become a valued tool in neonatal intensive-care units throughout America and abroad.

One of my favorite stories is about Dr. Ron Minson, a psychiatrist. One of his own children was having such dire emotional problems that all Minson's years of training and practice could not positively affect her. In exasperation, he went through the Tomatis Method with his daughter. Witnessing her profound turnaround, Dr. Minson dropped everything to study in Europe with Alfred Tomatis. He now runs the exemplary Center for InnerChange in Denver. Soundwork is at the heart of his clinic, augmented by attention to food allergies, nutrition, biofeedback, and neurotherapy (see appendix B and "Soundwork Resources").

Clearly, soundwork is infectious. Chances are that once you begin to use sound in your practice, it will naturally increase in value to you. At this point you may be considering your expensive certificate or professional license; are you about to start chasing after your long-lost love of music instead of paying your student loans or clinic mortgage? Before you put down this chapter in fear of financial ruin, rest assured that you are in control! Like any modality, the use of soundwork comes down to frequency and dosage.

Here are just some of the ways that soundwork is currently being employed in clinics and centers around the world:

- Office and treatment room ambience
- Relaxation techniques, stress reduction, auditory biofeedback
- Pain control
- Reduction of anesthesia and medications
- Correction of tonal processing difficulty
- Abatement of hearing sensitivities
- Correction of learning disabilities
- Birthing assistance
- Musical thanatology

So how can you initially employ sound without taking significant time off to study? Start off easy. Unprocessed sound (without sonic neurotechnologies) cannot harm. The worst you can do is irritate someone—

and don't worry, he or she will let you know. To begin, simply add sound as ambience. With proper attention to resonance (tone) and entrainment (rhythm), you can accomplish a great deal with minimal investments of time and money. It is the more sophisticated uses of sound programs—such as those using sonic neurotechnologies—that require more in-depth study.

A Brief Review of Psychoacoustics

Psychoacoustics is the study of the perception of sound: how we listen, our psychological responses, and the physiological impact of music and sound on the human nervous system.

The four basic ingredients of applied psychoacoustics for health and education are:

Resonance. The effect of one frequency vibrating another.

Entrainment. The process whereby internal systems speed up or slow down to match an external, periodic rhythm. (Review both resonance and entrainment in chapter 4.)

Sonic neurotechnologies. Sound processing techniques that have a measured neurological impact (see chapter 12).

Intention. Being clear about what you want to accomplish with sound.

Psychoacoustic Checklists

Thinking of the basic principles of psychoacoustics as checklists will help you apply them in your individual circumstances. Consider the following checklists as learning devices intended to let you view sound with a psychoacoustic filter.

Resonance: External sounds (simple tone or music)
Key question: *Do you want to stimulate or decrease activity?* High sounds charge the nervous system. Bass sounds can discharge the system.

Acoustic sounds are usually best.*

Complex sound or simple sound? Do you want to mentally stimulate (distract) the mind or create spaciousness? The density of sound—be it a four-part counterpoint or a single instrument playing out of time—can either absorb (and possibly tax) the nervous system or soothe and calm.

Entrainment: External rhythms

Key question: *Do you want to speed up or slow down the system?* Fast rhythms encourage beta brainwaves. Slow rhythms encourage alpha brainwaves. Very slow encourage theta and delta.

Sonic Neurotechnologies:

Key question: *What serves?* Programs with binaural beat frequencies can be used to facilitate brainwave states conducive to a specific health-related activity, be it self-directed healing sessions, pain reduction, or sleep. Sound stimulation programs with filtration and gating are generally appropriate in the psychotherapeutic and educational arenas.

Programs including sonic neurotechnologies should be used only after careful consideration and appropriate training.

Now let's look at a range of five circumstances in which soundwork would be applicable.

Office Ambience

Intention: Relax patients, soothe apprehension, calm harried staff.

Resonance: Midrange sounds bring calm. Think of sound as a nutrient in which high sounds charge and low sounds discharge the nervous system. In this instance, consider medium-speed harp music, acoustic guitar music, chamber ensemble classical music—music that breathes and has a lot of space.

Entrainment: Music at fifty to seventy beats per minute. This is the

---

* The harmonics of acoustic sounds stimulate the electrical fields of the body. In a healing context, I think of electronic, nonacoustic sounds as akin to iceberg lettuce—crunchy but with no nutritional value. In a healing environment, you want to feed the healthiest sounds you can to the nervous system. My rule of thumb: The only time to use electronic (synthesizer) sounds is if it is artistically congruent or therapeutically relevant. Otherwise, stay acoustic.

ideal relaxed heart rate. You don't want it to be too slow or people will get groggy and uncomfortable in your waiting room. Too fast, and they will get impatient and anxious.

Sonic Neurotechnologies: Not necessary unless your waiting room is equipped with headphones. If that is the case, use material created with binaural frequencies for relaxation.

Listen ⊙ to tracks 2 and 5 on the CD. See 📖 "Sound Remedies Catalog."

Treatment Room Ambience (bodyworkers, acupuncturists, and the like—anyone whose patients will spend thirty to sixty minutes having a treatment)

Intention: Deeply relax patients, facilitate release, encourage sleep.

Resonance: Do you want to charge or discharge the system? In this instance I suggest slow acoustic music or nature sounds—music that breathes and has a lot of space. Midrange to low-range sounds aid the slowing process.

Entrainment: Music at thirty to sixty beats per minute. Look for music that has little or no definable pulse or rhythm. This will help your patient leave the structures of time and move into the alpha and theta zones.

Sonic Neurotechnologies: If you are using a sound table, headphones, or speakers placed on either side of the patient's head, material created with binaural frequencies is very effective for deep relaxation.

Notes: Look for music that ramps down, settles at a bottom point, and then ramps back up. Your patients will entrain to the music. They will slow easily and gradually, stay deeply relaxed for the middle section, and come back up into gentle awakening and integration of your therapeutic services. You don't want to "pull" patients out of a deep state without their own normal reacclimation to faster brainwave states.

Listen ⊙ to tracks 4, 6, and 10 on the CD. See 📖 "Sound Remedies Catalog."

Pain Control

Intention: Deep relaxation. Brainwave state: alpha and theta.

Resonance: Midrange sounds bring calm. Choose music that breathes and has a lot of space.

Entrainment: Music at thirty to sixty beats per minute.

Sonic Neurotechnologies: Using headphones, binaural frequencies focused at alpha and theta. The accompaniment of guided visualizations can be very effective.

Notes: Is the pain control for an acute or chronic situation? Determine the length of time to be managed and adjust your sound protocol accordingly. This is a tricky area. It is best to teach patients the concepts of resonance and entrainment so they can determine how and what sound works best and for which part of the day.

Listen 🔘 to track 6 on the CD. See 📖 "Sound Remedies Catalog."

Correction of Auditory Tonal Processing

Intention: Tonify muscles of the middle ear that counterlever the three tiny bones (hammer, anvil, and stirrup).

Resonance: High-range, up-tempo sounds. Look at Mozart, then Gregorian chant later in the program.

Entrainment: Music at 100 to 130 beats per minute.

Sonic Neurotechnologies: Tomatis-oriented filtration and gating programs, headphones.

Notes: As discussed in chapter 12, this is a very sophisticated application of sound. Training is necessary. You could become a certified Tomatis practitioner or be trained in less intensive methods. Programs consist of sound processors to achieve the F/G effect; in the case of next-generation applications, prerecorded material may be all that is necessary. Auditory testing helps assess dosage and frequency of sound applications. Depending on the goal, the application may change as the effect evolves.

Listen 🔘 to track 1 on the CD. See 📖 "Sound Remedies Catalog."

Musical Thanatology (Music for the Dying)

Intention: Help the patient to unbind, to gently release and separate.

Resonance: To be determined by a trained therapist. Mostly harp and voice.

Entrainment: Probably on the slow side.

Sonic Neurotechnologies: Lots of pure love.

Notes: Therese Schroeder-Sheker's Chalice of Repose Project is extraordinary. Excerpts from Ms. Schroeder-Sheker's book can be found at www.thepowerofsound.com.

These examples should help you see a simple checklist for sonic assessment. Your primary questions should be: *What is called for and needed? What does the client prefer? What are my tools?*

In sound, everything keeps coming around to resonance and entrainment. All the tools—special recordings, vibroacoustic sound tables, filtration devices—are based on the psycho- and physiological effect of resonance and entrainment. (If you have questions about these two basic concepts, revisit part 1.) Even the simplest concept has a layer of complexity. In whatever ways you need to perceive and mentally file resonance and entrainment, I urge you to take the time to do so. These basic concepts will be the "filtering" mechanism used in your assessment of simple and advanced sound employments.

WHERE TO BEGIN? SOUND SPACE

Here are some simple ways to add sound to your practice. Appropriate sound in your waiting room sets a relaxing ambience, helping soothe anxiety or jangled nerves. With the addition of *intentional* sound, your clients' perceptions of the healing experience begin the moment they walk into your office. This will become part of the sense-memory they retain. A simple stereo system with warm sound can make a world of difference. A bonus: You will see the positive effect among your staff as well.

Use separate sound systems in each treatment room. I recommend this because your patients have different needs and treatment cycles. Portable desktop systems are of high-enough quality to suffice. The volume should always be kept low. If you can place portable speakers within a foot or two of each ear, you will see a stronger effect with material that uses binaural beat frequencies. BBFs are most effective with headphones.

When using music in the treatment room, always ask your patients what kind of music they prefer. If they don't care for your choice of musical style, it will be counterproductive. You may suggest they try something new, but remember that lacking earlids, we can't shut out unpleasant sounds. In some cases people prefer silence. In the cycle of tension and release, silence is a powerful tool. At the end of a session, build in perhaps five minutes of silence. This can create a valuable closure time.

As you add music to your practice, even on this most elementary level, you will see that it has a great impact. You are essentially enrolling a major sensory system into the healing process. You are becoming the disc jockey of that process. So gather a sound collection that you are familiar with. It can be overwhelming trying to do this all at once; I suggest beginning with music from companies that specialize in psycho-acoustic soundtracks. This will make your job easier. This does not mean that you cannot use your favorite flute meditation music . . . it's just that specially designed soundtracks ensure that the music takes resonance, entrainment, and sonic neurotechnologies into account. Fortunately, there is a substantial library of programs available.

Build your sound library a few selections at a time. This is a long-term investment. Get to know your soundtracks. They are important and individual sonic tools.

See 📖 "Sound Remedies Catalog." The catalog is compiled for easy accessibility and illustrates the breadth of sound programs currently available.

SOUND TOOLS

Based on resonance, soundwork creates change through vibration. As a neurologically based approach, applying music or sound can take many forms, from simple tuning forks to sound structures complete with computerized output of highly specific frequencies. The goal of the first tools I will discuss, vibroacoustic tools, is to vibrate the body.

BODY APPLICATIONS WITH SOUND TABLES AND SOUND CHAIRS

Vibroacoustics may be defined as "the process of hearing sound vibrations through the body." This is accomplished through specially constructed chairs, treatment tables, or beds (some with water) that are equipped with powerful speakers designed to vibrate the body with optimal psychological and physical impact. Dr. Drew Pierson, a psychologist with electrical engineering experience, notes that the purpose of vibroacoustics is to create tactile-soma integration. He says, "The body holds emotional events in cellular memory. The use of vibration from 4.5–1800 Hz (primarily 8–180 Hz) has the effect of disengaging those resonant patterns that seem to run in loops and fixate themselves in the body. Vibroacoustics change the bio-electrical signature of the emotional imprint."

Vibroacoustic music (VAM) resonates the body directly through nerves, skin, and bones. Based on multiple transducers built into the furniture—located under the back, buttocks, and legs—the sound is not directed to the ears. In fact, unless you wear headphones, the only sounds you hear with your ears are the lowest frequencies of the soundtrack. According to Dr. Pierson, the low sounds travel *up* from the vagus nerve to the reticular activating system, touching all internal organs along the way. This is in complete contrast to how sound, heard through the ear, travels down through the vagus nerve to the anus, attaching to almost all the internal organs along the way. The vagus nerve is a very important conduit of sound waves regardless of the direction.

Pierson became so impressed with the effect of vibroacoustics that he created his own line of sound chairs. His primary clients are healthcare professionals. "Professionals can use this chair for a number of modalities: sound therapy, biofeedback or neurofeedback applications—whether its binaural beats, monitoring feedback signals (biofeedback, neurofeedback, or any digital signal that can go into a RCA jack), or even your own musical instrument." Sound chairs are extremely versatile. Audio signals from any source (CD, electronic instruments, or microphone) can be input directly into the chair to produce the vibrational response.

Dr. Pierson explains that the principle of sonic induction through wood and metal is far more powerful than through the ear (and air). "The sound waves are added into the recliner via specially designed full-range-frequency, solid-steel transducers, which have been built into the structure of the recliner's frame. You become part of the sound through direct bone conduction." In order to distribute the sound waves more evenly through the whole body, Pierson places two 150-watt transducers in areas that have the greatest sound conductivity. (See "Soundwork Resources" for more information.)

While Pierson emphasizes the power of bone conduction, others consider skin absorption of sound equally important. Whole-body acoustic stimulation has been studied by Dr. Patrick Flannigan for more than thirty years. He believes that the human skin is a powerful sense organ: "Our skin is not just a covering; it is an enormously sensitive organ with hundreds of thousands of receptors for temperature and vibrotactile input. Every organ of perception develops ontologically and phytogenetically out of skin. In the embryo, skin folds and then forms our eyes and ears. Our skin may contain the latent capacity to perceive light and sound. I think that by stimulating the skin with energy in the right way, you can potentially repolarize the brain and charge it with energy."[3]

In a program evaluation conducted at the Clinical Center of the National Institutes of Health in 1997, titled "Effects of Vibroacoustic Music on Symptom Reduction in Hospitalized Patients," Dr. George Patrick reports, "We have seen statistically significant and clinically significant results in both tension-anxiety reduction as well as symptom reduction." The goal of the project was to determine the effectiveness of VAM in providing the relaxation response as an antidote to the stress of treatment and adjustment to the possibility of chronic or life-threatening conditions. Diagnostic groups included all chronic disease processes, such as cancer, AIDS, and heart, lung, blood, and psychiatric disorders. Data were gathered from 268 adult patients with varying diagnoses over a seventeen-month period. Cumulatively, a 53 percent reduction of symptoms following the program was reported.[4]

The sound researcher and chiropractor Jeffrey Thompson was so impressed with the effects of VAM that he created his own sound tables and the music to go with them. He explains why the sound tables have such a powerful effect: "A huge section of the brain stem and nervous system is devoted to sensing and processing vibration. The spinal cord is composed of nerve bundles carrying different kinds of sensation such as heat and cold, pain, pressure, vibration, et cetera." According to Thompson, two entire columns sense vibration and take up almost the whole posterior half of the spinal cord. In the primitive portions of the brain near the stem, large areas are devoted to the processing of vibration. "When you are lying on a sound table, powerful emotional information, in the form of musical vibrations, gets processed right in the part of the brain where our most deep-seated emotional programs reside."[5]

Given the emotional and physical effect of low bass vibrations through the skin, VAM is a valuable avenue of soundwork for mind or bodyworkers. Prices range from $1,500 to $45,000, with many models about $3,000. For a comprehensive listing of vibroacoustic delivery systems, I recommend *Mega Brain Power,* by Michael Hutchison (see the bibliography). These sound delivery systems (with or without headphones) will create a powerful experience for your patients. Many practitioners have discovered that VAM may be of as much value as the chiropractic, acupuncture, and other bodywork treatments themselves. To use this modality, your soundtracks are important.

Dr. Thompson recommends these titles for the following reasons (most will be optimally effective with the use of headphones as well as playback through the VAM):

- *Psychosensory Integration Series 1–6 (PSI)* (Jeffrey Thompson). This set of CDs is made specifically for Thompson's Sonic Induction Table. Each focuses on a different "emotional landscape" combined with brainwave entrainment frequencies for balancing the central nervous system. *PSI 2* is best for eliminating constant mental chatter. It has twenty-five layers of three-dimensional sound that will distract even the busiest mind. *PSI 3* is comforting and healing for the emotions. *PSI 6* can be a mystical journey.
- *Egg of Time* (Jeffrey Thompson). This CD was created as a general stress reduction, healing, and meditation soundtrack. It was also especially designed to play through the body on the sound therapy table.
- *Inner Dance* (Jeffrey Thompson). This CD was produced also for the sound table and centers brainwave entrainment frequencies in the theta and delta realms. It was produced primarily for physical and emotional healing and has been used by many people and practitioners for this purpose with great response. It is a constant flow of changing environments of multitracked, orchestrated musical soundscapes.

- *High Peformance Mind* (Anna Wise). Anna Wise is a longtime professional in neurofeedback training through the EEG Mind Mirror. Now she has produced an audio program of brainwave entrainment frequencies built into a musical soundtrack for boosting neural function.
- *Sound Body, Sound Mind* (Andrew Weil, Anna Wise, The Arcangelos Chamber Ensemble). Extraordinary binaural craftsmanship by Anna Wise in collaboration with Andrew Weil, M.D. This sixty-minute soundtrack of specially rearranged classical and world music is designed to facilitate self-directed healing, with thirty minutes directed toward theta and thirty toward delta brainwave states. Critically and popularly acclaimed, *SBSM* is one of the most extensive creative endeavors in the audio field of sound and healing.

See 📖 the "Sound Remedies Catalog" for these and additional selections.

TUNING FORKS

Another element of vibroacoustics comes in the compact form of tuning forks. Long used as an accurate tonal guide for tuning instruments, a tuning fork is a small steel instrument with two prongs that when struck sounds a certain fixed tone in perfect pitch. In the hands of sound researcher John Beaulieu, however, tuning forks represent a powerful new way to resonate the body, brain, and etheric fields: "Our bodies, like musical instruments, can be in tune or out of tune. When properly tuned, we have a sense of well-being and perfect self-expression." Beaulieu has pioneered a new musical form that can tune our bodies and nervous systems, with the purpose of creating greater harmony and balance. "When we listen to the tuning forks, our vestibular system—via the semicircular canals—reproportions our body based on the natural ratios of the tuning forks. During the listening process our physical body will reposture itself in alignment with the intervals created by the tuning forks. During the process, our nervous system via the right and left hemispheres of the brain comes into balance."

Dr. Beaulieu, a board-certified naturopath and polarity practitioner, tells an interesting story about how he came to see the value of tuning forks while sitting in an anechoic chamber at New York University. (An anechoic chamber is a completely soundproof room that resembles a sensory deprivation chamber.) "I had read about the experiences of the composer-philosopher John Cage and decided to conduct a similar experiment. While in the chamber, Cage heard two sounds, one high-pitched and the other low-pitched. The engineer who was working informed him that the high sound was his nervous system and the low sound was his blood circulating."

Inspired by Cage's experience, Beaulieu sat in an anechoic chamber for five hundred hours over a period of two years and listened to the sounds of his own body. "I began to correlate different states of consciousness with the different sounds of my nervous system," he says. "Being a trained musician, I noticed that the high-pitched sounds of my nervous system consisted of several sounds in different intervals. Then one day I brought two tuning forks and tapped them. Immediately I observed that the sound of my nervous system came into resonance with the sound of the tuning forks. It was then I realized that people can be tuned like musical instruments!"[6]

According to Dr. Beaulieu, author of *Music and Sound in the Healing Arts* (see the bibliography), there are two ways to use tuning forks to tune the body. One is to hold them by their stems, tap the ends lightly on your knees (or some other hard object), and then place each fork four to six inches from each ear (one tuning fork on either side of the head). You can then use your voice to harmonize with them. The second way is to strike them together gently (away from the head) to create harmonic overtones. You may also move them around your head or body in order to experience the effects of the interval they create.

As tuning forks have become increasingly popular with massage therapists and other practitioners to deepen relaxation and balance the body's energy fields, Beaulieu has developed a comprehensive product line he calls Pythagorean Tuning Forks. Numerous intervals are available based on ratios thought to have specific effects on the mind and body. (See "Soundwork Resources" for more information.)

Tuning forks and acupuncture points. An extraordinary approach to the use of tuning forks has been pioneered by Fabien Maman, founder of the Academy of Sound, Color, and Movement. Extensive trainings explore the field of vibrational medicine, qi movement, acoustic sound, and pure color. Tuning forks are an integral part of the Maman approach.

In his twenty years of research, Maman has found the exact frequency of each acupuncture Shu Point, Mu Point on the back, and Ear and Foot Reflexology Point. He uses tuning forks that match these frequencies on the acupuncture points of the body. As he explains in *The Body as a Harp: Sound and Acupuncture,* the tuning forks used on the acupuncture points act on the physical and etheric level (etheric acupuncture points). The tail of the tuning fork gives the message to the acupuncture point itself and then to the meridian. The fork itself vibrates in the etheric body and gives the same message to the etheric energy. When you put a tuning fork on the identified points, it balances the energy because the vibration goes exactly where it is needed.

According to Maman, the impulse is given by the vibration of the tuning fork. With the acupuncture needle, you send a message to the meridian. The tuning fork works faster because the vibration of sound travels faster than the vibration of the needle. Because the sound also touches the etheric points, the tuning fork vibration can work to dissolve the crystallization of energy in the etheric as well as the physical level. (See "Soundwork Resources.")*

OTHER INSTRUMENTS FOR SOUNDWORK

The precise ability to modulate or measure organs in the body with sound frequencies results from advances in high technology. However, traditional medicine has been using sound for a long time. *Ultrasound* is a

---

* Special thanks to soundworker Susan Alexjander of Aptos, California, for her reporting on the work of Fabien Maman and all her wonderful mentoring of this author.

common means of imaging. When high-frequency sound enters the body, it is reflected more strongly from the outside of organs than from their interior, and a picture of the outline of the organs is obtained.[7]

Lithotripsy is a profound medical usage of resonant frequencies. Acoustic shock waves, generated outside the body, are focused onto a kidney stone in the kidney or ureter, causing the stone to fragment. The technique has been used in hospitals since 1980. Currently more than two thousand lithotripters are in operation around the world and some five million treatments have been carried out. Approximately 70 percent of patients receive lithotripsy in conjunction with some other procedure. Thus, open surgery can be avoided in 95 percent of kidney stone cases. The procedure is used for the removal of pancreatic duct stones as well.[8]

In America the employment of frequencies to modulate the body—outside of the institutional uses previously mentioned—has been considered alternative medicine. Under the jurisdiction of the FDA, certain sound-oriented devices have been banned and confiscated in the past. These have included Radionics devices and the Audiokinetron (see chapter 12). Currently, however, sound devices and accompanying techniques are being used here and elsewhere. Here are two of note:

Infratonic QGM. From China comes a machine that produces qi energy. When a senior scientist at Beijing's National Electro Acoustics Laboratory discovered that qi gong masters emitted high levels of waves called secondary sound from their hands, she became professionally intrigued. So much so that Lu Yan Fang found a way to simulate this infratonic sound with a machine. Tests on eleven hundred hospitalized patients produced impressive results. Fang found that therapeutic benefits included headache relief, pain reduction, muscular relaxation, increased circulation, increased production of alpha waves in the brain, and alleviation of depression.

In China, Dr. Fang's Infratonic QGM is widely used as an effective tool for pain alleviation. Her work has been recognized by both the China Ministry of Health and the National Committee for Traditional Chinese Medicine. In the United States, use of the Infratonic QGM is pending FDA approval under the guise of a therapeutic massage device.[9]

Cymatic therapy. A computerized instrument transmits resonant frequencies of sound into the body. Unlike other sound therapy devices, audible sounds are sent not into the auditory canal but directly through the skin. Sir Peter Guy Manners, an English doctor and sound researcher of international distinction, asserts that his device and therapy use sound waves within the audible range to stimulate natural immunicological and regulatory systems, and to produce a near-optimal metabolic state for a particular cell or organ.[10]

"Every object, whether inanimate or alive, possesses a unique electromagnetic field that exhibits antagonistic, complementary (resonant), or neutral reactions when it interacts with other electromagnetic fields," says Dr. Manners. By transmitting precision sound frequencies into specific parts of the body, Cymatic therapy establishes equilibrium. Dr. Manners maintains that frequencies pass through healthy tissues and reestablish healthy resonance in unhealthy tissues.

Training is required to become a Cymatic practitioner. Cymatic instruments have been in use in the United States since the late 1960s. Throughout the world, these instruments are most often used by nurses, osteopaths, chiropractors, and acupuncturists. (For more information, see "Soundwork Resources.")

ADVANCED SOUND TECHNIQUES

I define *advanced soundwork techniques* as "prescriptive sound." These highly different modalities, such as Guided Imagery and Music or sound stimulation auditory training programs, require varying degrees of intensive training. Quite often this level of advanced sound technique moves from the realm of minor treatment adjunct into greater significance. In this section I will examine Guided Imagery and Music, binaural beat frequencies, and sound stimulation auditory training programs.

GUIDED IMAGERY AND MUSIC

The Helen Bonny method of Guided Imagery and Music (GIM) is a "depth approach" to psychotherapy. Specifically programmed classical music is used to generate a dynamic unfolding of inner experiences. This method provides experiential access to previously unassimilated facets of emotional material. Reported psychological outcomes of GIM include incorporation of previously unintegrated aspects of self, facilitation of insight and cognitive reorganization, enhanced mood, and increased sense of meaning.

A GIM session begins with verbal dialogue to determine issues, followed by a physical relaxation (such as progressive muscle relaxation) and mental focus (perhaps a scene). A specifically chosen program of music is then played, during which clients engage in spontaneous imagery and share their experience with the therapist.

In America, GIM is taught at three universities and accredited through the American Music Therapy Association. The method is also taught internationally.

An interesting research study was conducted in 1996 at the University of Miami. "The Effect of Selected Classical Music and Spontaneous Imagery on Plasma B-Endorphin" explored the efficacy of music and imagery. B-endorphin, one of the endogenous opioids, relates to immunomodulation, pain modulation, and altered mood states. In this research, certain music was found to buffer stress-induced increases in stress hormones, including B-endorphin. In a study of two hundred women in labor, researchers found that those who listened to anxiolytic music over a twenty-four hour period demonstrated significantly lowered plasma levels of B-endorphin and ACTH, two hormones released during stressful events. Although the effect of imagery on B-endorphin has not been examined, imagery has been shown to affect a wide range of physiological functions, including blood pressure, respiration, peripheral blood flow, muscle tension, white blood cell count, thyroid secretion, blood sugar level, brainwave patterns, and immune function.

What stands out from this study is that when three categories— music, imagery, and music and imagery together—were tested for their effect on B-endorphin, the third category (combined music and imagery) had a far stronger effect than did music or imagery by itself.[11]

The Bonny GIM method, evolving out of the human potential movement of the 1960s, is a profound tool for HCPs and psychotherapists to consider adding to their existing treatments. For more information, see "Soundwork Resources."

Sonic Neurotechnologies (SNTs)

As was thoroughly discussed in chapter 12, SNTs are sound processing techniques known for resonant neurological effects. There are currently two major technologies that define this field: binaural beat frequencies (BBF) and filtration and gating (F/G). They share only a few things in common:

- Both techniques use music and sound.
- Both techniques use psychoacoustic principles of resonance and entrainment.
- Headphone application is preferred.
- Sound processing is performed on a soundtrack (music, nature, or white noise). This generally involves adding or subtracting elements of sound to or from the original recordings. The BBF technique adds detuned pairs of frequencies; F/G subtracts large spectrums of sound and then gradually adds them back in.
- The two sound approaches of BBFs and F/G are very different in origin; they have diverse goals; and they are not used in tandem. The following extrapolation, geared toward educators and HCPs, refers to material contained in chapter 12.

Binaural beat frequencies (BBFs). This is an ancient sonic technology. A few thousand years ago, someone discovered that two minutely detuned sounds create a third sound in the brain, and that our brainwaves slow down or speed up to match this natural third sound. The technology of modern computers allows us to become extremely precise in the application of these tones. The question becomes: *What brainwave state is most conducive to a desired activity?*

- *Primary usages.* Enhanced mental focus, accelerated learning, relaxation, meditation, sleep.
- *Therapeutic applications.* The relaxation effect associated with BBFs has been shown to reduce anesthesia use in surgery, improve motor skills in neurologically impaired children, improve response to alpha biofeedback training, enhance hypnotizability, and manage pain, among numerous other applications.

- *Training.* Since the first programs were made available to the public in the 1970s, BBFs have traditionally been self-administered. You buy audiotapes or CDs with a specific matrix of BBFs already implanted in the soundtrack. Right now a sizable catalog of recordings use very sophisticated programs.

  I am not aware of any current program or curriculum for BBF design or implementation; nor have I heard of anything like this in the past. For the most part, this information is quite proprietary. Knowledge of neurology, psychology, and audio engineering is very much a consideration in the design and implementation of BBFs. Aesthetics aside, creating effective frequency combinations that deal with *all* of the brain waves at the same time is a complex task. We are never in just one brainwave state. Biofeedback experts can attest to the fact that all four brainwaves are active at any given point. Effective BBF matrices must take this into consideration.

  I have occasionally seen on the market inexpensive BBF machines. These devices are essentially sine-wave generators with individual settings for stereo channels. This capacity allows you to create separate detuned sound waves for each ear, thereby setting up your own binaural beat. Given the complexity of the brainwaves entrained with the BBFs, I highly recommend steering clear of this application. HCPs would be better advised to use existing recordings rather than to create their own. If you need very specialized BBF programs, I suggest you approach one of the companies listed below. For a fee, they may design or create programs to your specifications.

- *Equipment needed.* Cassette or CD player and headphones. BBFs are most effectively delivered through headphones. If this is not feasible, place speakers near each side of the head. The volume, in either case, should always be gentle.

- *Recommended resources.* In America, only a handful of individuals and companies specialize in the use of BBFs. The following is a short list. Additional companies involved in the use of BBFs are listed in "Soundwork Resources."

  1. *The Monroe Institute.* The Monroe Institute (TMI) is the granddaddy of this field. Thousands of research hours have been spent in study of the use of sound waves, resulting in its internationally

recognized trademark, Hemi-Sync (short for Hemispheric-Synchronization). TMI hosts an extensive professional division of licensed HCPs and educators. These volunteers research and network the use of Hemi-Sync programs in their various specializations and institutions. Annual conferences are conducted in which current results are presented. TMI also offers multiple in-house programs for corporate and public use of BBFs.

2. *Monroe Products* features a very extensive catalog of highly effective Hemi-Sync recordings evolving from research conducted at The Monroe Institute. The breadth of the following category list is a testament of the company's forty-plus years of development and application of the Hemi-Sync process: Allergies, Anger, Attention Deficit Disorder (hyperactivity), Blood Pressure, Breathing, Changing Behavior Patterns (addictive behavior/anxiety/depression), Death and Dying, Energy, Expanded Awareness, Financial Success, Fitness and Sports, Frustrations, General Wellness, Immune System, Learning and Memory, Meditation and Spiritual Development, Pain Management, Personal Growth, Pregnancy and Childbirth, Problem Solving and Creativity, Self-Confidence, Sensory Improvement, Sleep and Dreams, Stress, Surgery, Weight Control.

Many of these applications are extended programs. "Pregnancy and Childbirth," the "Surgery" series, and "Immune System" are comprehensive multicassette listening programs. Many series are created in conjunction with leading experts. "Going Home"—an extraordinary program for caregivers and those dying—is a twelve-cassette program. It was developed by Robert Monroe in collaboration with Elisabeth Kübler-Ross, M.D., the world-famous authority on death and dying, and Charles Tart, a renowned researcher of altered states of consciousness. The exercises provide direct, personal experience to release the fear of death, facilitate living fully in the moment, resolve unfinished business, and explore beyond the physical.

Hemi-Sync frequencies are barely audible and are accompanied by music or white noise (sounds such as distant ocean waves). Some programs include verbal cues or guided imagery.

3. *Brain/Mind Research.* Dr. Jeffrey Thompson is the founder and director of the Center for NeuroAcoustic Research at the California Institute for Human Science. He began researching the effects of sound in healing and changing states of consciousness in 1981. His recordings are used by the general public, psychotherapists, hypnotherapists, psychiatrists, physicians, and bodyworkers around the world. All recordings contain special modulated sound pulses that cause a sympathetic response in brainwaves to change consciousness into a deeply relaxed state.

Thompson's Psycho-Sensory Integration series (PSI) recordings are specially composed programs designed to bring the mind into the ultimate receptive state for deep relaxation and therapy while eliciting distinct emotional responses. Designed for use with headphones, the PSI series was originally created to be used through the vibroacoustic delivery of Thompson's PSI Sound Induction Therapy Table. The CDs and table together create what he calls the Psychosensory Integration Sonic Induction System (see page 197).

Dr. Thompson is a pioneer in acoustic vibration research. Most BBF matrices are laid under an existing soundtrack. Dr. Thompson's approach is different and quite creative. He creates the BBF effect by precisely detuning the stereo channel of each instrument. His BBF patterns are built into the harmonics of each instrument sound you hear, into the stereo field traveling spatially to the right or left hemisphere of the brain, into bird sounds, water, crickets, human voices, and NASA space recordings. Dr. Thompson conducts occasional workshops in the United States.

4. *Acoustic Brain Research (ABR).* Therapist-musician Tom Kenyon holds a master's degree in psychological counseling and has more than thirteen years of clinical experience. In 1983 he founded Acoustic Brain Research to document scientifically the effects of sound and music on consciousness and behavior. He is certified in NLP, Ericksonian Hypnosis, and Whole Brain Learning. He is the author of *Brain States* and coauthor of *The Hathor Material* (see the bibliography). He teaches extensively throughout the United States and in Asia.

Kenyon's use of BBFs runs the gamut. As with most providers of BBFs, his standard repertoire includes applications addressing body image, movement, healing the child within, creativity and intuition, and quick naps from jet lag. Examples of ABR's unique multitape programs illustrate a psychotherapeutic slant. ABR uses subliminal metaphors, visual imagery, and archetypal psychology in addition to the BBFs.

A sampling of ABR's programs: "Endorphin Trainer"; "Mind Your Health: A Cardiac Support Program," created with Dr. Bruno Cortis; "Psychoimmunology"; "Acoustic Supported Learning"; "Inspired: High Genius and Creativity"; and "Mind Gymnastiks."

Most BBF programs are widely available to the public. A standard warning is that BBF products should not be used when driving or operating heavy machinery. Likewise, people with seizure disorders are advised to have clearance from their doctors before use. Beyond these considerations, most BBF programs are considered over-the-counter sound, usable without prescription. As an HCP, then, your training in the use of these programs will come with your own experience. Use them yourself. This will help you position their application within your practice.

See ⬛ "Sound Remedies Catalog."

Filtration and gating (F/G). This represents the other pole of sonic neurotechnologies. The singular credit for the development of F/G technology rests with Dr. Alfred Tomatis While the concept of sound stimulation is not new, the use of filtration and gating techniques to stimulate the auditory system is.

Based on the belief that sound is a nutrient for the nervous system, Dr. Alfred Tomatis determined that the ability to interpret a full spectrum of sound is vital for overall health and well-being. (See chapters 5 and 12.)

A brief review: Tomatis developed a sound processing unit he called the Electronic Ear. The music of Mozart and Gregorian chant is filtered and gated by the Electronic Ear, then listened to through headphones. The by-product is a tonifying of the muscles of the middle ear that facilitates the efficient operation of its three tiny bones. Tomatis's goals were to repattern the hearing range and create active listening. He understood the link among hearing, the voice, and psycho- and physiological development.

Since the 1950s, another eight sound stimulation programs have evolved. More than half of these methods emerged in the 1990s. A full listing of known programs is found in "Soundwork Resources."

Filtration of sound involves the gradual reduction of low or high frequencies from a full-spectrum musical soundtrack. The term *gating* refers to audio processes in which definable sound circuitry routes a sound signal based on amplitude or pitch. Tomatis used this equipment in a way completely unanticipated by recording engineers, for whom gates serve the function of limiting or compressing sound. Tomatis used gating to create a random sonic event.

According to Tomatis practitioner Minson, the unexpected sound of gated Mozart "enhances active listening through novelty and unpredictability." Active and focused listening strengthens the auditory function of the middle ear. Filtration, according to Minson, charges (energizes) the nervous system. Between the filtration and gating of music, a new form of sound stimulation emerges. These processing techniques create a workout for the middle ear . . . auditory aerobics! The stronger the middle ear, the greater the spectrum that is sent to the inner ear and brain. Additionally, auditory tonal processing links directly with auditory sequential processing. The effects of limited tonal or sequential processing may have a definitive impact on learning and mental and or physical wellness. (See chapter 6.)

- *Primary usages.* As I discussed in previous chapters, sound stimulation auditory training has multiple applications. Learning disabilities (ADD, ADHD, dyslexia), stuttering, depression, sleep disorders, autism, brain injury, post-traumatic stress disorder, substance abuse, weakened immune function, chronic pain, tinnitus, and enhanced musicality are some of the reasons that people seek out sound stimulation trainings.
- *Therapeutic applications.* The Tomatis Method is an in-clinic therapeutic model. Sound stimulation is administered two hours a day for

thirty days over an eight-week period. Filtration goes as high as 8,000 Hz, and sound is delivered through headphones with bone and air conduction. Active and passive participation by the client is monitored by trained personnel.

The past two decades have seen new variations on the Tomatis Method. Some use equipment to perform F/G and include therapeutic support. Others incorporate CDs that use much lower levels of filtration and lighter gating intensities. These programs are designed for home, school, or office use and may or may not employ bone conduction. For the most part, they are not intended for the same degree of intervention as the stronger in-clinic applications. I refer to these at-home programs as sound stimulation auditory training.

- *Training.* In contrast to the field of BBFs—where there is no place to gain training in the methodology—training in sound stimulation is fully available for the professional educator or HCP. Currently, six organizations present trainings. Below are three examples. (See "Soundwork Resources" for further information on these and other programs.)

  1. The Tomatis Method. If you are interested in becoming a certified Tomatis practitioner, you will have to go to France. Tomatis International, the headquarters of the Tomatis Method, is located in Paris.

  2. Listening Fitness. You can be trained in a derivation of the Tomatis Method in which you see clients and have portable equipment for the F/G function with a longtime student of the Tomatis Method, Paul Madaule. The director of the Toronto Tomatis Listening and Learning Centre, Paul has created a training program to certify Listening Fitness instructors. Training includes a three-and-a-half-day course and work under supervision with ten clients (which takes between six and twelve months). Equipment is also available.

  3. The Listening Program (TLP). A leading example of the new generation of sound stimulation programs, TLP is an eight- to

sixteen-week program presented on eight CDs. The only equipment you need is a CD player and high-quality headphones. This is a modular program, easily adapted for specialized applications. Three series of TLP Extensions supplement and further refine The Listening Program—Sensory Integration, Speech and Language Integration, and High Spectrum.

TLP is produced by Advanced Brain Technologies and evolved from the National Academy for Child Development (see chapter 6). This is available only through authorized providers. Two-day training courses are conducted for therapists and health and educational professionals throughout the United States and Europe. Private in-service instruction is also available to schools and healthcare facilities.

- *Equipment needed.* Based on the programs you choose to study, your equipment needs will vary from Electronic Ears for the Tomatis Program to CD players and headphones for The Listening Program.
- *Recommended resources.* In addition to the three programs listed above, there are others available. Again, see "Soundwork Resources."

How to Use Sonic Neurotechnologies in Your Practice
- Buy prerecorded programs that incorporate filtration and gating or binaural frequencies.
- Purchase F/G sound gear, and become trained or certified so that you can create individual sound protocols for your patients.

CLINICAL MODELS USING SOUNDWORK

The following clinics all serve as examples of how other HCPs and educators have integrated soundwork—or built entire practices around the use of therapeutic sound techniques. In each case, sound occupies a different setting within the standard protocol. For more information on each clinic, see "Soundwork Resources" or (better yet) refer to its website. These clinics' online presentations give a fuller picture than space in this chapter permits.

- Center for InnerChange, Denver, CO
- Chalice of Repose Project, Missoula, MT
- Cymatics, England
- Davis Center for Hearing, Speech, and Learning, Budd Lake, NJ
- Hearing and Learning Center/Beth Israel Hospital, New York, NY
- Mitch Gaynor, M.D., New York, NY
- National Academy for Child Development (NACD), Ogden, UT
- New Visions, Faber, VA
- Pediatric Therapeutics, Chatham NJ
- Sound Listening and Learning Center, Phoenix, AZ

INSTITUTIONAL VENUES AND SOUNDWORK

In addition to clinics and individual practices, soundwork has been incorporated into institutional venues as well. From birthing to hospice, dentistry to surgery, psychotherapy to treatment of Alzheimer's, soundwork has been extremely effective. I have chosen a few research studies to demonstrate how it is being used.

BIRTHING

A study from Australia titled "My Room—Not Theirs! A Case Study of Music during Childbirth" addresses the use of music to minimize confusion during labor. Due to the exacerbating circumstances, especially for first-time mothers, the experience of hospital labor wards can be stress producing and difficult. This study determined that listening to music—especially familiar music—during the birthing process enhanced feelings of security and comfort as well as increasing the sense of self-esteem and personal control in what is often a disconcerting experience.[12]

DYING

The work of Therese Schroeder-Sheker is becoming legendary. She is an academic musicologist, religious scholar, and founder of the field known as musical thanatology. Schroeder-Sheker's descriptive, *musical-sacramental midwifery* speaks of the sacred quality of helping a dying person to "unbind" with the aid of music. Headquartered at St. Patrick Hospital in Missoula, Montana, the Chalice of Repose Project resides next door to the Oncology Department. Musicians trained in a two-year graduate-level program wear beepers and stethoscopes; their tools consist of a patient's medical records, harp, and voice. The work of the Chalice of Repose is based on eleventh-century French monastic practices for the dying. As a scholar, Schroeder-Sheker has painstakingly reconstructed the theories of medieval infirmary music and applied this wisdom to modern-day life transitions.[13]

DENTISTRY

Music has been used in dentistry and oral surgery for more than fifty years. According to an impressive 1960 study,[14] sound stimulation was the only pain reliever required in 90 percent of five thousand dental operations. Forty-five hundred dental operations were accomplished without drugs! The suppression of pain by sound may be due to the release of endorphins, which are the body's own natural painkillers. In the field of dentistry, soundwork is called audio analgesia. The use of sound in dentistry is widely documented.

SURGERY

A German study of ninety-thousand-plus patients in the peri- and post-operative phases of surgery found that 97 percent were significantly relaxed during recovery with the use of music. For some, the relaxing effects of music resulted in less anesthesia. Soft, tonal music was found to be most effective. Postoperative disorientation was also minimized when patients listened to classical or slow baroque music a few days prior to surgery and then had it piped into the operating room.[15]

PSYCHOTHERAPY

As early as 1954, medical research was being done on the effect of music in the mental health arena. Researchers documented the use of music to moderate feelings of depression or anger. They also found that music could evoke a range of emotions from joy to sadness.[16] Since that time, contemporary therapeutic pioneers—including Stanislav Grof, M.D., Helen Bonny, and Jean Houston—have shown that the combination of music, breathing, and guided imagery goes far beyond strong emotional releases to tap into the realms of the unconscious. Apparently, the use of all three elements allows entrance to subconscious regions that had previously been accessible only via powerful drugs.[17] One of the foremost pioneers in the use of music and guided imagery is Dr. Helen Bonny. Her method, Guided Imagery and Music (GIM), is used in conjunction with psychotherapy.

TREATMENT OF ALZHEIMER'S

Patients who are unable to initiate movement or cannot communicate verbally have increased needs for sensory stimulation. Such stimulation helps remote memory. Music therapy is widely used and quite effective with Alzheimer's patients.[18] Music therapy (as distinguished from the neurologically oriented soundwork) is psychologically based and used most often in hospital and group contexts. (See appendix F for a broad description of the definitions and applications of music therapy.)

WHERE DO I GO FOR RESEARCH?

Research into the effects of music and sound currently abounds. While concerted, coordinated efforts are not in place, clinical research is intensifying as a result of improved measurement techniques. As a global culture, we adore music. Much as if we discovered that candy actually has a function beyond sweet taste, to use music in an application-specific manner is a bonus appreciated by everyone.

Consequently, the American and European media frequently report on research results involving music. The following organizations are a good source for deeper explorations into the existing research base. Many hold conferences and coordinate research among their members.

Society for Neuroscience. At a 1998 meeting of this group in Los Angeles, no fewer than eight research papers were presented on the effects of music on different parts of the brain. From Hong Kong, Australia, Germany, the United States—research was abundant.

The International Society for Music in Medicine. Based in Germany, this group meets every few years. Two volumes of research and papers presented at its American conferences have been published. Sections include Music, Physiology, and Physics; Music, Specific Populations, and Therapy; Performing Arts Medicine; and Professional Issues and Theoretical Perspectives in MusicMedicine.[19]

First International Conference on Music in Human Adaptation. This meeting took place at Virginia Polytechnic Institute in 1997. A book representing interdisciplinary discussions and interactions of attending scientific, anatomic, physiological, medical, music, behavioral, and related human development communities has been published.[20] The stated purpose of the conference was to look at how and why the properties and elements of music uniquely synergize with basic physiological function to meet the organism's developmental, adaptive, and cenesthetic needs.*

MuSICA: The Music and Science Information Computer Archive. This, the mother lode of music research databases, can be found with a few keystrokes on the Internet (www.musica.uci.edu). MuSICA originates from the University of California at Irvine. Its extraordinary database (almost twenty-five thousand citations and abstracts of research publications, divided into 184 categories) contains scientific research (references and abstracts) on music as related to behavior, the brain, and allied fields. It is updated on a weekly basis. *MuSICA Research Notes*, a newsletter issued winter, spring, and fall, provides reports and critical analysis of research on music and behavior, including education, child development, psychology, cognitive sciences, neuroscience, clinical medicine, and music therapy.

---

* *Cenesthesia* is "the human sensation of normal and coordinated body function."

Music Intelligence Neural Development Institute (M.I.N.D.). Formed in 1998, the M.I.N.D. Institute is a community-based, nonprofit, interdisciplinary research institute devoted to using music as a window to understanding higher brain function, with the primary goal of enhancing children's reasoning and creativity. The M.I.N.D. Institute consists of the small team who did the original groundbreaking research (known as the Mozart effect) at the University of California at Irvine. According to physicist Gordon L. Shaw, the author of *Keeping Mozart in Mind* and a lead researcher in the Mozart Effect studies, "The M.I.N.D. Institute will be building on this research of the last ten years, including the structured trion model of higher brain function, its predictions, and the striking results of behavioral studies with both preschool children and college students."[21]

As you can see, there is absolutely no shortage of research in which to immerse yourself. Music, as a verifiably effective adjunct in health, education, home, or office, is now being examined at a dizzying pace. What is perhaps most exciting is the unabashed involvement of the scientific community. Music is first and foremost an art form. The division between art and science has been institutionalized over the last few centuries. The reunification of these two cultures is heartening and long overdue. Fascinating that it took an interest in accelerated learning to bring this about.

With the advent of the Internet, once isolated outposts of information are now available to all. Associations have been created. Conferences are regular occurrences. Communications and databases are but a keystroke away.[22]

CONCLUSION

Soundwork is a diverse field and growing all the time. So many professionals—be they music lovers or former musicians—are committed to incorporating music and sound into their professional endeavors. A familiar scenario goes like this: I receive a phone call from a doctor in Pennsylvania. He tells me that his wife is about to give birth for the first time, and he wants to know what music would be appropriate to keep down her stress level. In further conversation, he explains that he played the trumpet as a teenager but then abandoned it when he went to medical school. However, he has always known that music has a special effect. He is too busy to play an instrument at this stage of his career but has never forgotten what drew him to music initially—he loved the way it felt to be in that swirl of sound and harmony.

Flash-forward one year. The same doctor is now the father of twins, has attended a professional conference of an international medical association dedicated to the clinical study of music in medicine, and has enrolled his hospital in a research project involving music in the surgical environment.

Three years later, the doctor is applying for grants at the National Institutes for Health. He has created a standing committee at his hospital to add music to the environment in numerous ways. In his spare time, he is again playing the trumpet.

Epilogue

SHIFTING THE SOUND PARADIGM

This book suggests we hold sound in a new context:

- Sound and music are *nutrients* for the nervous system.
- The auditory mechanism is a mega-portal to the brain.
- Sonic *tools* empower health, learning, and productivity.

The overarching theme of *The Power of Sound* has centered on a new paradigm concerning the nature of sound and the vital importance of the auditory mechanism. Sound, hearing, and human communication are inextricably linked. The ability to perceive a full sound spectrum is a prime necessity for integrated living. With this understanding, sound awareness and intentional application becomes critical.

The writing of this book has encompassed a decade of my life. I believe the conscious selection of soundspace and the ability to accurately perceive it will represent an evolutionary shift. If we think of the human body as an "earth unit"—designed to house the heart, mind, and spirit—ears are standard equipment on all models. If sound is indeed *fuel*, and the ear the *portal*, why is it that our owner's manual is basically blank concerning this important energy component?

Regardless of the reason, those of us involved with pyscho-acoustics endeavor to shed light upon, and to invite further exploration into, this potent energy system. Intentional music and sound tools for the twenty-first-century human are on par with DNA strands, bio-engineering, nanotechnologies, and robotics. Mindfully, I have moved from the realm of sound enthusiast to sonic activist. And it seems that parallels between environmental and sonic activism emerge.

SONIC ACTIVISM

The sun provides power and heat *and* it can burn or debilitate us. We need water to survive yet too much can drown us. It all comes down to balance. Sound, like other elements, can fuel or deplete us. Given the necessity of increased sound awareness, what is the current state of sound? What are the politics of sound? Who controls the soundspace? Headlines from the Noise Pollution Clearing House[1] show that sound awareness is increasing all over the planet. In China, England, India, Korea, Kenya, and New York City, people and governments are taking healthy sound space into consideration as never before. Increasing noise pollution affects the planet's citizenry physiologically and psychologically.

Governments and industry will address the effects of noise pollution on health when sufficient economic factors arise. I predict this follows the trend of recent legal judgments against American tobacco companies. The impetus: spiraling healthcare costs for cancer-related treatments. I don't think that noise creates cancer, but I do believe that constant exposure to noise can wreak havoc on the immune system.

The visionary insights of Tomatis were 100 years ahead of his time. In the year 2000, people are just beginning to awaken to the *physiological* impact of noise pollution. Around the corner lies the awareness of the *psychological* impact of auditory dysfunction.

Sound is ubiquitous. How we use it is our choice. Sound is an ally; it always has been. The question is whether we are ready to embrace it as such. We talk of harnessing solar, wind, and other natural energies. For a fun thought, imagine cars running on energy created by singing drivers. Or cities powered by the recycled sounds of massive telephone networks. Basic physics impossibilities? Probably so. But sound is also quite low-tech. Sound as fuel for the human power grid is as close as your loved one's ear.

Appendices

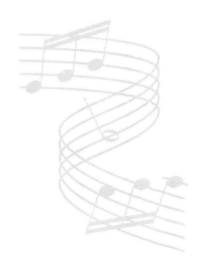

The Anatomy of Psychoacoustic Music Creation

As a music producer, I've developed some psychoacoustic techniques that may be of interest to producers and musicians who wish to expand into the territory of application-specific soundtracks. Because no one is born a "psychoacoustic producer," I'd like to share a little of my background. This brief story sets a context for what I've learned and why the instruction of both musicians and healthcare professionals in the use of psychoacoustics is of vital importance to the growth of the field.

In 1986 I left commercial composing. At that time I was living in Hollywood, and had acquired credits in radio, stage, corporate, and live musical production. I was gradually moving to the next level of TV and film composing. Yet something was personally incongruous in this pursuit; I didn't even own a TV! I couldn't tolerate the overarching violence, mindlessness, and commercialism of TV programming. There I was, though, chasing the money and prestige of the genre. While film composing was my goal, TV composition was part of the logical progression. Be it TV or film composition, however, I witnessed the intense hurry-up-and-wait, late-and-over-budget routine that plagues Hollywood composers. It just didn't add up to me.

At that time my path crossed with Louise L. Hay, a Science of Mind counselor. Louise is the founder and owner of Hay House, the world's largest publisher of self-help and human potential books, videos, and audiocassettes. She has written more than eighteen books, including the bestselling *You Can Heal Your Life*, which originated from a small pamphlet called *The Mental Causations of Physical Illness*. A believer in the power of affirmations to reprogram the mind and the simple use of love and forgiveness, she was available for private sessions in her Santa Monica apartment. As demand grew, she had also begun to release audiocassettes with her meditations and affirmations.

We liked each other on meeting and decided to collaborate. Between 1986 and 1989, I produced three albums with Louise. During that time I watched her work with large gatherings of people suffering from a new epidemic—AIDS. I observed groups chant and sing from the deepest part of their psyches. Many of the affirmations were from albums Louise and I created. Out of these experiences a major shift took place for me. As a musician, I saw and heard the difference between music written for entertainment and music written for healing. After that, I could never go back to chasing TV scripts.

In 1991 I placed an ad in a retail trade magazine for an album containing material I'd written with Louise.[1] The magazine's editor asked if I would be interested in writing an article about healing music. I declined. When asked why, I explained that I didn't really know what I was doing. I was "making it up" from instinct and intuition. Certainly this would not make for a credible article! The editor was intrigued, however. He called back a month later and asked if I was ready to write. Once again, I turned him down. At that point he became insistent. The following month he called again, this time offering to send a book that he hoped I would read. Then, perhaps, I would begin to write.

I am forever indebted to the obstinacy of editor Jeffrey Isbrandtsen, for through the book he sent, I was introduced to *psychoacoustics*, a term and a field I didn't know existed. *The Healing Forces of Music*, by Randall McClellan, Ph.D., is a seminal work and one that I highly recommend to this day (see the bibliography).

Deeply inspired and intrigued by what I read, I did write an article, and it sparked a voracious appetite to learn about psychoacoustics—so much so that I published another twenty-four articles in *New Age Retailer* in the following four years.

My column was called "A Sympathetic Vibration: Music and Sound in the Healing Arts," and I was given carte blanche to explore this widening field of psychoacoustics. I interviewed every leading psychoacoustic soundworker I could find. My agenda was clear: "I am a composer looking for the deeper meaning inside the notes. Let me ask every appropriate question I can think of and in exchange I can have your ideas published." It worked! Thus began my education in psychoacoustics. There was no place to study other than with the disparate individuals dedicated to working with sound.

One of the most interesting things I found was that most of these people were working in their separate laboratories of sound, absolutely committed and utterly isolated. Most did not know of each other's work, and many were leery of sharing. I was considered safe because I didn't have turf to protect: I wasn't a vocal toning adherent or a binaural frequency proselytizer. At the time, I didn't even know who Alfred Tomatis was. Many felt *their* way was the best way. But I was obviously eager and innocent. Almost every practitioner I visited took me in with an open heart and became a teacher. My first book, *Sonic Alchemy*, was the result of these years of travel and inspiring discussions (see the bibliography).

Because of the large amounts of time it took to transcribe and edit in-depth conversations, I had the opportunity to truly consider the words and ideas of my new teachers. As I did more and more interviews, I began to see both similarities and differences in approach among these practitioners. It was from the synergy of their combined thoughts that my theories began to germinate. I have stood on their shoulders, and now take what I've learned and make it publicly available. I hope to help propel the field of psychoacoustics to its next generation.

During my time with the magazine, a fringe benefit surfaced. Because I was writing about psychoacoustics, all products of this orientation that were submitted for magazine review were forwarded to me. Consequently, I also had the opportunity to survey everything coming to market. I unintentionally became an authority on commercial psychoacoustic products. What I found was a lot of good intention and technology—and, for the most part, extremely poor art. The aesthetic side of the music and production appeared to be a low priority of the creators, mostly because it's pretty tough to be both a scientific wizard and a brilliant musician. Most worked on a shoestring budget and were noble in their efforts to get something out to consumers.

So what has changed since 1991? I am pleased to report that a new generation of psychoacoustic products is coming on the market. The more information becomes available—and there have been numerous books published in the last decade—the smarter musicians get. As the marketplace begins to accept psychoacoustics as a genre (distributors refer to it as "Therapeutic Music and Sound," "Sound Tools," and "Psychoacoustics"), more musicians find they can afford to move their efforts into this arena. The net result is a marriage of art and science, advancing psychoacoustic refinements of music, and sophistication in production and presentation. These are goals that I support.

I foresee that soon there will be over-the-counter sound products and prescriptive sound therapies. As programs become more effective and pleasurable to use, the marketplace will embrace the concept of application-specific musical products. This should lead to mass distribution and greater utilization. Wide public acceptance and use of music and sound tools supports the field of soundwork as a bona fide therapeutic modality and life enhancer.

Following this train of thought . . . the better-sounding, more clearly explained, and more highly documented and researched psychoacoustic programs become, the greater will be their acceptance. Sonic neurotechnologies aside, it is the "sound" of the programs that will make all the difference. If something tastes bad, people don't put it in their mouths. Same thing with the ears. It is up to the musicians and producers to create soundtracks that host the technologies but are also wonderful enough to warrant repeated listening. In this conviction—of the necessity for combining high art with substantial science—I share what I've learned about psychoacoustic music production.

WHAT'S GOING ON IN THAT RECORDING?

The enclosed CD, *Music for The Power of Sound*, contains selections performed by The Arcangelos Chamber Ensemble. This music was produced by Richard Lawrence and myself between 1996 and 2000. I greatly appreciate the award-winning and patient players of Arcangelos, who served as the "workshop" from which these techniques derive.

I am assuming that by this point in the book, you have a solid grasp of the three cornerstones of psychoacoustics—resonance, entrainment, and sonic neurotechnologies. If not, please review the appropriate chapters. Knowledge of resonance and entrainment is necessary if you are to understand the purpose of the following techniques. I will be referring to these components often.

INTENTION

The starting place of any psychoacoustic production is intentionality. *What do you want to accomplish with your sound program?* Is the intended recording designed to aid falling asleep or is it for accelerated learning? Let's briefly examine these different poles of activities.

Sleep, beyond meditation and stress reduction, is as slow and low as you can get. Accelerated learning, on the other hand, is bright and active. So what brainwave state and heart rates are most conducive to these particular activities? What is the best combination of resonance and entrainment to achieve these goals? If you are interested in beta brainwave states for accelerated learning, the music will be faster and the orchestration will be higher (⊙ tracks 9, 11) (see "Music for Focus, Concentration, and Learning" on page 121). If a delta brainwave state is the goal, go for slow tempos and lower orchestrations (⊙ tracks 3, 5, 8, 10).

Entrainment and resonance at play: These are the tools for naturally influencing the pulse systems of the body (brainwaves, heart rate, and breath). The balance and alchemy of entrainment and resonance, with the possible addition of an appropriate sonic neurotechnology, is the psychoacoustic palette from which you will paint.

Psychoacoustic production is about common sense and conscious recognition of music's subtlety, which is what makes it so powerful. Most people do not realize what is taking place when they listen to music, so they are not psychologically armored against its impact. This makes it easier to influence them, and it also increases the importance of ethical intentionality. Once the goal and benefits of the music are defined, you can move on to other considerations.

CHOICE OF MUSIC

Our psychological response to any piece of music can enhance or negate the effect of a sound tool. If listeners don't like the sounds they're hearing, they won't want to listen. This is a simple fact. To facilitate effectiveness, you must determine a couple of things when you choose your music:

- Who is the intended audience and what kind of music will be best suited for its enjoyment?
- What kind of music is appropriate for the psychoacoustic treatment you will visit on it?

Let's examine the "intended audience" consideration. One of the lovely people I interviewed in *Sonic Alchemy* was Dr. Fred Schwartz, an Atlanta-based anesthesiologist and former saxophone player. In the operating room Dr. Schwartz has as many music CDs on his anesthesia cart as he has other medical tools. He is an innovator in the use of music and anesthesia and is highly respected for his work. Dr. Schwartz shares a poignant story: "I've always loved music and thought it had a lot of applications. Beginning in medical school, I used music with some of my patients. But what really affected me profoundly was when I was an intern, working in an intensive-care unit.

"I had a seventeen-year-old fellow who had a motorcycle accident. He had become comatose from the head injury. I was taking care of him and spending a lot of nights there. He wasn't responding to anything and it had been weeks already. So I started playing flute to him and his eyes would move when I played the music. So I thought, 'Gee, he is responding, there is something there.'

"We kept playing him music. His parents bought him a radio, and rock 'n' roll was what he liked. He woke up and made a full recovery three weeks later. And he remembered the music and it turned out that he didn't really like flute music at all!

"That's why he was moving his eyes! He was trying to tell me to stop. He came back from the near-dead to tell me, 'Let me die in peace, leave me alone, already!' That impressed me."

If the style of music is disliked, it will have a diminished effect. In the story above, the young man could not get up to turn off the CD player. But most people can and will. Let's look at another illustration of musical taste.

Rap music is now firmly entrenched in our American culture. Many wish it would go away; they find it offensive, monotonous, even irritating. In all likelihood it will not be looked on a hundred years from now as a great American innovation in art, such as jazz. Yet it is flourishing. Why?

Think about the structure of rap music. The basic elements are drums and bass. (This is your first tip-off to the entrainment and resonance effects.) Drum machines in rap put out a slow and steady 4/4 rhythm. The bass is predominant and turned up loud in the mix. What is the psychoacoustic effect of this sonic mixture? The slow rhythms entrain the nervous system down. The overabundance of bass frequency overloads the nervous system and causes a discharging effect. Put these entrainment and resonance elements together and you have a perfect prescription for sonic Valium. Psychoacoustically and physiologically, rap music is not an upper; on a pulse-entrainment level, it is a downer.

As an art form, rap has become prevalent in our culture because white youths— with the help of savvy advertising—want to musically emulate the African-American culture, *and* because it is great self-medication. If I were an inner-city teenager with family difficulties, friends in jail or dead, and little hope for the future, I'd be self-medicating however I could. The fact that music is such a strong tool in the arsenal of self-medication only reaffirms the belief in the power of music. Rap is a perfect example of psychoacoustic products as a tool in our lives.

A psychoacoustic exploration of rock or heavy metal music indicates that the characteristic tempos and timbres create a slightly different result. Rock, in its many manifestations, is usually more up-tempo than is rap. The consequent brainwave states will most likely be in beta rather than rap's low beta or alpha. Heavy metal relies on the distorted sounds of electric guitars. The primary audience for heavy metal is teenage boys. Something about the resonance of heavy bass, loud kick drum, and guitar distortion seems to soothe excessive testosterone. Venturing a guess: The heavy bass discharges while the distortions preoccupy the auditory function. (Imagine what the auditory system goes through to decipher and analyze, in real time, the sound of distortion.) The purpose of this conversation is not to judge, pigeonhole, or generalize different styles of music. Rather, my goal is to stimulate your analysis of the effect of tempo (entrainment) and tone (resonance).

Therefore, concerning the question of intended audience and musical choices, classical music would probably not be my top pick if my goal was sound tools for teenagers—too much generational resistance. I would instead go for music that they like to listen to, or find a way to entice them into something unusual and fun in other styles. Because musicians, let alone psychoacoustic producers, are not state subsidized, markets must be chosen carefully to ensure economic survival. Most likely, teenagers will not be first-line psychoacoustic record buyers. Thus, my choice is to cater to the adult or children's marketplace. For children, fun and engaging theatrical presentations create the perfect backdrop for sonic neurotechnologies. With adults, any of the musical styles can work, although I find classical music to have universal appeal. It is a known quantity, beautiful and rich in possibility for adaptation. This segues into the second consideration: What kind of music is appropriate for the psychoacoustic treatment you will be visiting on it?

When I speak of psychoacoustic treatment, I refer to the different processes of resonance and entrainment necessary to achieve your goals. You will most likely rearrange the music you are adapting in order to accentuate rhythmic pulse, raise or lower pitch, change orchestration, and simplify melodic content. (I will cover these areas in detail shortly.) *The main consideration is what kind of music is most easily adaptable.* I find that classically oriented music addresses both personal taste and adaptability. Still, I encourage you to try these principles in other musical styles to help diversify the field.

So our bottom-line questions about choice of music are:
Will your demographic like it?
Is it adaptable?

ENTRAINMENT

In this book I have extensively discussed entrainment and the role it plays in psychoacoustics. Entrainment is integral to any musical effect. Not only does it affect our internal landscape through external tempos, but it is also the vehicle by which our body pulses synchronize with each other. Given that rhythm is ubiquitous, entrainment is a vital influence.

So is this valuable tool used in production? I have an awareness of it at all times. For the most part I try to create in the music an easily distinguishable pulse. This makes it easy for the nervous system to latch on and take a ride.

An overarching concept in soundwork is trust. In my productions I do everything I can to win my listeners' ears. My goal is to help them feel so safe in the arms of my sounds that they will go anywhere the music takes them. I picture an escalator with very comfortable chairs in which listeners gladly recline. With such beautiful sounds and gentle rhythms, they have nothing else to do but to come along for the ride.

The only time I don't use easily felt entraining pulses in my production work is when I want no rhythmic movement at all. When I coproduced Andrew Weil's *Sound Body Sound Mind* (see "Soundwork Resources"), the purpose was to take the listener to a place most conducive to self-directed healing. The sixty-minute soundtrack started with a tempo of about 120 beats per minute. Over the first twelve minutes my coproducer, Richard Lawrence, and I gradually ramped down to the slowest rubato space we could create. We remained there for thirty-six minutes. Toward the end of this segment, we very gently added a slow tempo, gradually ramping back up to a waltzing pulse of about eighty beats per minute. In the rubato section, called "The Deep," our job was to create a sonic space that wouldn't disturb theta and delta brain waves. We had to make sure we did nothing to disturb someone in this space of delicate, subconscious access that had been achieved by our entrainment and the addition of binaural beat frequencies. In this section, rhythm would have been jarring and counterproductive. We made every effort to stay out of any form of pulse. To accomplish this non-entraining effect, we used non-Western instruments—sitar, Bansuri bamboo flute, tamboura, Tibetan bowls—all sounds that could fill the space yet be out of the world of rhythm. Yes, we could have used Western instruments, for any instrument can play rubato (without tempo). But we felt that because we had employed Western instruments in a classical context in the ramping down and then back up, something completely different would contribute to the sense of freedom from form.

One of the vehicles I employ when working with The Arcangelos Chamber Ensemble is pizzicato—lightly plucking strings, rather than using the bow. This provides a gentle rhythmic pulse. Quite often Richard and I will take an existing internal voicing and have the string players pluck each note instead of the normal legato bowing. The effect, especially with multiple players, is a wonderful round sound that provides an easily recognized rhythmic pulse.

🔘 Track 8 on the CD is our arrangement of Vivaldi's Largo from the Oboe Concerto in B Major. When listening to this arrangement, notice the use of the pizzicato. It creates an ongoing, nonobtrusive effect. Yet psychoacoustically, this gentle plucking becomes an escalator. Your nervous system locks on to this external periodic pulse and will match it. Volumes can become quite low, yet the nervous system is attuned to the rhythm.

Often, in the course of a piece we will either gradually speed up or slow down, depending on where we want to take the listener. Effective use of entrainment involves the periodicity of the tempo. Therefore, the goal is to stay as regular in pulse as we can. If we become too erratic, the entrainment will not be successful. Notice how on ● track 6, our rendition of Mahler's Poco Adagio from Symphony no. 4, the pulse is set by the pizzicato bass, then gradually slows, then slows even more. Using the iso principle, our goal was to sonically meet listeners near the tempo we imagined their body pulses would be when first lying down. The intention of the album is to facilitate falling asleep. Therefore, our destination, simply put, was to transport the listener into as slow a zone as we could. By the end of the piece, notice how we reach almost a non-tempo state. In the process, the bass pizz comes in and out. But because we established this as the pulse initially, we assume that each time it returns it is recognized as the *rhythmic escort*. With entrainment, that is essentially what we are doing. We are merely a body pulse escort service!

The Mahler arrangement on ● track 6 comes from the Arcangelos album titled *De-Stress*. The selection that follows it starts with ocean waves that match the tempo of the ending Mahler. Using waves as the entrainment device, we set up a continued slowing pattern. Our hope was that referentially, people would equate the sound of slow ocean waves with deep relaxation. The sounds of the distant water resonate in the lower frequencies. This also serves to discharge the system.

In listening to this piece now as I write, what occurs to me is that you don't need to be a rocket scientist to figure out that the slower a piece of music, the more it will make you fall asleep. My goal in these explanations—beyond the obvious—is to point out the architecture that allows for subtle application of these principles.

Notice in my descriptions I often state "we hope" or "we assume." Many things can be proved with precise high-technology measurement. Other things are left in the province of intuition and experience. Remember, we are talking about the *art* of psychoacoustics in addition to the science. In that realm, boundaries are always being stretched. This is how innovation takes place. We try things, see what kind of feedback we receive, and either embellish or discard. I urge you to do the same.

A brief word about entrainment and habituation. One of the ways the brain conserves energy is by determining patterns in things. Once this takes place, an event can be filed away. The brain has habituated to the incoming pattern and decided it is safe; active awareness shifts elsewhere. This takes place with many of the senses, not just sound. When it comes to rhythmic entrainment, there are two paths to consider with habituation.

If you *want* habituation to occur—no ongoing (active) listening—keep rhythms nice and steady. Habituation is a good thing in less active brainwave states, such as alpha, theta, and delta. However, if you want to keep the listener in a beta state, you will be more successful by avoiding habituation. You want the brain to stay tuned, to actively listen. Think of *listening* as active, focused attention and *hearing* as passive sound awareness.

To keep the brain in a highly focused mode, don't allow habituation. The way that I achieve this is by subtle changes in ongoing tempos. This is a little tricky, because entrainment is based on periodicity, which is ongoing and non-erratic rhythm. To accomplish subtle changes that remain within the bounds of periodicity, I recommend prerecorded click tracks with the musicians in the studio. Rather than a steady eighty beats per minute, a click track gradually moves between seventy-eight and eighty-two beats per minute. These subtle tempo changes, although not necessarily decipherable to the ear, serve the purpose of keeping the auditory system alert. Because tempos do not fit an ongoing pattern, active listening is kept in place. This requires beta brain waves.

Other entrainment devices include the use of anything percussive that can establish an easily listenable sound. Drum machines, however, are my least favorite entrainment tool and probably the least effective. Periodicity is necessary, but nothing in the human body beats at the perfection of a machine. The result is a rebellion of listeners' bodies. They get irritated and simply say, "Shut that damn thing off!" Once they do that, you are out of luck. Entrainment is never a forced event.

RESONANCE

A core concept in soundwork, developed by Dr. Tomatis, is that sound is a nutrient for the nervous system. Tomatis believes the ear should be considered differentiated skin, that actually the entire surface of the body perceives sound. He believes the body *hears*. This takes place through the perception of vibration.

This concept pervades my psychoacoustic producing. As with entrainment, the effects of resonance and tone are ever present in my artistic and psychoacoustic judgment calls. Listen to 💿 track 10 on the CD, Bach's Largo from Concerto no. 3 for Two Violins. The purpose of this piece is to enhance accelerated learning via the body relaxed–mind alert state described by Georgi Lozanov. Rhythmic entrainment was used to slow the heartbeat to fifty to seventy beats per minute for the body-relaxed state. This is known as the ideal relaxed heart rate. To achieve the mind-alert side of things, we relied on resonance.

To accomplish this, a few psychoacoustic refinements were put into place. This means we changed something from the original to make it more application specific. For increased concentration, we wanted to stimulate the nervous system. Therefore, we changed the orchestration. Originally, Maestro Bach voiced this beautiful piece for two violin lead instruments. We used flute and clarinet instead. Why? Because we felt that the high woodwinds would cut through the background voices a bit more. We wanted the high register of the clarinet and flute for "charging" purposes. To ensure this, we considered changing the key to a higher register. We ended up not doing so because we found it to be more artistically pleasing the way it was written. This makes sense; Bach was a genius. We are never out to try and *improve* these mas-

terworks, but, rather, we respectfully *adapt* them so they are as psychoacoustically efficient as possible. Bach's motivation was different from ours. Most of his music was
written with a seventeenth-century church audience in mind. In this instance, with
due deference to God, we are thinking mostly about increased productivity in the
classroom or office.

Let's take the example of high and low frequencies in the other direction. If our
goal is to slow down the nervous system, Richard and I will lower a key if necessary
and use midrange instruments (viola instead of violin, French horn instead of trumpet, alto flute, and the like). If we are using a piano, we might instruct the pianist to
keep most of his work in the midrange.

We often use nature sounds in our work for resonance purposes. If you look at the
sound of crickets or wind on an oscilloscope, each is in the 5,000 Hz range, with a
visible first harmonic at about 10,000 Hz. This is a "charging" frequency range.
Therefore, it becomes easy to pick nature sounds for their resonance factors as well as
their creative, entraining, or psychological impact.

SIMPLIFIED MELODY LINES

When picking a repertoire for a particular project, my coproducer and I will go
through exactly one hundred pieces on the first pass. We then each pick the twenty
movements we think best suited for the purpose. From our secret ballots, we look for
joint selections and hope there will be ten or twelve. Somehow, like old card collec-
tors, we can swap a Vivaldi for an Albinoni and end up with the right mix.

Often, we both love a piece of music that completely works for the application,
but it might include a sixteen-bar phrase that absolutely does not work. Remember,
our vision of the music's end use is almost always different from the composer's original assignment.

We use a lot of slower movements in our work. Interestingly enough, largo selections can usually be used as is, but we often find that the adagio and andante movements contain sections that become more dissonant or busier than the rest of the
piece. Clearly, tension is integral to creating release. The composers didn't want their
audiences to fall asleep or get too relaxed in the original environments. Remember
that in a symphony, usually only one of the four movements is on the slower side. If
they got too relaxed, listeners would be snoozing in the pews or concert hall.

Given that psychoacoustic refinements might be warranted for our applications,
what can two conservatory-trained arrangers do? One of three things: Completely
omit the section that is not appropriate, keep in the section but take off the lead line
and allow the inner voices to take the forefront, or run for the hills—because in America, playing the piece exactly as written is sacrosanct. However, Scottish concertmaster
Richard Lawrence reassures me that it was common practice for seventeenth- and
eighteenth-century European composers to riff on each other's pieces. They were
improvising and changing the masterworks much the way today's pop and jazz artists
create new renditions of older classic tunes.

So what is the effect of editing out a section that is not psychoacoustically relevant? If we do it right, listeners don't even know it's gone. Such is the case in our rendition of Mahler's Poco Adagio (● track 6). In many instances we are looking to soothe the psyche. If too much tension is in the original piece, it will not work. Because we have our own chamber ensemble and record all our albums from the ground up, we are able to make these changes. Much classical music on the market—in the "Lifestyle" marketing category—cannot duplicate this. Its producers are dependent on existing archived recordings.

The effect of deleting just the lead line is most interesting. On ● track 12, you will find the Bach Allegro Assai from the Violin Concerto no. 2 in E Major. This is a good example of inner voices brought to the surface. Notice how we start off with a low pizzicato arrangement of the inner voices with everything else omitted. In the second stanza, we bring in the melody line; in the third, we return to the inner voices in pizzicato. For the fourth and sixth stanzas, we play the inner voices legato without any lead line. They are as beautiful and fulfilling as any aspect of Bach. The interesting thing is that with a sixteenth-note lead line usually above them, unless you are reading a score, you would not be able to focus on them—they are background and subservient. But brought to the surface to shine on their own harmonic merit, they are wonderful undiscovered gems. The reason we pulled the lead lines in these instances was because the music became too busy for our purposes. We felt that it would cause distraction when we wanted to create unobtrusive soundtracks for focus and concentration.

By the way, I first fell in love with the elegance of inner voicings while studying classical piano. Because I couldn't play very fast, I had the opportunity to hear every note clearly. When played at normal speed, the inner voicings are usually obscured, because the mind focuses on the melody, which is usually the highest-pitched line.

Here's an exaggerated yet interesting illustration of the effect of extraneous auditory information coming into the brain: Play two different recordings of music at the same time. Try to just sit there for a minute before reaching for the volume dial or sledgehammer. Chances are your reflex will be to immediately change the sonic environment. Why? Your brain gets confused with too much information at the same time. Even our most highly evolved personal computers will crash with too much random input.

A final thought on this process of "weeding." I have been told on numerous occasions that the pieces that feature inner voices seem to speak to listeners' inner voices. As trite as it may sound, there have been too many correlations between our listeners' favorites and the pieces we have "thinned out" to be coincidental.

SONIC ISOMETRICS

Sonic isometrics is a term I've created to explain the process of alternating simple and complex auditory data to the brain. I use the term isometrics for two reasons. First, its definition pertains to having equal quality of measure. Second, its popular connotation is the use of our own strength against itself to build muscle or create release. Psychoacoustically, I attempt to accomplish both goals with this sonic technique. Alternating simple and complex auditory data to the brain can be done in numerous ways. Let me explain the rationale behind the concept.

When I began working with The Arcangelos Chamber Ensemble, in 1996, it was my first opportunity to apply psychoacoustics to a classical music environment. I immediately noticed the harmonic richness of vibrating strings and woodwinds. They sound dense and rich, like the best European chocolate. Additionally, I found the intricacy of classical contrapuntal harmonies to run the gamut from elementary to ultimate complexity. When harmonics and harmony are combined, a significant amount of complex information is being sent to the cortex for translation and interpretation.

From my study of the brain, I know that it is the quintessential computer. Awake or asleep, the brain constantly deciphers millions of bits of minutiae. Music and sound are perceived in many different areas of the brain. Rhythm is tracked by the cerebellum, melody is handled by the temporal lobes on both sides of the brain, and the interpreting of notes takes place on the right side of the brain (corresponding to areas on the left that handle language).[2] The *whole* brain is working as it interprets incoming auditory streams of information. What occurs to me is that this data stream can be filled to the brim—or it can be thinned out a bit. Why lessen the amount of data? Fatigue.

You might wonder, *Can the brain can get tired?* Have you ever suffered a sense of brain fade or brain fatigue? I certainly have, especially after intensive thinking. This is the time when someone says, "Let's take a break for ten minutes."

I've learned that the reason we sleep is not necessarily because the body is in need of rest. Rather, the mind needs to slow down. Think of a gigantic network computer system that must go off-line for a period of time every day to update and houseclean . . . doesn't it make sense that the brain would do the same? The brain is an unfathomably powerful organ. We could probably think ourselves to oblivion given half the chance!

Because the brain can fatigue from too much too fast, maybe we should lessen the load. What takes place when we send a lot of sound and then a little, and then a lot and then a little? *A lot of sound* can be defined in terms of density of orchestration or arrangement, amplitude, or complexity of harmonic structure. *Density of information* is the key concept here.

I believe that by alternating complex sound (that has abundant material to be processed) with simple sound, multiple reactions take place:

- *The brain is energized.* The process of tension and release affects all organs and muscles. Why would the brain be different?
- *Habituation is broken.* When the brain deciphers patterns, simplistically speaking, it goes onto autopilot, turning greater attention to other activities. Sonic isometrics helps us focus by not allowing a pattern to emerge. In baseball, the

change-up pitch keeps the batter off balance, unhabituated. Habituation diminishes alertness.

- *The muscles of the middle ear are exercised* by continually readapting. Strengthening these muscles helps cantilever the three bones of the middle ear, thereby increasing the delivery of a full spectrum of sound from the eardrum to the cochlea. The fuller the spectrum of sound we hear, the more stimulation the brain receives.

How to achieve sonic isometrics? Richard Lawrence and I have experimented endlessly with this concept. We have arrived at two different approaches.

- *Interludes.* Here we sandwich nature sounds and simplified, rubato melodies played by one or two instruments between fully orchestrated movements—we are alternating simple sound and complex sound data. In ⊙ track 4 of the CD, Vivaldi's Largo from the Viola d'Amore Concerto in D Minor, notice how the melody of the movement is played in rubato—nonstructured spaciousness prior to the regimentation of the movement's rendition. We think about contrasts: open/closed, dense/spacious, tension/release. After the movement is played, we go back to simple sound space and close the piece with nature and simplified melody.

- *Rearrangements.* For an example of this second approach to sonic isometrics, go to ⊙ track 3, the Adagio from the Concerto Grosso op. 6, no. 8 by Corelli. Everything is kept in the musical domain without the simplicity of nature sounds; instead, *arrangement of instrumentation* and melody are used to accomplish the same thing. In this selection, the first three minutes of Corelli's concerto is played by the full chamber ensemble. We then segue into piano, violin, flute, and cello. Notice the lightness and spaciousness of the sound. We have attempted to create a big breath, a lot of air around each line and instrument. This provides room to think, feel, rest, fall between the cracks. When there is a wall of sound—regardless of its beauty or melody—another function is served. Complex sound, for me, is all-encompassing; it demands fuller attention. With simple sound, there is room for other things to occur. (Also refer to to ⊙ track 7, Interlude from Dance of the Blessed Spirits.)

Notice that at minute five, the entire ensemble returns. Now there is much more information for the brain to process. This is therefore an example of complex-simple-complex.

The technique of sonic isometrics is based on intuition. I know of no scientific basis for the concept. Judging from the feedback I have received, however, it is an effective device—and I believe that this effectiveness ultimately will be clinically verified. I eagerly await and welcome your innovative arrangements of this concept in the future.

CONTOURS

Gradual changes in tempo and shifting dynamics (amplitude, panning) help offset the brain's process of habituation. I call this process *contours*.

As I discussed under "Entrainment" in this chapter, Richard and I go out of our way not to have our ensemble play metronome perfect. The human body doesn't have a metronome, and that level of rigidity in rhythm sets up a subtle conflict with our organic inner rhythms. The entrainment tug-of-war is between our desire to go to the music and, conversely, to resist it. To win the tug, it is best to match the body's natural tempo. While we need to stay periodic and regular, to be entrainment effective, we often create a click track that the players work to in the studio. Very gradually, we speed up and slow down. The purpose is to keep the brain actively involved. If it senses a pattern that it can count on, it will turn its attention elsewhere. As I have discussed, habituation is a desirable state for deep relaxation applications. However, for attention and mental enhancement, look to maintain rapt attention.

We do the same with volume or panning dynamics as with rhythmic contours. *Subtlety* is the best way to maintain musical integrity without sounding contrived. Again, the purpose of contours is to keep the brain engaged in the process of active listening. Is your goal an active brain or a sleepy brain? Pick the times you want to influence the brain through rhythmic or dynamic contours accordingly. (⦿ Track 1 is a great example of dynamic panning that encourages active listening.)[3]

NATURE SOUNDS

I often use the sounds of nature in my work. If used sensitively and with intention, they can enhance any project. If used sloppily, they sound fabricated and will cheapen your efforts. Incorporating nature sounds into a psychoacoustic soundtrack can be a time-intensive project. I've discovered that in order to use these sounds effectively, I must commit as much time as it takes to manicure every sound on a multitrack recording. To do anything less creates a product that sounds substandard. What's the appeal of these sounds to me? They serve a number of psychoacoustic purposes.

Refer to ⦿ tracks 1, 4, and 12 on the CD.

- *Psychological.* Underneath our stylish clothes, we humans are animals too. We respond on a very primal level to the sounds of the earth, sky, and water. The use of gentle nature sounds makes us feel both safe and familiar. They're also fun—a great duck at the right place can be very funny! These are good states to create when working with music for healing.
- *Resonance.* Nature sounds, like all other sounds, have definite frequencies. I find that they cover the spectrum of sound. I use them mostly for high-frequency effect. Crickets, wind, and rain can help create the sonic environment that charges the nervous system. I do this in a very dronelike way so it fades into the background and listeners hardly even know it is there. Yet the frequencies are

still being perceived by the brain. There are low-frequency sounds as well. You will have to build your own library of sounds by either recording them yourself or buying them from sound companies that specialize in licensed sound effects.

- *Entrainment.* Nature sounds can be used to entrain or to take a listener completely out of time. The sounds of ocean or lake waves are very effective in creating a rhythmic trance. You must thus pick your waves carefully for their speed. Conversely, nature sounds are wonderful in creating a totally rubato effect if you are looking to take your listeners out of time. This depends on the intention of the project. Think of nature sounds as part of your sound palette.
- *Drone.* Because of the drone quality of many nature sounds, they are perfect for masking binaural beat frequencies or other sounds in your track that are not necessarily pleasing to the ear. Also, as drones, these sounds help in interludes when I want lots of space between rubato, simplified melody lines.

A final note on nature sounds: Take the time to do them right. Otherwise, leave them outside.

SONIC NEUROTECHNOLOGIES (SNT)

After reading chapter 12 you should have a good understanding of the two basic avenues of application-specific sound processing. When considering binaural beat frequencies or filtration and gating for your project, two questions arise. *Which SNT serves your purpose?* And, more important, *Who will you collaborate with?*

As an ethical musician, I urge you not even to think about creating the protocols of these technologies yourself—unless you are a psychologist, neurologist, and licensed therapist. These psychoacoustic sound treatments can have profound effects. Just because we can create these effects as musicians does not mean we are equipped for the outcome. SNTs fall into the category of frequency medicine and should be honored as such. Rule of thumb: Collaborate with experts in the field.

When I work with these technologies, they become an integral part of my project plan. Everything creative is planned around the SNTs. This is the only way to emerge with a congruent product. When I coproduced *Sound Body Sound Mind*, our binaural frequency composer was the internationally respected brainwave biofeedback authority Anna Wise. Before we began our musical structure, she created a literal blueprint of four binaural frequencies that changed at regular intervals. Her graphic layout took twenty feet of horizontal paper. It was against this backdrop of her planned brainwave journey that we orchestrated the rest of the album.

Likewise, we worked hand in hand with the protocol team that created The Listening Program. This eight-CD program, designed to retrain auditory tonal processing, uses Tomatis-oriented filtration and gating techniques. It took us months to create an integrated program of music, nature, and F/G. Our SNT technical protocol team consisted of one psychiatrist clinically trained in F/G by Tomatis, one neurodevelopmental expert, and one speech and language pathologist.

Some SNTs should be relegated to the category of prescriptive sound programs. This means they are sold only in conjunction with therapeutic support. This is especially true with F/G work. On the other hand, I find that binaural beat frequencies are more adaptable to over-the-counter sound. By this metaphor, you see that the effects of these auditory treatments should be taken with the utmost seriousness and sense of responsibility. Use them with caution in your work. Remember, you do not know who will end up with your album in their hands. Therefore, the onus of responsibility rests with you.

SUMMARY: THE ANATOMY OF PSYCHOACOUSTIC MUSIC CREATION

Intention: What do you want to accomplish?

Choice of music: Intended audience? What kind of music is apropos?

Entrainment: Creating pulse in music; being a *rhythmic escort.*

Resonance: High frequencies *charge;* too many low frequencies *discharge.*

Simplified melody lines: Does the arrangement serve?

Sonic isometrics: Alternating simple and complex auditory data to the brain.

Contours: Using rhythm, amplitude, and stereo placement to break habituation.

Nature sounds: Tremendous value; take the time to do right!

Sonic neurotechnologies: What serves? Who will you collaborate with?

In the application of psychoacoustic principles, think:

- Entrainment/Resonance/SNTs
- What brainwave state is most conducive to a particular activity?
  Beta: fast and high; delta: slow and low.
- Use common sense and conscious recognition.
- Think about subtle distinctions.
- Think sonic alchemy.
- Remember the cornerstone of psychoacoustic orientation:

  R
  E
  S
  O
  N
  A
  N
  C
  ENTRAINMENT

The following acronym will help you remember the four basic elements:

I R E S T	
Intention	(thought, heart)
Resonance	(tone)
Entrainment	(rhythm)
Sonic neurotechnologies	(precision)

To the community of musicians: I look forward to the collective breakthroughs in psychoacoustic music production. This field is positioned for great innovation and recognition. The finer the combination of art and science, the more effective we all will be.

Stress-Induced Auditory Dysfunction

9

INTERVIEWS WITH
ROBERT J. DOMAN JR., RON MINSON, M.D., AND BILLIE THOMPSON, PH.D.

In chapter 7, I began an inquiry into the effects of stress and trauma on the auditory system. There is very little written information about this concept. However, I believe a direct correlation between stress and auditory function exists.

I am a musician and producer specializing in psychoacoustics—not a psychologist or doctor. Therefore, I have turned to professionals who have active clinical experience with adults and children. My interest is in furthering exploration of the topic of stress-induced auditory dysfunction. Just as other conditions may have a root in inadequate tonal processing, so might the effects of stress. Physical health, mental productivity, and emotional balance suffer from extreme stress. This is not new information. But is it possible that the auditory system holds a key to remediation and rebalance? Might sound and the ear play an important role in this equation? As a journalist, I am following up on a lead. I think there may be a story in the making here . . .

I prepared a list of questions and submitted them to three authorities in the therapeutic use of sound. Robert J. Doman, Ron Minson, M.D., and Billie Thompson, Ph.D., have varied backgrounds and approaches. Sound plays a crucial role in the practices of each. Independently, Doman (a neurodeveopmental specialist), Minson (a psychiatrist), and Thompson (an educator) have come to see soundwork as pivotal in the clinical populations they attend to. As you will see from the following interviews, each has a different way of approaching my inquiries. Here are the questions I posed to each of them:

- Is there an effect of stress or trauma on the auditory system?
- What kinds of stress do you see and what are the symptoms?
- What are the psychological issues that manifest themselves in the ear?
- How do they manifest?
- Do stress and trauma have effects different from psychological or physiological issues?
- What is the effect of mixed laterality?
- Is there a scientific basis for this?
- What are the solutions for mixed laterality?
- Success rate and time?
- What causes mixed laterality?
- Do many adults have mixed laterality due to stress or psychological trauma?
- What are their symptoms?
- How are they usually treated?
- Why is stress-related auditory dysfunction rarely spoken about?

INTERVIEW WITH ROBERT J. DOMAN JR.

Robert J. Doman Jr. is the founder and director of the National Academy for Child Development and the creator of NACD's Neurodevelopmental Therapy. He received his initial training with his father, Robert J. Doman, M.D. Dr. Doman was highly respected for his work in physical medicine and rehabilitation for brain-injured children and adults for more than forty years.

Robert Doman has continued this pioneering work and is a world-renowned educator and lecturer specializing in the development and use of eclectic treatment techniques. These include neurological sequential processing methodologies and advanced sound therapies. Doman's work ranges from the treatment of severe brain injury to accelerated programs for the gifted. He has personally designed more than fifty thousand individual home-based neurodevelopmental programs. The results of this work have led to his recognition as a leader in early childhood and accelerated education, as well as in the treatment of learning and developmental disabilities. For contact information, see "Soundwork Resources."

This interview was conducted in April 2000.

JL: Bob, I would like to talk to you about a subject I call stress-induced auditory dysfunction (SIAD). Let me give you the context in which I am exploring this . . .

From the Tomatis vantage point, one of the functions of the auditory system is to serve as a battery; sound comes through the ear portal to charge the nervous system. With noise-induced hearing loss (NIHL), not only do we lose the ability to take in sound in relationship to communication, but we're also limiting the amount of energy available to energize the nervous system. We know NIHL is an inner-ear function having to do with damaged cilia cells and that it is not repairable at this time.

As I have explored Tomatis's thoughts about the psychological impact on the middle ear, I wonder about additional layers that take place around stress and trauma. In an article you wrote in 1982 titled "Dominance and Emotionality," you made a reference that has caught my attention. "Abnormal neurodevelopment may be caused by psychological, physiological, or environmental problems in child-hood, deviations of a normal auditory development may also occur later in life due to stress or trauma."[1]

I'm quite interested in the effects of stress and trauma on auditory function. I have a personal investment in this investigation. After a few years of compacted emotional stress, I have noticed some uncomfortable personality changes. Men-tally, I have become mildly dyslexic. Emotionally, I have to keep a tighter aware-ness of not taking life too personally. My balance in these areas is different from how it used to be. I never would have made a link between these new mental and emotional patterns until I came across your article concerning auditory cross dominance.

Is it possible that a consequence of stress overload is an auditory cross domi-nance? Perhaps this takes place in addition to "shutting down" our middle-ear function? And from auditory cross dominance, neurological dysorganization and emotional overreactivity occur?

It seems very few people are talking about this. What is occurring here? When we go through traumatic and stressful loss, how does that manifest in auditory function and what is the broader impact?

RD: From my experience, if you're functioning dominantly in an organized neuro-logical fashion, your dominant hemisphere is in control. Your dominant hemi-sphere is logical thought, analytical thought, and long-term memory. If you're functioning subdominantly because you're developmentally mixed dominant or if you're functioning subdominantly because of emotionality, then the dominant-hemisphere functions of logical and analytical thought are diminished and you're functioning more with the emotional part of your brain.

The prevailing thought on dominance has gone into a bit of a misperception in terms of "you're functioning in either your right hemisphere or your left hemi-sphere. If you're functioning in your left hemisphere, you're dominant; if you're functioning in your right hemisphere, you're subdominant." From the way I see it, it's more of a hierarchy where we all start off life being subdominant.

When we perceive preschool children, they're all subdominant. They're develop-ing language skills, they tend to be emotional, they're very much into creativity, very much into music, not yet developing logical and analytical thought. Then if devel-opment occurs as it should, they later develop dominance and don't lose any of those things they had (creativity, emotionality, et cetera) but they begin to overlay the sub-dominant functions with this dominant-hemisphere specialized function that per-mits higher-level language function, analytical thought, and logical thought.

Now, if the dominance doesn't occur as it should, then they lack that special-ization. They lack logical, analytical thought and they react emotionally rather than analytically and logically. If we create a situation with any human being in which they are too immersed in subdominant function—and that could be music (typically vocal music) or stress and emotionality—what tends to happen, from my experience, is that even though they might have been dominant or close to dom-inant, utilizing and having access to that dominant-hemisphere control, they tend to just go subdominant, and the longer they're in this emotional state, the more the system begins to fall apart.

Your experience of suddenly becoming dyslexic could demonstrate itself in auditory or visual problems, visual reversals or auditory reversals. . . . These symp-toms are essentially a reflection of your functioning so much in a subdominant mode that you essentially broke the system that existed.

JL: What is an auditory or visual reversal?

RD: A visual reversal is the classic "dog forgot." You are seeing it backward. An audi-tory reversal is where you would put the last syllable before the first syllable, or you would switch numbers; somebody says *725* and you hear *527*. Most people wouldn't be terribly aware of that except like when somebody gives them a telephone num-ber and they have to dial the number and they get someone else.

JL: So what happens when that takes place?

RD: What happens is that because you're functioning so much in the subdominant . . . the dominance or the close-to-dominance that you had established begins to dis-integrate. Where you might have been right-handed, right-eyed, right-eared, you're functioning so subdominantly that you begin to lose the dominance that you established and you're no longer completely right-sided or completely left-sided. If I see someone who suffers a stroke, or suffers a traumatic injury to the brain, we see these things get changed and shaken up. It also seems that emo-tionality can produce essentially the same effects as physiological trauma.

JL: So when you say "emotionality," is it possible that when we go through serious levels of emotional stress it can create auditory cross dominance?

RD: Yes.

JL: What do we do about that when it happens?

RD: Well, if we are aware of it, we can reinforce what should be, which would involve plugging or occluding the ear just to knock it back over to where it belongs. As a matter of fact, we have many kids who lack dominance and are emotional and have behavior problems. We often plug that subdominant ear, or patch that sub-dominant eye, and their behavior changes within minutes.

JL: Bob, your son Alex first suggested that I had an auditory cross dominance. This came about after he observed me for a long time.

RD: Yes.

JL: When I inquired as to what I could do to reestablish right-ear dominance, he sug-gested that I don't ever talk on the phone with my left ear again. Consequently, I have made it a point not to do that. At the same time, I started to occlude my left ear for about an hour a day with a foam earplug. I also went through The Listening Program. I don't know whether it's just a placebo effect, but it feels like I'm returning to a right-ear dominance. My thinking has been clearer and my emotional-logical balance feels more in sync.

RD: Good.

JL: The question that surfaces from my own personal experience is that if stress can indeed cause an auditory dominance switch to occur, is it possible that millions of people in this country suffer from the repercussions of cross dominance? Those repercussions manifesting themselves neurologically and emotionally?

RD: Yes, it is. Undoubtedly, we have the stress. And we also have telephones that are contributing to the problem. Most people, unfortunately, tend to put telephones to their subdominant ear (usually the left ear) so they are free to write with their dominant hand (usually right). Adding cell phones to the mix has created a situation where the majority of us are spending more time on the phone than we ever have before. Those of us who listen to the phone and drive tend to drive with the right hand and use the left hand to put the phone to the left ear.

JL: Therefore, it's possible, even without increased traumatic stress, that just by the overuse of the left ear one can actually create a cross dominance?

RD: Absolutely.

JL: Do you hear anybody else talking about this? If not, why?

RD: No. The dominance issue is something that was actively discussed back in the 1960s. It was presented as the primary cause of learning disabilities and was overstated. The reaction of the professional community was to discount it because it was overstated. Since that time, it has been pretty much ignored. When it's not ignored, it has become an area of controversy. As a matter of fact, one of the areas of controversy right at the moment is relative to which ear should, in fact, be the dominant ear.

The Tomatis people disagree with me in that my work has pretty much demonstrated that if you're right-sided, everything should be lined up on the right side; if you're left-handed, everything should be lined up on the left side. Where the dispute comes in is with the auditory channel, wherein the majority of people have their language center in the left hemisphere. . . . [It] is perceived by many, including many of the Tomatis people, that most people should be right-eared regardless of what their dominant hand is. My experience says that's wrong.

JL: So in terms of the treatment of auditory cross dominance, can we revisit how that can be switched back and what people can do to ensure that they stay dominant?

RD: The function determines structure. Essentially, if you're right-handed, you'll be right-ear dominant. Let's say you're a neurologically organized, efficient person, and you're all left-sided or all right-sided . . . if you don't have any problems with your ears—like having sinus problems and fluid developing in your dominant right ear, which would tend to throw your dominance over to the left—just making sure under normal circumstances that you're emphasizing the right ear with the telephone is sufficient to maintain it.

JL: Really? Just that in and of itself?

RD: Yes. It's a controversial area and most of the professional community won't even acknowledge the existence of dominance. But having tested the dominance on twenty thousand people and worked at establishing a change in it, I tend to disagree.

JL: In the overall scheme of things, how important do you rate the process of dominance?

RD: It's person-specific. It's everything from people who have significant mixed dominance that doesn't seem to affect them to any great degree to kids who begin to stutter at the beginning of soccer season because they're kicking with both feet. Part of the influence of dominance tends to be relative to how efficient the rest of the system is. For example, if I have someone who is physiologically in good shape, who has superior sequential processing skills, lives a pretty successful, not terribly traumatic life, and if their dominance is off a bit, it's probably not a big deal. But when things change, it becomes a more significant deal. For example, a lot of the problems geriatrics experience [are] largely a reflection of dysorganization that has existed throughout their entire lives but was not a tremendous factor. But when they get old and things start falling apart physiologically, those little neurological inefficiencies become more significant. So you see a lot of older people whose long-term memory seems to be affected dramatically. I think a lot of that is a reflection of dominance. In older people who have difficulty controlling their emotionality, I believe dominance is an issue. When they were physiologically in good shape and everything else was running, the system was able to compensate.

Maybe in your case, when all systems were go and things were going pretty well, maybe that dominance has always been off. But when you got in a situation with a divorce and all that goes with that, where stress levels increased that adversely affected you physiologically, then possibly a minimal preexisting cross dominance became a significant issue.

JL: Do you think that sound stimulation auditory trainings are helpful in restoring proper auditory dominance? For example, The Listening Program features a mild level of right-ear reinforcement. It starts off evenly balanced between both ears and then reduces the volume to the left ear by three decibels. By the middle of the program, TLP is reduced six decibels in the left ear and concludes there. This is a very mild volume difference to each ear. Yet do you think this can have an effect?

RD: I think so, assuming we're talking about right-sided people who want a right-ear dominance. If someone were left-sided and wanted a left dominance, they could wear the headphones switched with the right headphone on the left ear, et cetera. This would have the same effect of retraining the dominant ear.

Our brain has a level of attention that is significantly beyond our conscious awareness. I think the brain responds to a whole lot of subtle variations that we are not aware of perceiving. I think those variations tend to have a pretty significant impact on the system. If you think about it, there's a great deal that goes on in the brain on many different levels that you're not aware of.

For example, I can be sitting on a plane and two hours into my flight, out of nowhere, my brain says, "Hey, dummy, you forgot to pack your alarm clock," and somewhere in the back of my head for some reason my brain was going through my packing scenario and realized I didn't pack my alarm clock. I wasn't consciously thinking about packing, let alone thinking about whether I packed my alarm clock, but my brain's working on that. So on those kinds of levels, things are occurring and I think on levels where we're just processing data, be it visual or auditory data, there's a level of awareness of often very subtle variations that some level of our brain is picking up on. By the way, I hate it in the middle of a flight when I think I did forget something like that because I can't find out until I land.

JL: Bob, is it true that ninety percent of your work is essentially with the neurodevelopment challenges of children? With the other ten percent, do you find adults also who come in and say, "Hey, I'm on top of my game and then all of a sudden I find myself looking up from the ground and what's going on?"

RD: Yes, I think ninety percent is pretty accurate, but I see a lot of people, so that ten percent ends up being a significant number of people. That adult population is everything from stroke patients to entrepreneurs who just want to function better. By the way, relative to stroke patients, they're some of the best illustrations of the significance of dominance. If I have someone who is a right-sided person with a stroke in the left hemisphere, they lose their language function and they tend to become very emotional. If they have the stroke in their right hemisphere, they don't lose their language function and they don't become overly emotional. What I typically have to do to get language function back and control of emotionality is to reestablish dominance, and in some cases that means moving everything over to the other hemisphere.

If you have someone who has that left-hemisphere stroke and the right arm is so impaired that you can't reestablish dominance on that right side, they start using their left hand, and to get that cortical function back again, I have to move the visual and auditory dominance from the right eye and ear over to the left eye and ear.

JL: Let's take it back to somebody who is not in that dire of a situation. What do you do when you are dealing with an adult who says, "I want to be able to function better," and you realize that they may have a dominance issue going on? In addition to occlusion or switching the telephone, what other auditory means do you use? Are there other methods in addition to the auditory?

RD: Auditorily speaking, we start by just plugging an ear.

JL: And how long would you do that?

RD: Typically, it's the whole waking day for most people.

JL: For how long?

RD: Well, it depends on how long it takes to get it switched over. It can be a matter of a couple of months to a year.

JL: And the principle behind that is what?

RD: Essentially, when you're plugging the ear, you're not totally occluding the sound.

You are just diminishing and creating a variation between how much is going in one ear versus the other ear.

JL: So by doing that you're basically forcing the right ear to acclimate or reestablish its dominance?

RD: Yes. Basically what is occurring is: Stimulation produces organization, which essentially is a reflection of stimulation of the growth of connections between neurons. So if there's more input going in one ear, the other ear is basically growing more connections through that route.

JL: And this growth can take place at any time in our lives?

RD: Yes. So essentially, if you will, we are growing connections.

JL: If, for example, I have moved into cross dominance, does that mean that I will always have an open bridge between the two, or is it possible for me to move it back over to the right? What do I need to do to maintain that? Am I always prone to crossing over again? How do I look at that in the running of my life?

RD: I think the longer dominance has been established, the stronger it is. If I have a child, for example, who just established his dominance six months ago and he tested pretty right-eared . . . but he gets fluid in his ear, an ear infection, and essentially is occluding that ear because of the fluid for a period of a few weeks, that's sufficient to knock his dominance off. If it's been established for a few years, and he gets fluid in his ears for a couple of weeks, that very possibly is not enough to knock the dominance off.

Part of what creates the controversy in this auditory dominance area stems from the fact that there's no great way to test auditory dominance. Actually, when we are working with kids, we rely largely on evaluating the function to determine if the dominance has been established.

JL: I don't quite understand it.

RD: We largely look at the general function of the individual to try to make the determination of whether or not dominance has been established.

JL: How would adults know if they have a situation with auditory cross dominance?

RD: Well, I think most people start experiencing an increase in emotionality and greater difficulty in controlling emotionality. A few simple examples: They find themselves bawling at a movie that they would never have shed a tear over before, they experience auditory reversals as we had discussed earlier, problems with auditory long-term memory.

JL: Please define that for me.

RD: Auditory long-term memory is simply memory past immediate short-term or intermediate-term memory. When someone would normally tell you their name or their telephone number and you would remember it, if your auditory dominance slips, essentially you misfile the information and you don't remember it anymore.

JL: So actually a person can determine whether or not he has a cross dominance based on a checklist of symptoms.

RD: Right. Part of what we do to try to ascertain whether or not we've got the dominance established in children is looking at their function.

JL: And with adults?

RD: Same thing. Actually with adults, before I would even consider treating something, we would look at their function first to see if it's in fact creating a functional problem for them. Now, if you came to me and said, "Bob, I listened to your tapes and after listening to your tapes I think right-handed, right-eyed, and left-eared, should I fix that?" I for sure wouldn't necessarily say yes. I would question you about your emotionality, about your auditory long-term memory, and if functionally you didn't see a particular problem, I would tell you not to worry about it.

JL: Let's briefly go back to auditory long-term memory. What the criteria would you use for that? In other words, if somebody is introduced to somebody else, or there is a phone number or other piece of information involved, in a normal case how do you determine whether there is appropriate long-term memory function?

RD: Well, if we're dealing with a child, we can question the parents relative to forms of instruction and how well the information sticks. If you're giving visual input and the kid remembers the visual information and doesn't remember the auditory information, that pretty much tells us what is happening there in terms of long-term memory.

Most adults—if you bring it to their attention and start paying attention to their function—they'll be aware of it. Most of us know if we're generally being good at remembering names and all of a sudden we can't remember names or telephone numbers anymore, or our work situation is where we've got a boss who is giving us a string of directions and we used to be able to remember them and now we can't.

I had dinner tonight with one of my friends and her aunt is in a nursing home. This poor gal's long-term memory is such that she can't remember if she ate a meal or not. She's in one of these nursing homes where they have a dining room where residents come down to the dining room and have their meals or they can call and have their meals delivered. My friend can talk to her aunt and say, did you have dinner? And her aunt says, "I don't remember if I had dinner."

JL: So long-term memory is anything over an hour or two?

RD: There's some discussion about that. Short-term memory is immediate in and out. Intermediate-term is a few minutes to hours, and then it's long-term memory. However, there is some disagreement in terms of this definition.

JL: In terms of other ways that auditory cross dominance would be treated besides occlusion and switching the telephone, are there other auditory methods that you would suggest, or other methods that are not tied to the auditory mode?

RD: To some degree it's a matter of controlling the overall situation. If I have a child, for example, who is in a very emotional and stressful environment, I can pretty much plan on not being able to establish their dominance because there is just too much subdominant action going on. My father had an opportunity to evaluate the first group of Suzuki kids who came over to the States. These kids were really immersed in music and he found dominance problems in virtually one hundred percent of the kids.

JL: Because they were immersed in music?

RD: Yes. Music is a subdominant-hemisphere function.

JL: Let me just make sure I understand this. If I am right-handed, that means my left hemisphere would be my dominant hemisphere?

RD: Yes.

JL: Are you are saying that because music is such a right-brained function, the effect of that is it causes people to become left-ear dominant?

RD: Well, more that if children are immersed too heavily in music at the time when their dominance should be established, which is four to six years, it can be enough of an influence that their dominance does not get established.

JL: And you are saying the majority of the Suzuki kids had that?

RD: Yeah, back in that group, the first group that he brought over to the States to demonstrate what he did.

JL: Well, that works at total cross purposes if we understand that musicality demands proper dominance.

RD: Right. Normal amounts of things in proper balance is fine, it's just when things get too far out of kilter that problems arise.

INTERVIEW WITH RON B. MINSON, M.D.

Dr. Ron B. Minson brings a unique background in public health, family practice, and psychiatry to his position as founding physician of the Center for InnerChange (located in Denver, Colorado). He received his medical degree from the UCLA School of Medicine in 1964 and is board-certified in psychiatry and neurology.

After completing psychiatric residency at the University of Colorado Health Sciences Center, he worked at the Arapahoe Mental Health Center and established a private practice. He later served as chief of psychiatry for Presbyterian Medical Center and as director of behavioral sciences at Mercy Hospital. In 1989 Dr. Minson began researching the effects of sound on the psyche, becoming certified in the Tomatis Method in 1990 in Paris, where the revolutionary method originated. He has trained in both the Berard Method and Samonas Sound Therapy. In 1995 he also became trained in biofeedback and neurofeedback. Dr. Minson is a leading protocol designer of The Listening Program, a new sound stimulation auditory training method based on the work of Tomatis and Robert J. Doman Jr. For contact information, see "Soundwork Resources."

The following interview was conducted in May 2000.

JL: Ron, do you know anything about auditory cross dominance?

RM: When you say cross dominance, do you mean a left-ear-directed person in a right-dominant organization?

JL: Yes, in other words, what seems to have happened with me. I'm right-handed and -footed and apparently I ended up with a left-eared dominance (presumably a cross dominance) that I'm trying to revert back over to the right.

You see, I never had this before. I went through the whole Tomatis Method with you, and I imagine you would have told me if I was left-ear dominant at the time. Something happened to my ears between 1995 and 1999. During this time I went through an inordinate amount of stress. I am interested in knowing what you see in your clinic concerning stress-induced auditory dysfunction.

RM: I see a lot. Let's start with how it may show up. There are several ways that, in response to psychological or emotional stress, we defend or protect ourselves with regard to the auditory system. This involves different ways of tuning out. Using a listening test, we can show this protective response. For example, by lowered thresholds of perception, you actually decrease your ability to perceive and process sounds coming in from your environment—communication or any sound.

For example, if a child were in a home where the other children were yelling or fighting or saying negative and critical things to the child, one way of decreasing that painful stimulus would be to lower his ability to perceive the sound, which shows up as a lowered auditory threshold. This is one way to tune out painful incoming information. Another way is to close your selectivity. Selectivity is a pitch discrimination test that I also perform when doing a listening test.

The test of selectivity is done by asking the person when they hear two sequential tones to tell if the second tone is higher or lower than the one they first heard. A person should be able to quickly and easily differentiate the pitch or tone changes throughout the entire spectrum of sound on a standard audiometer, which would be eight thousand to one hundred twenty-five hertz. Actually, a person after age eleven should be able to do this test quickly and easily. It is a developmental test, and that ability gradually emerges from early childhood to eleven years of age.

When there is repressed emotional pain, people's selectivity is not fully open. This is a response to psychological and emotional pain that inhibited full development of the self and is reflected in a person's auditory processing abilities. Interestingly, I also see many people with mild traumatic brain injury such as a whiplash—which causes a kind of cortical disruption of connections—who often have closed selectivity, and this improves remarkably when we use the Tomatis Method. These head-injury clients often complain of difficulty with sound sensitivity, often hyperacusis, which is a painful response to sound, as well as difficulties with word finding and other memory problems. As we do the Tomatis Method, the selectivity opens up and there are other changes in the listening test. This is concurrent with cognitive improvement as well. Unfortunately, I do not have the privilege of having this test done on clients prior to their coming to the Center for InnerChange for comparison to see what their auditory processing was like prior to and after a particular trauma. As you know, most of the adults that we see have some long-standing depression, anxiety disorder, or a recent head injury, and children are brought in with learning disabilities and attention and behavioral problems. In these groups of people, there is usually a difficulty with their selectivity or their ability to discern pitches that does improve during the treatment process. Invariably, people then talk about being able to process and perceive auditory information more easily.

So that's another way they can respond to stress; one is by lowering their threshold and two is by closing their selectivity. A third way would be that the auditory threshold may be in a normal range, but they develop dips and valleys in listening tests. Instead of being a nice, smooth, ascending curve from the low to the high frequencies that is maximum around two to three thousand hertz, there are breaks in the curve, often in the language range. This is also a kind of tuning out and a response to stress.

Finally, the one we're speaking of this afternoon, relative to the ear and dominance as in your case, is the person who goes left-ear dominant in a right-dominant organization. This is a form of cross dominance. In general, this assumes they have language in the left brain and they should be right-ear dominant.

The impact of emotional information is farther away. The person feels more distant from incoming information that might be negative, critical, judgmental, condemning, or loud. So it's a dampening effect. Again, another defense, a psychological defense and a response to stress as well. I have not seen many people who are right-ear dominant who went left in response to a stress. I'm sure it occurs, but I've seen people for the first time after they have already experienced their stressors and don't have information regarding their dominance prior to seeing them. The majority of people I see are left-ear dominant. I think they're left-ear dominant in response to stress.

JL: The majority are left-ear dominant?

RM: Yes.

JL: Even though the rest of them is right dominant?

RM: Correct.

JL: In terms of the use of sound stimulation retraining, do you find that it's successful in being able to resume right dominance?

RM: Yes, definitely.

JL: Do you think that The Listening Program is also strong enough to do that in some cases?

RM: Yes, in some cases, but in general we were careful in The Listening Program to not use the laterality so strongly with our decibel levels that we would switch dominance. However, we want to nudge it in the appropriate direction. If someone were at one time right or rather in the middle, meaning sometimes they will switch back and forth where they are neither fully left nor fully right, probably TLP is strong enough to help them integrate or strengthen that right dominance.

JL: What is the difference in the way it is done with the Tomatis Method versus The Listening Program?

RM: In the Tomatis method during the latter phase of listening, we remove the majority of sound from the left ear headphone so there is very little sound coming in through the left ear, thus encouraging a right ear dominance through increased stimulation to the right side. In TLP, the sound is decreased by only three decibels in the left ear for weeks 3 and 4 and by six decibels for weeks 5 through 8. This is not enough to switch dominance, as some sound is still coming into the left ear. The strength of the input to the right ear is much stronger in Tomatis. What do we see when a person becomes right-ear dominant from a previous left-ear state? The person experiences more fluid speech with easy expression of ideas whereby hesitation and pauses are gone or diminished. Psychologically, people state they feel more present, grounded as opposed to being disconnected from life. This switching to the dominant ear must be done in a timely manner. If done prematurely, clinical discomfort can ensue.

When a child is prepared and ready to really be in the world—meaning his learning problems have gotten better, for example, and he feels better about himself—his emotional reactivity is down and then we move him to the right ear. Parents note that he is very present, very much in the world, as opposed to being distracted and disconnected. He is very connected, very here and now. If, however, we move him to the right ear before he is ready—prematurely, let's say, when he is still struggling with his self-esteem around a learning difficulty—what we may see would be an emotional reaction of upset and whining or complaining, again about the struggle he is having with his learning problem. It is as if that left ear was keeping him somewhat protected from the full impact of his difficulty. When children become right-ear directed, the problem is right in their face, the problem is just so present they cannot push it away or ignore it. So the timing of that shifting to the right ear can be very important. This example shows how dominance affects listening and our experience of ourselves in the world.

With an adult, as they move to right-ear dominance, they'll say things like, "Everything is so much more crisp, not only in how I hear but even in what I see, the light on trees, the shimmer, the colors, the sky, the clouds. Everything is brighter and more crisp." Of course, partly they will sometimes say that in response to the overall auditory training or the auditory stimulation of Tomatis as the brain wakes up, so to speak, as they feel more alert and more clarity. So this may happen in response to stimulation with high-frequency sound as well as with moving to right-ear dominance.

I can talk more easily about the auditory responses due to stress from what I see when people come in, as mentioned, with left-ear dominance, a lower threshold or closed selectivity. But I have not had the experience that you describe of people having done the Tomatis program, done well and had a good response, followed by huge stresses in their lives and then coming back to me and saying, "I need a tune-up because I have had difficulty in my life and I would like your help getting me back on track." That just has not happened for me, but it makes sense that this can happen.

JL: I had a Tomatis listening test done about two months ago, before I did The Listening Program. I compared it to my last listening test that was done after I completed the Tomatis work with you in 1995. I'm sorry to say there was a big degradation.

RM: Yes, and I imagine this degradation was due to the stresses you experienced. Another change often reflected on the listening test that also corresponds to stress and emotional reactivity is elevated bone conduction. Both cross dominance and elevated bone conduction result in increased emotional reactivity and irritability. The listening test shows an inverted curve where the bone conduction is elevated over the air conduction, whereas it should be the other way around.

JL: And that is due to?

RM: It appears to be due to stress and anxiety as well as other causes, and when the bone conduction is higher than air, invariably depending on where that is occurring, the person feels more stressed (to use a general word). To interpret elevated bone conduction along these lines, it is necessary to first rule out physical causes of inverted curves such as middle-ear infections, ear wax, or other problems with the middle ear. When this elevation occurs in the body zone, let's say from two hundred fifty hertz to seven hundred fifty hertz, people often describe feeling more anxious in their body, more tense, more physical distress, the kind of tension we might describe as performance anxiety or test anxiety, a stage-fright kind of feeling, just more tension in the body and more on edge.

In the zone from seven hundred fifty to four thousand hertz, when it's elevated there, the voice is often very tense, they feel mentally stressed, easily overwhelmed, and emotionally reactive or short fused, quick to fly off the handle. A person feels overwhelmed; little things feel like big things.

JL: Yes.

RM: It's as though our emotional reality is taking precedence over our thoughts or our ability to judge and discern what's truly going on. There is an emotional over-reactivity. What I see is people's perceptions are distorted. What they hear they start reacting to emotionally without really processing what is truly going on. They start reacting to their overwhelmed perceptions, their sense of just being over-driven. And all this is reflected auditorily.

JL: So if somebody is overdriven, the ear is not the cause—rather, the ear is a reflection?

RM: Yes, that is how I see it.

JL: Does it then actually turn into a loop? If we are overdriven behind too much stress, then the ear responds to it? The ear is one of the physiological responses that takes place?

RM: In lay terms, that would be one way of expressing it. However, when you say "the ear," I don't think there is that much going on in the middle ear or the cochlea per se. Is it the ear, Joshua, or is it the brain's interpretation of what is coming in due to stress reflected back to our auditory perception? Although there is certainly the closed selectivity, changing a threshold, but where is that occurring? I think it is occurring in the brain and is reflected as a measure of what we hear and how we process what we hear.

JL: Therefore, this level of auditory dysfunction manifests from the eardrum all the way up into the different auditory sensors in the brain?

RM: Yes, I think it's more central than peripheral. That is why some of your questions were hard to answer. I don't think it's happening totally in a peripheral mode.

JL: So an overstressed auditory function causes us to perceive sound in a different manner?

RM: Absolutely.

JL: Consequently, the way we perceive sound at that point serves to just deepen the sense of stress. It is a loop!

RM: Yes, exactly. Here's a personal example. My hearing changed relative to stress from listening very intently to some new therapeutic CDs I'm helping to create as part of The Listening Program. I listened at night after a very stressful week and I was making all kinds of notes about my dissatisfaction with the gating, blending, and frequencies. I then listened to the exact same sections the following day and they sounded fine. The next morning, I was not stressed.

So there is a really good example of how my auditory interpretation of my world was influenced by my level of stress. I was overreactive, I was unable to interpret accurately what was truly happening. I was overinterpreting my environment, in this case the music coming in, from a level of irritability or fatigue and giving it a false judgment.

This is what we do with our relationships. In relationships we overinterpret, misinterpret, overreact to a tone of voice, to what is said, coming from the place of having an overdriven sympathetic nervous system, overstressed, overwrought, overwhelmed.

JL: Overdone.

RM: Yes. Overcooked. All of that.

JL: So we know that this stress response takes place with the auditory system, and that once we get to a certain point, it starts to affect our perception of sound. And then that overinterpretation of sound serves to keep us in the loop of overdoneness.

RM: When you say "overinterpretation of sound," I like that. However, if we look at the auditory system as being a sense organ like an antenna that is tuned to frequencies in our environment—and depending on the health of our system—that antenna is picking up really clear interpretations when a person is whole, centered, and grounded, or that person is picking up a lot of static-like irritation when stressed. The sound is not only the words people say, but their tone of voices misperceived and misinterpreted.

Another good example was with my daughter, Erica, prior to going through the Tomatis Method. This also happens with many children I see who have difficulties with closed selectivity or discrimination and poor self-esteem issues resulting from learning disabilities. Erica frequently said, "Why are you mad at me?" and, "Why are you yelling?" when I was neither yelling nor angry. She had difficulty with the emotional content of language, often thinking people were yelling or angry when in fact they were not. I might have been excited, I might have been emphatic, speaking in an excited or slightly louder voice. I might have said, "Wow, did you see that?" and she says, "Why are you mad?" This is a good example of a cross auditory dominance problem.

So when there is a misperception of environmental sounds, I think you have to include the emotional content of the sound. The voice is a carrier wave, not only of thought but also of feeling.

JL: Therefore, once the process of perception goes awry, misinterpretation runs rampant.

RM: It sure does. We see this in relationship difficulties in couples, parent-child relationships, and in the work environment. I see this stress reflected much more commonly in the auditory system than in the visual system. (I use the word *see* as a visualized metaphor.) We don't look at someone and say, "Gee, they look fuzzy and unclear." We are much less likely to make misinterpretations from visual filters than with the auditory filters. This is why we have so much miscommunication in society.

JL: If we understand that this loop gets set up, then what can I tell my readers about remedying this situation? When somebody is in a situation where they have selective auditory loop, where can they go, what can they do?

RM: To get appropriate help, the first step is to recognize that there is a problem—too much stress and the symptoms we mentioned earlier. To deal with excess stress via the auditory system is new to most people, as most do not realize how stress affects how we hear and how we process and react to what we hear. Therefore, simple things to do to minimize stress would be to get adequate exercise and sleep and to get involved in stress reduction approaches such as biofeedback, yoga, meditation—even a vacation may help. But it is important to realize that we can use sound therapeutically to reduce stress and to improve our sense of well-being and to balance our autonomic nervous system.

The next step is to listen to gentle, soothing sounds: sounds of nature, oceans, things that are calming and soothing that do not require a lot of mental processing. The Sound Health Series does that because you changed it in ways that a person does not have to think about what they are hearing so much. They do not have to process. It is not complicated, not complex. It is not a Bach three-part invention. It is simple, easy, relaxing sound. It is important to decrease noise and chaotic sound in our environment that adds immeasurably to our stress levels, and to increase harmonious sounds.[2]

I'm speaking to you right now and there's a water fountain in the house. I have it on all the time. I find that very helpful and relaxing. When a person becomes stressed to a certain level, it's almost as though the stress system gets locked in and even though they're doing things to relax, they can't seem to find the switch to turn off the overdriven system. They cross a threshold, being overwhelmed and overstressed. They go see a therapist and talk about all the things that are bugging them, and all that does is work them up more. They can't find that switch to turn off or settle down their nervous system.

Therefore, you need something more—and something that addresses stress in the auditory or central nervous system. You might do The Listening Program or a Tomatis listening program. Certainly listening to Gregorian chants, sacred music of different kinds, helps also. I have to put a plug in here for Dr. Tomatis's genius in recognizing the importance of how we hear through bone and how this root can be used to decrease stress. As you remember, when you did the Tomatis program, the music you listened to was delivered by air as well as bone conduction. When people come in with a lot of stress and do the Tomatis work, their stress levels drop rapidly. We see decreases in anxiety and stress levels with the Tomatis Method often within the first three to five days.

JL: And this is with the sound coming in through bone?

RM: Bone and air both are used in the Tomatis Method, but usually we're using the full spectrum of frequencies, not just filtered high frequencies. In a stressed person, too much filtered sound, too early, may increase their stress as they resist what high frequencies may be bringing up. So if I see someone who is really stressed with closed selectivity and elevated bone conduction, for the first five days they will do Tomatis using unfiltered, full-spectrum sound and Gregorian chants. The unfiltered sound is the music of Mozart. We may even emphasize the lower frequencies in the body by removing some of the high-frequency sounds. Once they are grounded and relaxed, then I will filter the music. That's when I want the high frequencies to promote mental alertness and clarity of thought and to increase physical and mental energy. It is important not to use filtered music too soon in a stressed person.

JL: Explain this more, please.

RM: Let's say you're really exhausted after a long day or from physical work outside and I say, "Hey, Joshua, let's go to the club and work out. It will be good for you." You say, "No way. I need to rest and then I can work out."

It is the same thing with sound. If you're going to give them a workout—that is, high frequencies—and they're already overdriven, you're going to overdrive their system. They need full-spectrum sound first. They need a lot of space in the sound like you do in the Sound Health Series. They need space like what's found in Gregorian chants.

JL: Understanding how sound stimulation programs that use bone conduction will serve this, what about programs like The Listening Program that do not use bone conduction?

RM: I think TLP is good because it does have full-spectrum sound in the beginning and end of every fifteen-minute segment. Also, it starts slowly with the filtration so when we start the first three weeks, the level of filtration is not terribly high. If someone were very stressed and found the filtered or gated sections too intense, The Listening Program lends itself to being individualized. They can stay at weeks one and two longer or skip the more intense gated tracks until their nervous system has settled down. Finally, I should mention that the vagus nerve also gets a lot of stimulation from sound, and stimulation of this nerve is an important pathway in stress reduction. It is to calm the overdriven system. The stimulation of this biggest nerve increases a sense of well-being. The name given to this part of the autonomic nervous system is *parasympathetic*. It is the balancing, relaxing side of the flight-fight system that is called the sympathetic. So people feel much calmer.

Joshua, I hope this discussion on stress and the auditory system is useful to you and your readers.

INTERVIEW WITH BILLIE THOMPSON, PH.D.

Dr. Billie M. Thompson founded the Sound Listening and Learning Center in Phoenix, Arizona, in 1987 and in Pasadena, California, in 1994. She directs these centers and also provides outreach programs in other parts of the United States. She has worked with several thousand people of all ages, gifted through learning disabled, assisting them to expand their potential and to achieve their educational, personal, and career goals. She has trained in and integrated a number of innovative and effective educational programs with the Tomatis Method, including the Rubenfeld Synergy Method, Structure of Intellect, Accelerated Learning, and Neurolinguistic Programming. Dr. Thompson trained and worked closely with Dr. Alfred A. Tomatis, founder of the Tomatis Method, before his retirement in 1994. She actively promotes Tomatis's work by publishing articles and giving presentations. She is the coeditor of *About the Tomatis Method* and editor-publisher of the English translations of Tomatis's autobiography, *The Conscious Ear*, and his first book, *The Ear and Language*. For contact information, see "Soundwork Resources."

This interview was conducted in April 2000.

JL: Dr. Thompson, I'm looking at the effect of sound and listening on human function. In my efforts to explain the importance of the ear, what needs to be done to safeguard it, and the various maladies that may harm auditory function, I have looked at the physiological effects of NIHL. Additionally, I have begun to examine what is taking place on a psychological level with stress and trauma.

In the course of my research, a few small references have caught my attention. For example, in your article in *IEEE Engineering in Medicine and Biology* magazine, you say, "Poor listening can begin at any age and for any number of reasons. It might result from a health problem, an accident, a major lifestyle disruption, or from stress." Robert Doman, similarly brief, says, "Deviations of a normal auditory development may also occur later in life due to stress or trauma." I noticed that you and Doman contained your thoughts on the effects of stress on auditory function within very small references. Can you share your current thinking about stress and the ear?

BT: A real visible example of the effects of stress on adults is that kind of hearing loss called Executive's Ear. It is one that gradually declines. It seems similar to the impact that too-loud sound has on some musicians' ears, in which they lose their high frequencies. As I understand it, we don't know why this loss occurs other than a problem with stress in the lives of men in their forties and fifties who seem to experience it. It seems to gradually worsen as years pass.

JL: Aside from the physiological effects of NIHL, I'm quite interested in exploring the psychological impact on our auditory system.

BT: We can observe a tuning out from disuse, just like in anything else. For example, if you sit in a chair for three weeks without getting up and then try to get up and walk, your legs are not going to work. The effects can be far reaching. Suppose you broke a leg and you didn't do therapy to reestablish your muscle strength and rhythm; you could have secondary problems such as getting a scoliosis caused by an imbalance in the muscle strength in both legs. This imbalance can occur in all kinds of scenarios with the human body, including the ear.

Tomatis says that when you tune out for a while or have never developed your listening and language abilities, the ear muscles have to be retrained and conditioned to work well. The ear and voice have to be integrated to work together for communication and learning. Working with the ear precedes working with the voice, because the voice produces only what the ear can hear, a law known as the Tomatis Effect. Tomatis observed that people tend to tune out at least some incoming information when they suffer a trauma from an accident, illness, or some type of physical or emotional abuse. Over an extended period of tuning out some sounds, they're more difficult to attend to, and you have to work to regain tuning in to them. Though they don't just automatically come back, they can be trained to work well. And that is what we do. I think people can understand that when they're in an environment and they don't want to hear something, something physiological occurs that's rooted in a psychological response or reaction. For example, consider the engineer who has just spent three years installing a new computer system and then is told by the boss that he has to start all over next Monday because his system is already outdated. Does he want to hear that? Probably not!

What about the adult who has no idea that when she tunes out what certain people tell her, she tunes out specific ranges of sounds, not just the specific voices? In tuning out the frequencies of those sounds, that person may make her personal, professional, and educational communication more difficult, and hence more stressful. Mostly people think, "I'll tune out my dad's voice," or maybe it's their mom's or child's voice, but the effect actually goes beyond that. Now you come to the broader effect of poor listening, including not knowing that you do not know what is coming in to you and not picking up the information you need. When we don't get some information, our brain begins to fill in the gaps. Now our imagination becomes the basis for our feelings and our actions.

In many cases people can change and tune in later if they work through the stress or trauma. We can observe on a Tomatis listening test that the person more easily listens to certain sounds than before. In other words, they do not resist the sounds, and probably not the person or event that initiated the closure of listening. I have observed enough people making this kind of change over the years that I have no doubt that auditory laterality can change and even quickly when their body and psyche release the resistance.

An interesting example occurred in my training with Dr. Tomatis in Paris. We were using a technique whereby we determine the dominant ear and then determine how strong the dominance is. I was working with a woman who was born in Romania, spoke Romanian as her first language, and who had moved at the age of five years to France, where she learned to speak French and English. Her early life in war-torn Romania was traumatic, and when she spoke in Romanian, she was left-ear dominant. But she loved French and English, preferred to speak them, and was right-ear dominant when she spoke them. She showed me how significantly speaking impacts our processing and how much language holds emotional weights for us. With this kind of cross auditory dominance, we are observing a very complex relationship among the ear and voice and psyche.

JL: I had an experience in the earlier part of the nineties that was very stressful for a couple of years. It had to do with a move from Los Angeles to New York, a marriage that was breaking up, the premature birth of my daughter, and loss of employment. They all occurred suddenly over a short time and fortunately did not end up as catastrophic as they might have. After that time, however, I began to notice I was getting a little dyslexic at the keyboard, something I had never experienced before. Concurrently, I noticed that I was becoming highly emotional, more so than I ever remembered. It felt like something had shifted, something had changed inside of me. Now fast-forward a few years, and I am working on a professional training where I am a presenter. One morning, before the morning session, I put my head under water to rinse my hair when I was in the bath. My left ear got plugged up. This made my presentation extremely difficult. The process of thinking was like moving through concrete.

Later that morning, a colleague said to me, "Look, I've been working with you fairly intensively for the last few years, and may I share my perception of what may be taking place. You're a right-handed guy and everything you do seems to be right dominant, but given the fact that you just had a plugged left ear, you had to work very hard to put your thoughts together so you could teach. If you were right-ear dominant, having a plugged left ear would not have been such a big deal in your performance. Consequently, I think you may have a mixed auditory dominance."

From that experience, I began examining the possibility that a by-product of previous trauma and high stress was a state of auditory cross dominance. In addition to the emerging dyslexia, an indication of mild neurological dysorganization, my highly increased emotional reactivity pointed to the cross dominance issue. Have you seen anything like this in your practice?

BT: Sure. Anytime you are working with your own psyche, your own integrity, your relationships with people, your mind wants to be right. We have our own thoughts and beliefs about what we should and shouldn't do. Sometimes we do things that don't seem logical, but we're driven to do them anyway. Then we have to figure out how to handle any communication or relationship problems based on the way we handled our action. We have to clean it up, and until we do, a lot of confusion comes in. Once you clean up any broken agreements, you go through an integration period during which things get clear again. The lack of clarity or confusion has to do with being out of integrity with yourself and/or with some other people.

I've come to this insight from my own personal experience and from working with thousands of people over the years.

One of the most difficult things to do is to say to someone, "I've been making you wrong, and I apologize." Whatever the situation is about, you have to be willing to listen to whatever someone is willing to say to you and say what you are thinking. Both are necessary to have an open communication. You have to be willing to have the other person say to you what they want or don't want, what they are thinking, and what they are feeling. And then observe what is beyond that conversation in that relationship that you can support for yourself and for other people. Listen to know what another thinks, keeping a safe listening environment by how you receive what is merely someone's view. I have learned to work with people to develop agreements that allow for this open listening environment to be created. It is essential to have both good auditory functioning and good listening strategies. All of these changes take time and usually require at least some facilitation or coaching. If the stress is reduced, then right auditory dominance can be supportive of an efficient control by the right ear. Confusion is created by having your left ear dominant, your attention focused inward, your flipping back and forth in how you are processing the information inwardly and externally, and by having no clear sense about the spatial location where the sound is coming from. I address these with the Tomatis Method.

I think that to complete communication, we require a combination of being able to say what you need to say to someone and being willing to hear back what they need to say to you. There is this flow of information, and each person is being his or her best and supporting the other person to be his or her best, too.

Many different ways exist to create a relationship that is supportive of a person with or without having the same view. Developing agreements is an integral part of the work that I do with people.

JL: So you have noticed that people who have suffered from high emotional stress, a death, divorce, or whatever it happens to be, can manifest in a cross dominance effect?

BT: Yes, I think that happens more than we realize. It's what I experience when on some occasions I find myself typing the keys backward. I'm either tired or working to resolve what seem to be two opposing beliefs that are both true. I work diligently at keeping my relationships clean and pacing myself so I don't get tired, even though I do work a lot. It's a matter of inner listening and outer expression not jibing; [of] not having our body and mind being congruent. So my job is to support each person to have the functional ability to listen, the desire to tune in, and the strategies to maintain a safe listening environment. That's my work at the Sound Listening and Learning Centers.

Stress-Induced Auditory Dysfunction is the first in a series of exceptional soundwork-related interviews and excerpts compiled by me. These and future interviews will be posted online at www.thepowerofsound.com.

Core Principles
of Alfred Tomatis

- The primary function of the ear is to convert sound waves to electro-chemical impulses that charge the neocortex of the brain.
- Sound is a nutrient; we can either charge or discharge the nervous system by the sounds we take in through both air and bone conduction.
- There is a distinction between *hearing* and *listening*. The two are related, but distinct, processes. Hearing is passive; listening is active. This corresponds to the difference between *seeing* and *looking*. Listening and looking are active focusing processes.
- The quality of an individual's listening ability will affect both spoken and written language development; listening ability also influences communication, thereby shaping the individual's social development, confidence, and self-image.
- The active process of listening can be enhanced or refocused by auditory stimulation using musical and vocal sounds rich in high frequencies. This entails the use of filtered and enhanced audiotapes employing the music of Mozart and Gregorian chant. Additionally, Tomatis has invented a device known as the Electronic Ear. One of its functions, accomplished through the effect of electronic gates and filters, is to reestablish the right ear as the dominant ear of hearing.
- Communication is a process that begins in utero. The unborn child hears as early as the fourth month after conception. Sound actually helps grow the fetus's brain and nervous system.
- We can duplicate only the sounds we can hear. This is known as the Tomatis Effect.

Tomatis: Revising the Map of the Musician's Odyssey*

I've often wondered why I feel unmoved by a musician's perfect technical performance—and, conversely, why I can be transported to the heights of ecstasy by a less than perfectly articulated performance of an impassioned talent. Is it the player's exuberance for life? Is it the performer's connection with her spirit? Is it the artist's access to his pain and joy that excites the audience? Many artists struggle to communicate through their instruments beyond the dynamics and notes.

I believe the difference between a sterile performance and one that conveys an electric charge lies in the artist's ability to connect. To connect with yourself and with others is to communicate. To communicate is to listen. To listen is a learned skill. It is through the extraordinary work of Dr. Alfred Tomatis that we may recover the lost art of listening.

As a music producer and composer, I am especially interested in the effect of the Tomatis Method on musicians. I have read widely, spoken with experts in the field, and interviewed musicians who have undertaken the method. I have also participated in a thirty-day Tomatis program that introduced me to the benefits of full-spectrum audition. Tomatis has identified the profile of the perfect "musical ear." His auditory retraining program takes a quantum leap toward tapping the full resources of the artist's talent.

---

* I gratefully acknowledge the Center for InnerChange in Denver, Colorado. It was here that I had the opportunity, under the kind and wise guidance of Ron Minson, M.D., to begin the process of inner tuning. Within the walls of this listening center, Minson's love of music and healing is pervasive.

EAR TRAINING FOR MUSICIANS

Although I have discussed the use of the Tomatis Method to repair damage caused by the psychologically induced shutdown of parts of the hearing function, I believe this technology also has tremendous applications as an enhancement technique for musicians. Speaking of his early years as an ENT specialist, Tomatis says, "My dream was to somehow aid singers who damaged or lost their voices."[1] His love for music and for the people who compose and perform it has never waned. According to Paul Madaule, Tomatis has "investigated the influence of certain auditory modifications on the vocal qualities of singers and on the instrumental performances of musicians."[2]

Tomatis believes there is a perfect musical ear. This specific listening profile reflects the following aural perceptions: the attuning of the entire sound spectrum and the ability to analyze this spectrum with maximum speed and precision, most specifically in the range of 500 to 4,000 Hz.

Tomatis also believes that the optimal analysis of music involves:

- An ascending curve up to the frequencies of 3,000 to 4,000 Hz
- An open "auditory selectivity"
- A precise auditory spatialization
- A right-sided auditory dominance

According to Madaule, "These narrowly overlapping and complementary functions of the ear constitute the listening act. . . . The failure of one or several of these parameters provokes a disharmony which translates into impaired listening and consequently into deficient musicality."[3]

Selectivity refers to the ability to distinguish the difference between tones and their relationship—in other words, which tone is higher or lower than the preceding. *Spatialization* is the process of isolating where a sound comes from, such as in front of, above, or behind you. *Dominance* refers to which ear is your stronger one and is similar to being, say, right-handed. Tomatis believes that right-ear dominance is paramount for singers and musicians. This relates to the location of specific functions in the right and left hemispheres of the brain.

It is through the application of filtered music and the use of the gating mechanisms of the Electronic Ear that a Tomatis practitioner essentially *tunes up* a musician's ears. According to Timothy Gilmor, "As the sound reaches the individual's ear, it is further modified by the Electronic Ear, which presents the sound in two rapidly alternating forms. In one form, the lower frequencies of the incoming sound are accentuated and the higher frequencies are diminished; this provokes a state of nonaccommodation (passive hearing). In the second form, the higher frequencies of the incoming sound are accentuated and the lower frequencies are diminished; this provokes an accommodation or focusing response (listening)."[4]

The goal is to come as close to the Tomatis model of the perfect musical ear as possible. When I asked Chris Faddick, a longtime Tomatis technician at the Center for InnerChange, if he had ever seen a perfect musical ear, his reply was that he hadn't;

they are very rare. A Tomatis practitioner in another center repeated the same sentiment. The specifications, however, of a perfect musical ear are used as the goal when retuning the ear.

Tomatis practitioner Gilmor states, "After listening repeatedly to music and speech sounds modified in this way, the muscles of the inner ear are conditioned to attend to sound in an improved manner."[5] The bottom line is that the two tiny middle-ear muscles get lazy from blocked receptivity. The use of the filtered, gated music is meant to tonify and return these muscles to optimal performance. It trains them to attune to the higher harmonics of any sound source. The net effect of this is to "help the musician control and remedy the color of the sounds produced by his instrument," and help the singer control the timbre of his or her voice. Moreover, the progressive filtering out of low and mid-frequencies (and then their gradual return) trains the ear to listen for the entire harmonic range of sound information.

Amazing changes occur through the retraining of the ear. The charging of the nervous system with high-frequency sounds seems to cause (or reawaken) a vigorous and energetic approach to daily life. These high frequencies aid breathing, enhance memory, increase concentration and attention, lower susceptibility to fatigue, generate greater motivation in everyday activities, and require less time for sleep. Madaule states, "All of these factors, but particularly the increased abilities of concentration and of memory, can help the person considerably in the acquisition of musical expertise. Following a series of filtered music sessions, the singer or the instrumentalist realizes that the whole integration of a piece of music becomes faster and easier."[6]

Additionally, the motor functions are affected by the frequency infusion of filtered sound. Madaule says that "for string players, pianists, and percussionists, greater awareness of body image translates into more control of arms, wrists, hands, and fingers." Because the vestibular system has a monitoring action on equilibrium, "better vestibular control improves the temporal-spatial awareness required for rhythmic sense."

After completing the thirty-day Tomatis process in Denver at Dr. Ron Minson's Center for InnerChange, the changes in my musicality were quite noticeable. Charts for pieces I had been playing for many years but never bothered to memorize were suddenly unnecessary. With new music, my learning speed accelerated significantly. My ability for sustained concentration has been amplified. My preference in sounds has totally shifted; I have no taste for electronics—if anything, I want little to do with them. I believe this relates to my gaining a different orientation to higher frequencies and harmonics. In my composing, I find myself pulled toward much simpler compositions. My ear is hungrier for the purity of harmonics than for intellectual complexity. The simplicity seems to allow the overtones more room to breathe.

MUSICIANS TALK ABOUT
THE TOMATIS METHOD

I interviewed five musicians who had completed the Tomatis program: two pianists, two singers, and a violinist. Three of these musicians are also composers. Just as we have individual fingerprints, so our voices and ears reflect singular journeys. Therefore, experiences of the method will be unique. Yet note the similarities among these five musicians and their Tomatis experiences.

MM, Concert Pianist

"It's not fun, it's miserable. I hated it! But something told me that I needed to do it, and I wanted to experience it. I had read so much about it. It's a big investment of time: driving over there, sitting for two and a half hours, driving home—doing this every morning. That's a lot of time and money to listen to scratchy records.

"But the rewards have been well worth it. I find the quality of the sound I produce on the piano is richer and deeper. It seems to me, on an intuitive level, that it is because of what I am doing with Tomatis. You know, as a musician, that your ear is more important than your hands. If I can hear something, then I know I can play it. The problem is always in the hearing it. If you can't quite hear it, then you certainly can't reproduce it. After the Tomatis, it was much easier for me to hear; I had a great deal more facility. I was amazed. I thought this was a quantum leap. This was the first effect that I noticed and it continues. Prior to the program, I wasn't totally right-ear dominant, and almost all musicians are. Part of my work was moving more into right-ear dominance.

"There were other effects: I have less insomnia, less depression, and I feel that it has really assisted me in growing physically and spiritually. But the very striking differences are in the way I play and the way I speak and sing. It is dramatic.

"If you deepen your ability to hear, the music itself has much more depth, meaning, energy, purity, life. In a certain way, it is comparable to . . . When we are growing spiritually and emotionally, what we are doing is getting rid of obstacles and blocks. We are into purer and more open spaces. In alchemy, they say 'getting to neutral.' It is getting to that open, multidimensional place that has space and life, an aliveness to it but not content. Maybe what is happening is the abuse that we undergo—naturally, as part of our education—that produces barriers and obstacles and limits . . . Maybe what we are doing, as we go through therapy, is these barriers are pushed, those obstacles are removed. We get more and more to our natural being, our natural mind, our natural heart. Maybe by clearing out the hateful sounds, and making the whole ear clearer, we can hear and make purer sounds. And those purer sounds certainly affect you. If I can come from a purer place in me, it will open that place in you."

BH, Singer

"There were so many times that my teacher would sing a line and want me to repeat it. And what I repeated was not the same as what he sang. He figured that it was either because I wasn't hearing him or I wasn't hearing me, or both. After the first Tomatis session, that changed.

"I am a recovering alcoholic and have been part of Alcoholics Anonymous for twelve years. From that, I understand dysfunctional families of origin and the idea of tuning things out and not listening. So I have a real extensive track record of tuning things out and not listening, not wanting to hear things that you don't want to hear.

"I am singing a lot better for several reasons, but I think that the main impact of the Tomatis has been on the way I hear myself. I could be doing all these other things, but if I can't hear me, then what difference does it make? And the main thing is that I haven't wanted to hear me. This is what I have had to overcome and I think the Tomatis has helped that. It has given me a different feel for checking what my sound is like. I am trusting the way that it feels. The earphone work in the booth has done a lot for that. When I talk into the microphone and then I hear it back from the phones, it forces me into a different perception of my voice."

BB, PIANIST AND RECORDING ARTIST

JL: Using frequency to vibrate frequency, Tomatis has a specific objective: He is looking to create a musical ear. What do you think after going through the method?

BB: I have a different opinion. I don't feel that the basic purpose is to necessarily develop the perfect musical ear. The goal is to enhance the life force in its full spectrum of aliveness. With our medical model, we are so pathology oriented: "Here's a problem. Let's go in and fix it. And then let's measure from here to here to see if we got the results."

How do you measure quality of life? How do you measure tenderness and compassion? How do you measure sensorial perceptions of beauty? It is at this other level of humanness that Tomatis's work is actually affecting people. But it also has the effect of fitting into the medical model, of having research data that can be measured. That is the male model.

JL: What are you noticing with your playing?

BB: Subtlety of touch is much more refined. My expressiveness is tremendously improved when I play for people. I would say the level of reaching people's hearts is more profound.

I also notice that there has been a cross catalytic force, a cross pollination of sensorial stimuli that is affecting my musical creations. There is a deeper, more profound serenity. Everything is more alive, deeper, more tender. All the emotions of compassion, reverence, devotion, even exultation, intimacy, [have] just reached another level. And that is where art comes from. I am a perfect research subject. I am an artist who wasn't able to practice because of trauma, severe injury, and stress. But I have not lost; I hardly notice any loss. The motor coordination that affects learning, for a musician, is very powerful.

The whole time I went through the Tomatis training, I had to go to the ladies' room constantly. Every half hour. Then I realized that the kidneys are where we hold emotions. So I was literally flushing out all this stuff. It was almost as if I was getting my brain washed out and then it was going through my kidneys. I feel that washing effect has an effect, on all levels of creativity, imagination, and originality.

MD, SINGER

"After all the passive work, I started getting a lot of energy. I was also remembering dreams that I had as a child.

"With the singing, I noticed a difference with the toning in the second phase of the method. I used to talk with a constriction in my throat, as if I was holding back. After the second phase, that started to roll back. I can't even reproduce the way I used to sound. Between the second and third phase, I made some amazing vocal breakthroughs. With this new relaxation in my throat, something changed in how I place my resonance in my head. I was able to produce much more sound, much more forward sound, hitting higher notes.

"It seems the Tomatis Method works on a lot of different levels. Physically, because you are concentrating on specific things like resonance and sound, there is this *feeding* and input of energy. And emotionally, to tap into the childhood memories that I did makes me really believe that some part of my brain is getting stimulated. This allowed me to release something that I would not have been able to release otherwise. Deep issues were surfacing for me and I was able to deal with them.

"I really think my releasing of emotional issues allows me now to sing much more open and broader. It is very difficult to sing when you have a lot of tension. And when you let go of the tension, it is so freeing and easy. There are so many parallels between singing and being in a good place, a free place with the self."

DF, Orchestral Violinist and Recording Artist

During the first two-week session. "When we realize how the ear controls balance and dyslexia, and then apply this to the problems that musicians face—related to coordination, the sense of rhythm, and the awareness of the sound we're making—one sees the tremendous impact this work has.

"I've been practicing Mozart violin concertos. They have to be so perfect by their nature—and they have so many passages that are rhythmically intricate. I have found that this work is starting to take care of some of the problems that I've had in the past. It doesn't just wipe them away, but it opens them up, provides enough change that it is an impetus to then really work at them. Some of Mozart's fast passages, with a lot of sixteenth notes with demanding bowing patterns, require rhythmic evenness and position changes. These technical factors can interfere with the lovely natural feeling of the music. This work is having a direct impact on those problems. This is due to increased coordination.

"I've found myself talking like a baby when I get in my car."

Four weeks after the first sessions. "I have a high energy level, clear focus and intent. The changes in my playing: Things known subtly are now coming out, I'm focusing on the music inside and allowing it to come through the instrument, there is an increased ability to think intensely in mind about fast parts and therefore the muscles seem to just follow.

"My personal power feels stronger than before. My power of imagination is increasing. I've been bowling after many years. By imagining the pins down, I bowled over two hundred for the first time. By changing the way I focus, it seems to change how I play.

"How does the Tomatis work effect that? This work increases interior focus by working on the brain and its ability to focus. It brings great clarity—like a huge booster shot or like adding memory to a computer."

Six weeks after completion of the full program. "I've realized how subtle this work is. It is like going for a walk, very slowly uphill. You don't notice that you're moving uphill. But after a long time, you notice that you are at the top of the hill."

AB AUDIRE

The Tomatis Method is a highly unorthodox yet powerfully effective process for change. Learning disabilities, depression, and energy-related problems are the most common reasons people seek treatment. As public awareness of the Tomatis concepts grow, many are utilizing this sonic process for reasons other than the curing of maladies. Increasing numbers come to Tomatis for consciousness exploration, inner healing, brain enhancement, and increased musicality. However, I believe that none of these four goals is actually separate. In the same way as brain-mind-body-spirit are seen as a unified whole, exploration, healing—and then enhancement—all occur in a natural sequence. We cannot become more-proficient musicians if we are unable to hear our deeper selves. This requires us to look at what has caused our listening to diminish.

Certainly musicians can achieve increased flexibility, better reading, higher concentration, and faster memory skills through the Tomatis Method. This alone is of great professional value. I believe, however, that the mother lode lies in the personal opening to the inner muse. And in order to cross this gate, you must be willing to release old survival patterns that no longer serve a purpose, in order to dispel the shadows that obscure the flow of the creative self. Without this step forward, technical proficiency will be just that—technical and proficient.

Tomatis speaks repeatedly of the active process of listening. He says, "To reach out towards that to which one listens is *ab audire* in Latin, which translates in French as *obeir*, 'to obey.'" Dr. Tomatis believes that if we truly listen, we begin to hear on such a deep level that we come into obedience. That true listening allows us to connect to such a high degree with our own higher source that it becomes a privilege, an honor to obey. Tomatis concludes, "*Obeir* is to let oneself go completely in listening. Who is it that speaks? It is the Logos that speaks. It is the universe that speaks, and we are the machines to translate the universe."[7]

The Birth of a Sound Therapy: Alexander Doman

In an effort to improve treatment programs for children with neurodevelopmental impairment, Robert Doman Jr. and his staff have investigated every sound therapy method that has come to prominence.

Robert's son, Alex, was executive director of the National Academy for Child Development from 1993 through 1999. During that time, he supervised sound stimulation auditory programs for fifteen hundred children and adults from around the world.

Very few practitioners have broad-based experiences with multiple sound programs. Alex Doman does. He has studied numerous approaches and designed individual applications. After observing the work of Tomatis, Berard, Joudry, and Steinbach on the NACD client base, Alex ultimately created a new sound training called The Listening Program.

The following statements are Alex's professional opinion. I've included this excerpt from The Listening Program Guidebook *because it sheds a very interesting perspective on the continuum of this particular branch of soundwork— sound stimulation auditory training.*

Throughout my father's career, NACD researched and utilized every promising auditory methodology of which they became aware. Prior to the time I joined NACD in 1993, they had been recommending the *Tomatis Method* to those for whom it was practical, accessible, and affordable. My father oversaw hundreds of families' use of Patricia Joudry's *Sound Therapy for the Walkman*. In addition, he utilized and developed many other techniques for enhancing auditory and listening functions. These included listening to nature, environmental sounds, white noise, classical music, Gregorian chant, auditory bombardment methods, ear dominance methodologies, as well as his original development of techniques to improve auditory sequential processing.

When I joined NACD in 1993, I immediately began an education in sound therapy. The NACD staff clearly understood the importance of establishing effective auditory processing of the full dynamic range, from 20 to 20,000 Hz. Most people gradually begin to lose their ability to perceive high frequencies, even as children, and much more severely as they age. We can also lose low and mid-range frequencies, which affects us adversely too. Voids, gaps, or hypo-perception may appear in the form of missing frequencies—frequencies which are simply not effectively perceived. Conversely, hyper-perception (hypersensitivity) to certain frequencies can also appear and become a problem. These imbalances impair auditory processing and a wide range of related neurological functions. NACD had been recommending and monitoring sound therapy programs which can effectively address these imbalances for over two decades. I'd like to briefly share with you our experiences with a number of these sound therapies.

Tomatis

Dr. Alfred Tomatis is the father of sound therapy. His groundbreaking work has influenced everyone who came after him. He established the first scientifically based sound therapy system. My father has always had great respect for Dr. Tomatis's work.

However, most of the Tomatis centers were located in Europe and—particularly in the 1980s—there were only a few Tomatis Centers in the US. Tomatis therapy also required regular office visits to a Tomatis Center many times a week over the course of several weeks. Although it was valuable, it was often inaccessible, usually requiring travel and many incidental expenses. Therefore, Tomatis therapy could help only a minority. It was simply impractical for most NACD families.

Joudry

A writer named Patricia Joudry created a very practical alternative for the families that couldn't access the Tomatis Centers—a set of tapes and a book she called *Sound Therapy for the Walkman*. The whole process could be conducted safely on portable equipment at home. This fit the NACD model, which emphasizes parental involvement in home-based programs.

The Joudry tapes were not high fidelity and had to be listened to for several hours each day. The quality of sound made listening quite difficult. They represented a simplified and incomplete version of the Tomatis therapy. Nonetheless, they put it within reach of thousands of people who could not use *true* Tomatis therapy, and, more often than not, they worked! They produced important gains in auditory tonal processing for hundreds of NACD families. However, they did not work in all cases, and *Sound Therapy for the Walkman* never represented a comprehensive, scientifically grounded system of sound therapy.

Berard

Immediately on hearing about *Auditory Integration Therapy*, we found it attractive: its theories made sense, it had a scientific basis (based on Tomatis' work) and it required just two 30-minute sessions per day for ten days! Dr. Guy Berard had noticed correlation between auditory sensitivity to particular frequencies with particular patterns of psychological disturbance. By listening to music through special equipment, clients got rid of the "peaks" in their audiogram, and, consequently, much psychological distress. AIT is not a home-based system; it requires people to attend therapy sessions at locations possessing expensive proprietary equipment. However, it promises (and often produces) extremely fast results. A ten-day vacation for sound therapy might be inconvenient, but it was not beyond the reach of many NACD families.

NACD recommended AIT to all the families for whom we thought it was appropriate. We were seeing very good results with most of our children, but AIT produced more negative reactions than we had seen with the Joudry tapes. It needed closer supervision, but it represented a distinct improvement. Soon, the demand exceeded the capacity of the existing AIT therapists. In fact, the waiting lists became too long. In 1993 Dr. Berard came to the USA, and an NACD trainer was certified to conduct Auditory Integration Therapy.

Ironically, as one of the first individuals to make use of it, I happened to be among the minority who had problems with AIT. All of my auditory problems actually worsened. I knew my experience wasn't typical, because the AIT system was working pretty well for most NACD clients. However, the results were not always consistent, and even when it worked, the benefits often began to fade after as little as a few months. We had another major problem: with many of the more severely hurt children who needed sound therapy most, we could see that it was impossible to get an accurate audiogram, which was the basis for establishing the AIT protocol.

Then NACD encountered a number of children who were progressing better than most of our AIT clients. They were being treated by practitioners of *Auditory Enhancement Training* (AET). AET was also based on Dr. Berard's work, but lacked his official blessing. AET practitioners used different equipment than AIT therapists used. We investigated it and found that it was more consistent, adjustable and had less distortion. At that time we arranged for an AET trainer to fly to Utah and train two NACD staff members, including myself. NACD also purchased the AET equipment. We were happy with it; the sound quality was better, and it allowed the therapist to make more choices about filtering specific frequencies. Perhaps even more importantly, our AET trainer introduced us to two other treatment innovations.

The first innovation she taught us was the use of *voiceprints* instead of audiograms. Voiceprints analyze the frequencies present in the spoken voice. Missing or predominant frequencies generally correspond to frequencies at which auditory processing is also compromised. Voiceprints made absolute sense to us, based on the *Tomatis Effect:* "The voice can reproduce only the sounds the ear can hear." Voiceprints seemed to offer us a more consistent and accurate picture of auditory functioning than we got from audiograms, especially for more severely hurt children, whose audiogram results were unreliable. Although we still sometimes utilized audiograms, voiceprints became our primary tool for designing protocols. As we hoped, our clinical results improved significantly.

The second innovation involved lengthening the treatment sessions and lowering the volume of the music. The standard AIT protocol involved listening to treated music for 30 minutes twice every day at high volume. Our AET trainer said she was getting better results with a single one-hour session every day, with the treated music played at a reduced volume. We tried both approaches, and found that the single one-hour session worked better. Some other therapists questioned us for making this change, but our clinical results were getting better and better.

A New View of Sound Therapy as an Ongoing Process

Again, I used these protocols on myself, and again I did not get significant benefits. My own condition did not improve, but it did not worsen. Clients were getting helped more effectively than ever before. But there were exceptions, and as an "exception," I was keenly aware of the gap. I was puzzled, so I discussed the various approaches with my father.

The Tomatis approach concentrated on retraining the voice through the ear and stimulating the brain with high-frequency sounds. The Joudry program put some of the most important gains within the reach of many more people. Berard emphasized how peaks in the audiograms (hypersensitivity to certain frequencies) created psychological problems. There was value in each approach, especially Dr. Tomatis's work. Yet none of the approaches provided all of the answers.

We just took what we thought made sense for our families. Our hypothesis was that all these interventions had value and offered important benefits. Each held parts of the puzzle. We had long understood that restoring auditory tonal processing was the basis of it all—normalizing perception from 20 to 20,000 Hz.

At this point, we had tracked thousands of children for many years during and following various sound therapy programs. We were seeing the benefits diminish after a few months to a year or more with a good majority of the kids, no matter what program they were doing. Dr. Berard originally said his program should be done once and never repeated, but then he revised that recommendation and suggested people could do the program again after a year or more. Even before he said that, however, we had seen the need, and for certain clients we had started doing *booster programs.* For less involved clients, we also started having people do a shorter series, as little as two or three sessions.

All of these deviations from the prescribed system reflected a shift of view on our part. We began to see that therapeutic auditory stimulation was an ongoing process. As soon as you leave a listening session, you're exposed to leaf blowers, traffic, loud thumping bass music, and countless other buzzes, hums, and whooshes. Many factors work to undo the benefits of the sound therapy. When kids are not so well organized, neurologically, they're especially susceptible. The therapeutic improvements involve laying down new neurological pathways, which need to be reinforced. With practice, they get easier to reinforce, but it's unrealistic to believe that reinforcement will never be necessary again.

So we knew we needed an ongoing program. The only cost-effective way was to make it home based. We didn't want to go back to Joudry, because we knew that Tomatis/AIT/AET produced stronger results, but we saw that a home-based approach was by far most practical and accessible for the majority of our clients.

Samonas

In late 1995 an NACD family alerted my father to *Samonas Sound Therapy* CDs from Germany. I experimented with several discs that could be purchased publicly (Samonas level-one discs) and was very impressed by the CDs' technical excellence and by the quality of the music itself. I improvised a protocol based on my knowledge of other therapies and had positive results. I regained all the ground I had lost while doing AIT therapy plus much more. In fact, each of my auditory symptoms improved decisively: my sensitive hearing, the tinnitus, and my difficulty hearing voices over background noise.

In May 1996 I attended a training program in Samonas Sound Therapy with Ingo Steinbach in Great Britain. My own experience with his CDs had already been so positive that I emerged from the training full of enthusiasm. However, the training itself was incomplete in some respects. It focused on an education about the foundational and primitive nature of audition in human neurology, a review of some of Tomatis' most important discoveries, and a discussion of the possible applications of each of the Samonas CDs to specific conditions (tinnitus, depression, ADD, etc.). It emphasized the intuition of the therapist, rather than offering specific, tested protocols based on a body of clinical experience.

Nevertheless, I was happy with the Samonas recordings. Although fairly expensive, they were of much higher quality than the Joudry tapes, and even improved on the subjective experience people derived from classical music played through Tomatis's *Electronic Ear* at the Tomatis centers. The recommended recordings we had used with AIT and AET had been a broad mix of genres—primarily pop and rock—with only two pieces of classical music. And, most important to us, Samonas could be used at home, making it practical for many NACD families. So Samonas offered many important advantages.

However, formal protocols were clearly necessary. I consulted with my father and NACD staff members and designed seven basic protocols for seven distinct categories of individuals, based on our experiences with the other sound stimulation methods. As we applied them, we adjusted them as necessary. Over the following three years, we modified them continually, as we continued to learn from experience. Ultimately, we developed over fifty separate protocols for the Samonas recordings, and utilized them with over 1,500 people. It became obvious that we were leading the way in this process. We had far more clinical experience and were doing much more to formalize protocols than any other therapist using the Samonas recordings, including its originator.

Our therapeutic experience using Samonas was excellent. Because it was a home-based program, it reached many more families, and the therapeutic process was very effective. We had many successes with a wide range of individuals. We developed a guidebook, materials for monitoring compliance, written descriptions of the protocols telling clients exactly what to listen to for how long on what days. For the most part, it worked. But not always.

There were several times when CDs needed by our clients were unavailable and remained back-ordered for months, hampering their progress. Sometimes, despite our attempts to prevent it, clients would get confused. They would use the wrong CD for a period of weeks. They'd just make mistakes. The CDs were strong enough that sometimes that caused problems. On some occasions, the CDs seemed to have provoked emotional episodes. This could be avoided by limiting exposure, which Steinbach recommended. But this was not a satisfactory resolution; we knew the very short exposure times he was suggesting were not sufficient to produce a reasonable rate of therapeutic progress. The only way to account for all these issues would be to establish a pattern of very frequent interactions with each Samonas client, but this would make the program even more expensive. We concluded that, although we still believed in home treatment, we no longer felt Samonas was the optimal solution.

Conceiving a New Approach to Sound Therapy

NACD had a need for a rigorously conceived, expertly-produced, home-based sound therapy program that could be used for ongoing auditory stimulation. Over time, our conversations led us to consider developing our own program. I investigated creating a new company to support this development, which eventually I did. *Advanced Brain Technologies* emerged from this consideration. Our organization had a need for a rigorously conceived, expertly-produced, home-based auditory training that could be used on an ongoing basis.

I knew our goal: restoring tonal processing through the entire range of audible sound, from 20–20,000 Hz. Every one of our 50 different Samonas protocols had been directed at accomplishing this single goal. The differences in the protocols accounted for differences in what individuals could tolerate, techniques for creating variety, or differences in emphasis. Ultimately there was one primary objective. The approach just had many variations. It was clear that in designing our recordings and protocols we wanted to observe certain simple principles.

Recordings needed to exercise the ears and brain through the full spectrum of audible sound. Each individual may have a unique problem, but the goal for everyone is to listen effectively to the full tonal range. The music, the filtering, and the gating needed to address this. We wanted to provide stimulation that reached from the lowest bass notes that human ears can hear to the highest overtones.

The treatment of the music needed to be strong enough to be effective, but mild enough so that even if used incorrectly it would not create negative reactions. We planned for it to be available only through therapists who would supervise its use, but we knew that people can easily get confused. We wanted the recordings themselves to be inherently safe, so the whole system was, to a significant degree, mistake-proof.

We required protocols that specified the right schedule for listening. People need to listen to therapeutic music long enough but not too long. The auditory stimulation had to have adequate frequency, intensity, and duration. This applies to every session, to every day, and to every week. It even determines the duration of the entire course of sound therapy. Time structure was one of the most essential decisions we had to make.

We also knew that people would need musical variety; otherwise they would *habituate* or *tune out* what they were hearing and it would cease to be effective. The brain gets tired of whatever becomes too familiar, and it's very good at identifying patterns. So we knew we couldn't use any one CD for too long a sustained period of time. We wanted to provide novelty in the soundscape to avoid habituation.

Of course, we knew we would train the therapists. But the education had to get to the clients too. We wanted to include educational materials with the CDs, elucidating the clients, not just the therapists. From our experience, we know that if people understand the program, it will be easier for them to complete it.

The Listening Program we have released is the result of an intensive effort by a multi-disciplinary team, committed to excellence on every level. Every second of music on each CD has been edited and crafted for aesthetic refinement as well as therapeutic efficacy.

Music Therapy

The Power of Sound has been an exploration into the therapeutic applications of sound. Quite often, this will be sound manifested as music. This book has not explored music therapy. As I previously discussed, the difference between the two applications is the approach. Music therapy is primarily a psychological approach; soundwork is neurological, based on the effect of sound waves on the nervous system. Certainly there is overlap in the two approaches. The field of music therapy is held by me, the medical establishment, and the general public in the greatest of esteem.

The following description of music therapy comes directly from the American Music Therapy Association's website.

> Music therapy is the prescribed use of music by a qualified person to effect positive changes in the psychological, physical, cognitive, or social functioning of individuals with health or educational problems.
>
> The American Music Therapy Association is the largest professional association which represents over 5,000 music therapists, corporate members, and related associations worldwide. Founded in 1998, its mission is the progressive development of the therapeutic use of music in rehabilitation, special education, and community settings. AMTA sets the education and clinical training standards for music therapists.

What do music therapists do?

Music therapists—Assess emotional well-being, physical health, social functioning, communication abilities, and cognitive skills through musical responses. Design music sessions for individuals and groups based on client needs using: music improvisation, receptive music listening, songwriting, lyric discussion, music and imagery, music performance, and learning through music. Participate in interdisciplinary treatment planning, ongoing evaluation, and follow up.

Who can benefit from music therapy?

Children, adolescents, adults, and the elderly with mental health needs, developmental and learning disabilities, Alzheimer's disease and other aging related conditions, substance abuse problems, brain injuries, physical disabilities, and acute and chronic pain, including mothers in labor.

Where do music therapists work?

Music therapists work in psychiatric hospitals, rehabilitative facilities, medical hospitals, outpatient clinics, day care treatment centers, agencies serving developmentally disabled persons, community mental health centers, drug and alcohol programs, senior centers, nursing homes, hospice programs, correctional facilities, halfway houses, schools, and private practice.

What is the history of music therapy as a healthcare profession?

The idea of music as a healing influence which could affect health and behavior is as least as old as the writings of Aristotle and Plato. The 20th century discipline began after World War I and World War II when community musicians of all types, both amateur and professional, went to Veterans hospitals around the country to play for the thousands of veterans suffering both physical and emotional trauma from the wars. The patients' notable physical and emotional responses to music led the doctors and nurses to request the hiring of musicians by the hospitals. It was soon evident that the hospital musician needs some prior training before entering the facility and so the demand grew for a college curriculum. The first music therapy degree program in the world [was] founded at Michigan State University in 1944 . . . The American Music Therapy Association was founded in 1998 as a union of the National Association for Music Therapy and the American Association for Music Therapy.

Who is qualified to practice music therapy?

Persons who complete one of 69 approved college music therapy curricula including internship are then eligible to sit for the national examination offered by the Certification Board for Music Therapists. Music therapists who successfully complete the independently administered examination hold the music therapist–board certified credential (MT–BC). The National Music Therapy Registry (NMTR) serves qualified music therapy professionals with the following designations: RMT, CMT, ACMT. These individuals have met accepted educational and clinical training standards and are qualified to practice music therapy.

Is there research to support music therapy?

AMTA promotes a vast amount of research exploring the benefits of music as therapy through publication of the *Journal of Music Therapy, Music Therapy Perspectives*, and other sources. A substantial body of literature exists to support the effectiveness of music therapy.

What are some misconceptions about music therapy?

That the client or patient has to have some particular music ability to benefit from music therapy—they do not. That there is one particular style of music that is more therapeutic than all the rest—such is not the case.

What are some of the ways music therapy techniques can be applied by healthy individuals?

Healthy individuals can use music for stress reduction via active music making, such as drumming, as well as passive listening for relaxation. Music is often a vital support for physical exercise. Music therapy–assisted labor and delivery may also be included in this category, since pregnancy is regarded as a normal part of women's life cycles.

How is music therapy utilized in hospitals?

Music is used in general hospitals to: alleviate pain in conjunction with anesthesia or pain medication; elevate patients' mood and counteract depression; promote movement for physical rehabilitation; calm or sedate, often to induce sleep; counteract apprehension or fear; and lessen muscle tension for the purpose of relaxation, including the autonomic nervous system.

How is music therapy utilized in nursing homes?

Music is used with elderly persons to increase or maintain their level of physical, mental, and social/emotional functioning. The sensory and intellectual stimulation of music can help maintain a person's quality of life.

How is music therapy utilized in schools?

Music therapists are often hired in schools to provide music therapy services listed on the Individualized Education Plan for mainstreamed special learners. Music learning is used to strengthen nonmusical areas such as communication skills and physical coordination skills which are important for daily life.

How is music therapy utilized in psychiatric facilities?

Music therapy allows persons with mental health needs to: explore personal feelings, make positive changes in mood and emotional states, have a sense of control over life through successful experiences, practice problem solving, and resolve conflicts leading to stronger family and peer relationships.

Describe a typical music therapy session.

Since music therapists serve a wide variety of persons with many different types of needs, there is no such thing as an overall typical session. Sessions are designed and music selected based on the individual client's treatment plan.

For contact information on the AMTA, see "Soundwork Resources."

Glossary

Acoustics. The science of sound.

Acoustic Nerve. The eighth cranial nerve, concerned with hearing and balance.

Acoustic Trauma. When a loud sound strikes in an instant, causing damage to the auditory mechanism.

Air Conduction. Sound waves, transferred through the air, that vibrate the ear drum, setting the auditory mechanism in process.

Ambient Noise. The total of all noise in the environment, other than the noise from the source of interest.

Amplitude. The volume of a sound.

Anechoic Chamber. A room in which the boundaries absorb nearly all the incident sound, thereby effectively creating free field conditions.

Arcangelos. The chamber ensemble featured on the enclosed album, *Music for The Power of Sound.*

Audiologist. A person trained in the science of hearing and hearing impairments.

Audiometer. A machine used to test hearing.

Auditory Cross Dominance. A process whereby a person with right-sided dominance, i.e., with a leading right hand, right foot, right eye, has a left leading ear (or vice versa if left handed).

Auditory Integration Training (AIT). A sound stimulation program developed by Dr. Guy Berard of France.

Auditory Nerve. The nerve carrying electrical signals from the inner ear to the base of the brain.

Auditory Perception. How the brain understands and uses the sound it receives.

Auditory Sequential Processing. The ability to link pieces of auditory information together, to remember the order of things heard.

Auditory Tonal Processing. The ability to differentiate between the tones utilized in language.

Basilar Membrane. A thin sheet of material which vibrates in response to movements in the liquid that fills the cochlea.

Binaural Beat Frequencies (BBFs). A neuroacoustical phenomenon which takes place when the brain hears one tone in one ear with a slightly detuned tone in the other. As a means of measuring the difference between these two tones, the brain creates a third "phantom" tone, unheard elsewhere.

Biological Rhythm. Self-sustained cyclic change in a physiological process or behavioral function of an organism that repeats at regular intervals.

Bone Conduction. The transference of sound waves through reverberations of bone to the inner ear.

Bony Labyrinth. The cavity in the skull which contains the inner ear mechanism.

Brainwaves. The electrochemical activity of the brain which produces electromagnetic wave forms. Beta waves (14–35 Hz); Alpha waves (8–14 Hz); Theta waves (4–8 Hz); Delta waves (.5–4 Hz).

Central Auditory Processing. The processing of sound along the auditory neural pathways from the cochlea to the brain and using that sound in the brain's auditory centers.

Cilia. Delicate sensory cells, resembling hair-like projections, located in the organ of Corti portion of the cochlea. Connecting with nerve fibers, cilia cells transport airborne vibrations from the inner ear to the brain.

Circadian Rhythm. A self-sustained biological rhythm which in an organism's natural environment normally has a period of approximately 24 hours.

Cochlea. Shaped like a snail's shell, this organ of the inner ear contains the organ of Corti, from which eighth nerve fibers send hearing signals to the brain. (See Inner Ear.)

Compression and Rarefaction. A process involving the alternating density of molecules in the air and how information is passed.

Contours. Gradual changes in tempo and shifting dynamics (amplitude, panning, etc.) to offset habituation of the brain.

Cortex. That surface of the brain where sensory information is processed.

Decibel (dB). The measurement of the volume or loudness of a sound.

Detuning. A process used in the creation of binaural beat frequencies whereby simultaneous stereo tones are slightly changed, i.e., sound frequencies differ by a prescribed number of Hz from each other.

Drone. A long, uninterrupted sound, or set of sounds, underneath music.

Eardrum. The membrane, known as the tympanum, that separates the outer ear from the middle ear.

Earmuffs. Special ear protectors designed for protection from loud sound.

Earplugs. Noise protection made of foam, silicone, or wax.

Earlids. Something we ain't got!

Electronic Ear. An essential component of the Tomatis Method created by Alfred Tomatis. This device, interconnected between a tape or CD player and the listener's headphones, has the capacity to filter the sound through two channels with different settings. A gating mechanism alternates the sound between the channels when it reaches a specific intensity. The Electronic Ear is designed to educate the ear to its full functions as a receptor, a mechanism to make subtle discriminations, and an energy generator.

Entrainment. In the context of psychoacoustics, concerns changing the rate of brainwaves, breath, or heartbeats from one speed to another by matching an external periodic force (rhythm).

Filtration. A removal of specific frequencies.

Filtration/Gating Techniques (F/G). A methodology devised by Dr. Alfred Tomatis to retrain and strengthen the auditory mechanism.

Form. The structure underneath all other elements of music.

Frequency. The periodic speed at which an object vibrates; the number of vibrations per second of a sound.

Gating. Refers to a random sonic event. This is accomplished by electronically processing a soundtrack (i.e., Mozart) so it unexpectedly jumps between high and low frequencies or variances in amplitude.

GIM. The Helen Bonny method of Guided Imagery and Music.

Golden Section. A specific geometric proportion seen in Egyptian pyramids (thirteenth century B.C.) and the Parthenon at Athens (fifth century B.C.), as well as artwork and nature.

Harmonics. A series of tones that vibrate above a fundamental note. Known as overtones or partials, these softer tones are pure and clear sounds.

Harmony. The result produced when tones are sounded simultaneously.

Hearing. The subjective and passive response to sound.

Hearing Loss. Any reduction in the normal way a person hears.

Hertz (Hz). The international standard term for a unit of frequency or cycles per second (cps). Named for the German physicist, Heinrich Hertz.

High Frequency. Any tone that has more cycles per second; generally anything over 1000 Hz.

Infrasonic. Sound waves below 20 Hz.

Inner Ear or Cochlea. Here the vibration of sound is converted into electrical signals. The vestibular system also resides here. The semicircular canals and the vestibular sacs are the upper part of what is known as the bony labyrinths of the inner ear.

Instrumental Colors. In Western music, the study of instrumental color is known as orchestration.

ISO Principle. "Iso" means equal. Applied to therapeutic music, initially matching the mood of the music to that of the listener and then slowly changing that mood, tempo, or timbre.

Laterality. Lateral preference is the predominant use of one side of the body over the other.

Listening. Active (vs. passive) hearing.

The Listening Program (TLP). A sound stimulation program developed by Advanced Brain Technologies.

Lithotripsy. The dissolution of kidney and pancreatic duct stones with acoustic wave bombardment.

Loudness (amplitude). A perception of sound strength; a psychological impression.

Low Frequencies. Any tone that has fewer cycles per second; generally anything up to 1000 Hz.

Melody. A succession of single notes. The primary element we hear in a composition.

Middle Ear. A hollow region directly behind the eardrum preceding the inner ear. The middle ear is only about 2 milliliters in volume and houses three small bones known as the hammer (malleus), anvil (incus), and stirrup (stapes), and two tiny muscles—the tensor tympani and stapedius.

Music Therapy. Using familiar music to enhance relaxation, comfort, and enjoyment. Primarily psychologically oriented.

National Academy for Child Development (NACD). Headquartered in Ogden, Utah.

Neurodevelopment. The development and organization of the central nervous system.

Noise. Derived from the Latin word *nausea*, meaning seasickness. Any loud, unmusical, or disagreeable sound.

Noise-Induced Hearing Loss (NIHL). A diminution of hearing capacity due to repeated or extended exposure to dangerous noise levels resulting in damaged cilia hair cells in the cochlea.

Non Periodic. A non-regular pulse and frequency.

Organ of Corti. Located in the cochlea, the region containing hair cells that transmit sound waves from the ear through the auditory nerve to the brain.

Ostinato. An accompaniment figure that is repeated. Also known as pedal point.

Outer Ear. Consists of the pinna (auricle), auditory canal (meatus), and eardrum (tympanic membrane). Also known as the external ear.

Oval Window. The membrane that vibrates, transmitting sound into the cochlea. Separates the middle ear from the inner ear.

Perilymph. The watery liquid that fills the outer tubes running through the cochlea.

Period. The time that elapses before a rhythm starts to repeat itself.

Periodicity. The quality of repeating precisely the same pattern on a regular basis.

Pink Noise. Noise with constant energy per octave band width.

Pitch. Signifies how high or low a tone sounds to the ear.

Psychoacoustics. The study of the perception of sound, including how we listen, our psychological responses, and the physiological impact of music and sound on the human nervous system.

Resonance. The effect of one vibration on another. The frequency at which an object most naturally vibrates.

Resonant System. When two or more objects have similar vibratory characteristics allowing them to resonate at the same frequency.

Resonate. To re-sound. Something external sets something else into motion or changes its vibratory rate.

Rhythm. Periodic movement. The organization of music in time using long and short note values.

SIAD. Stress-induced auditory dysfunction. Term coined by author.

Semicircular Canals. Curved tubes containing fluid, the movement of which makes us aware of turning sensations as the head moves.

Sensorineural Hearing Loss. Hearing loss resulting from an inner ear problem.

Sonic Isometrics. Term coined by author to explain the process of alternating simple and complex auditory data to the brain.

Sonic Neurotechnologies (SNT). Phrase coined by author to describe the precise mechanical manipulation of soundwaves to bring about desired changes in psyche and physical body.

Sonorous Body. Anything capable of producing sound.

Sound. A sensation caused by an object or objects that vibrate. Anything that creates the sensation of hearing.

Sound Stimulation. The excitement of the nervous system by auditory information.

Sound Stimulation Auditory Training (SSAT). A precise application of electronically processed sound, through headphones, to retrain the auditory mechanism to take in a wider spectrum of sound frequencies.

Sound Therapy. Using the principles of resonance, entrainment, and vibration to effect changes in tissues and organs. Primarily neurologically oriented.

Sound Wave. Alternating low and high pressure areas, moving through the air, which are interpreted as sound when collected in the ear.

Soundwork. The use of sound as a therapeutic modality.

Sympathetic Vibration. The natural ability of a substance such as metal, wood, air, and living flesh and bone to vibrate to a frequency imposed from another source.

Spectrum. A sound wave's resolution into its components of frequency and amplitude.

Stapedius. Tiny middle ear muscle that pulls the stapes sideways.

Tectorial Membrane. Located in the organ of Corti, a thin strip of membrane in contact with sensory hairs, which is moved by sound vibrations producing nerve impulses.

Tensor Tympani. Tiny middle ear muscle attached to the malleus that increases the tension in the eardrum.

Timbre. Tone color or quality, e.g., trumpet vs. violin.

Tinnitus. Ringing in the ear or noise sensed in the head.

Tomatis, Alfred A. (1920–   ) French ENT, sound researcher, inventor, author. Creator of the Tomatis Method. Considered by many to be the "Einstein of the ear."

Tomatis Effect. "The voice can only reproduce sounds that the ear can hear," is the basis on which the French Academy of Medicine and Academy of Science named one of the many discoveries of Alfred Tomatis.

Tomatis Method. A noninvasive program of sound stimulation, audio-vocal activities, and consultation. It is used to enhance abilities or overcome problems that are listening-related, such as speech and language, learning, attention, and communication, among others. The method was developed by Alfred Tomatis over fifty years ago and has been used throughout the world with both children and adults.

Tone. A sound of definite pitch.

Tuning Fork. A small steel instrument with two prongs, which sounds a certain fixed tone in perfect pitch when struck.

Tympanum. Also known as the eardrum. Membrane separating outer ear from middle ear.

Ultrasonic. Sound waves above 20,000 Hz.

Vagus Nerve. The pneumogastric or tenth cranial nerve. It is called the vagus (wandering or vagabond) nerve because it meanders through the thoracic and abdominal cavities.

Vibration. An oscillatory motion of solid bodies.

Vestibular Apparatus. A part of the cochlea concerned with maintaining balance.

Vestibulo-Cochlear Nerve. The eighth cranial nerve.

Vibration. A rapid rhythmic motion back and forth.

Waves. Rhythmic alternations of disturbance and recovery in successively contiguous portions of a fluid or solid mass.

Wave Motion. The phenomenon of a transfer of energy (or information) from one source to another.

Wave Length. Distance between the peaks of successive sound waves.

White Noise. Noise whose energy is uniform over a wide range of frequencies. Analogous in spectrum characteristics to white light.

Sound Remedies Catalog 📖

The focus of the Sound Remedies Catalog is the emerging field of sound-work, broadly defined as the intentional creation and employment of music and sound for specific applications. The catalog contains categorized lists of music and sound programs, recommended reading, and resources in the following categories:

- Children
- Concentration/Accelerated Learning
- Creativity
- Exercise/Fitness
- Healing and Balance
- Massage/Bodywork
- Office/Treatment Room Ambience
- Relaxation/Stress Reduction
- Sleep
- Therapeutic Applications
- Transitions: Cradle to Grave

New programs are constantly being reviewed and added. Categories will continue to grow as psychoacoustic programs of high aesthetic value and effective sonic technologies are produced.

Most programs in the catalog have *not* been created for entertainment purposes. Rather, they've been produced with highly specific methodologies and outcomes in mind. Be it for health, learning, or productivity, these "sonic tools" are designed for the enhancement of human function.

HOW DO I ACCESS THE CATALOG?

Due to space limitations and constantly updated resources, the Sound Remedies catalog is not included within *The Power of Sound*. However, the complete catalog can be viewed online at www.sound-remedies.com. Printed catalogs are available for a nominal fee, and can be ordered by visiting the website or by calling 800-788-0949.

Music for The Power of Sound
CD Track Listing

Music for The Power of Sound is specially orchestrated classical music selected from the Sound Health Series. It is performed by The Arcangelos Chamber Ensemble, under the music direction of Richard Lawrence. The purpose of this CD is twofold: to provide sonic ambience conducive to relaxation and learning and to illustrate concepts contained within this book (see referral page numbers in Track Listings below).

While there are no sonic neurotechnologies (filtration/gating or binaural frequencies) used in these selections, the natural principles of resonance and entrainment inform all arrangements. Putting technical explanations aside, *Music for The Power of Sound* is a modern embodiment of the age-old musical goal: beautiful sounds for enhancement, balance, and well-being.

TRACK NO.	REFERRAL PAGE NOS.	TITLE (COMPOSER)	(TIME) (SOUND HEALTH ALBUM)
1	192, 235	Divertimento #1 in D Major K136 with Interlude (Mozart)	(5:10) (Motivation)
2	191	Clarinet Quintet in A Major K581 Theme and Variations (Mozart)	(5:55) (Motivation)
3	225, 234	Adagio from Concerto Grosso Opus 6, No. 8 (Corelli)	(6:19) (Relax)
4	191, 234, 235	Largo/Viola d'Amore Concerto in D Minor with Interlude (Vivaldi)	(5:36) (Learning)
5	191, 225	Gymnopedie #1 with Interlude (Satie)	(5:17) (Inspiration)
6	191, 192, 229, 232	Fourth Symphony, Poco adagio (Mahler)	(7:55) (De-Stress)
7	234	Interlude from Dance of the Blessed Spirits (Gluck)	(2:10) (Inspiration)
8	225, 228	Largo from Oboe Concerto in B Flat with Interlude (Vivaldi)	(4:10) (Learning)
9	225	Oboe Quartet in F Major K370 Allegro (Mozart)	(4:17) (Motivation)
10	191, 225, 230	Largo from Concerto No. 3 for Two Violins (J. S. Bach)	(5:52) (Concentration)
11	225	Sunshine Suite, 3rd Movement (Lawrence)	(1:49) (Productivity)
12	127, 232, 235	Allegro assai from Violin Concerto No. 2 (J. S. Bach)	(5:15) (Learning)

Soundwork Resources

(Author's note: The following resources represent an unfolding universe of institutes, programs, schools, and commercial organizations dedicated to application-specific utilizations of music and sound. This listing should be taken as a starting point. Kindly pardon omissions.)

Within you will find the following categories:
Tomatis Centers
Music Therapy
Guided Imagery and Music
Music and Sound in Education
Binaural Beat Frequencies
Sound Stimulation Programs Using Filtration/Gating Techniques
Clinical Soundwork Models
Soundworkers Referred to in *The Power of Sound*
Soundwork Services and Organizations
Soundwork Products Referred to in *The Power of Sound*
Internet Research Resources

TOMATIS CENTERS

There are about 250 Tomatis Centers in the world. Below is a list of centers that use the Tomatis Method in Canada, the United States and Mexico. These are the only centers that are accredited by Dr. A. A. Tomatis. To access the home page of each of these Centers, use the Internet: www.tomatis.com.

CANADA
Regina
Toronto

UNITED STATES
Arizona—Phoenix
California—Greater San Francisco Area; Pasadena
Colorado—Denver
Louisiana—New Orleans

Maryland—Bethesda
Massachusetts—Amherst
Texas—Dallas
Washington—Seattle

MEXICO
Garza Garcia, Nuevo Leon
Guadalajara, Jalisco
Mexico City, DF
Monterrey, Nuevo Leon
Torreon, Coahuila

OUTSIDE NORTH AMERICA CONTACT:

Tomatis International Headquarters
Christian Tomatis, Director
144 Avenue des Champs Elysees
Paris 75008, France
Tel: (33) 1-53-53-42-40

MUSIC THERAPY

The American Music Therapy Association
8455 Colesville Road, Suite 1000
Silver Spring, MD 20910
Tel: (301) 589-3300
Fax: (301) 589-5175
Email: info@musictherapy.org
Website: www.musictherapy.org
Over fifty schools nationwide offer degree programs in music therapy.

Temple University
Dept. of Music Education and Therapy
Attn: Kenneth Brusca, Ph.D.
938 Park Mall, TU 298 00
Philadelphia, PA 19122
Tel: (215) 204-8314

Arizona State University
Department of Music Therapy
Attn: Barbara Crowe, MNT, RMT-BC
Tempe, AZ 85287
Tel: (602) 965-7413

The World Federation of Music Therapists, Inc.
P.O. Box 585
01080 Vitoria-Gafteiz, Spain
Tel: (34) 45-143-311
Fax: (34) 45-144-224

GUIDED IMAGERY AND MUSIC

Association for Music and Therapy
Attn: James Rankin
331 Soquel Avenue, Suite 201
Santa Cruz, CA 95062

The Bonny Foundation
2020 Simmons Street
Salinas, KS 67401

Mid-Atlantic Institute
Attn: Carol A. Bush
Box 4655
Virginia Beach, VA 23454
Tel: (757) 498-0452

MUSIC AND SOUND IN EDUCATION

The American Orff Schulwerk Association
P.O. Box 391089
Cleveland, OH 44139
Tel: (216) 543-5366
Website: www.aosa.org
Offers training in the Orff method in the U.S. and abroad, featuring xylophones, glocken-spiels, poems, rhymes, games, storytelling, songs, and dances.

The Suzuki Association of America
1900 Fulsom Street, #101
Boulder, CO 80302
Tel: (303) 444-0948
American headquarters for the Suzuki method and training.

Life Sounds
Attn: Chris Brewer
P.O. Box 227
Kalispell, MT 59903
Tel: (406) 755-4875
Resources and training in accelerative learning.

American Association of Kodaly Educators
1457 South 23rd Street
Fargo, ND 58103
Tel: (701) 235-0366

BINAURAL BEAT FREQUENCIES

Acoustic Brain Research (ABR)
Producer: Tom Kenyon
Share Foundation / S.E.E. Publishing Co.
1556 Halford Avenue #288
Santa Clara, CA 95051-2661
Tel: (408) 245-5457
Fax: (408) 245-5460
Email: lovecorp@ix.netcom.com
Website: www.tomkenyon.com
Natural and electronic sounds with verbal and non-verbal input.

Brain/Mind Research
Producer: Dr. Jeffrey Thompson
204 N. El Camino Real, #E116
Encinitas, CA 92024
Tel: (800) 349-7358
Email: bmrinc@hotmail.com
Website: www.body-mind.com
Electronic music-based research with cutting edge applications and effectiveness.

Brain-Sync
Producer: Kelly Howell
P.O. Box 3120
Ashland, OR 97520
Tel: (800) 984-7962
Email: braininfo@brainsync.com
Website: www.brainsync.com
Emphasis on meditation, relaxation, mind expansion, weight loss, and fitness.

The Monroe Institute
62 Roberts Mountain Road
Faber, VA 22938-2317
Tel: (804) 361-1252
Fax: (804) 361-1237
Email: MonroeInst@aol.com
Website: www.monroeinstitute.org
Leading-edge research and applications for forty-plus years—the granddaddy of the field. Recordings span wide spectrum of application.

Synchronicity Foundation
Producer: Master Charles
P.O. Box 694
Nellysford, VA 22958
Tel: (804) 361-2323 or (800) 962-2033
Fax: (804) 361-1058
Email: synch@synchronicity.org
Website: www.synchronicity.org
Emphasis on "meditative awareness."

SOUND STIMULATION PROGRAMS USING FILTRATION/GATING TECHNIQUES
(* denotes training programs for professionals)

The Tomatis Method*/France
Developed by Alfred Tomatis, M.D.
See page 288

Auditory Integration Training*/France
Developed by Guy Berard, M.D.
USA contact: Society for Auditory Intervention Techniques (SAIT)
P.O. Box 4538
Salem, OR 97302
Website: www.teleport.com/~sait/

Digital Auditory Aerobics*/USA
Developed by EARliest Adventures in Sound, L.L.C.
P.O. Box 18776
Fairfield, OH 45018-0776
Tel: (888) 257-9516
Fax: (513) 674-9935
Email: info@digitalaerobics.com
Website: www.digitalaerobics.com

Hemispheric Specific Auditory Training*/Denmark
Developed by Kjeld Johansen, Ph.D.
Ro Skolevej 14
DK-3760 Gudhjem, Bornholm, Denmark

USA contact: A Chance To Grow, Inc./New Visions School
1800 Second Street NE
Minneapolis, MN 55418
Tel: (612) 789-1236
Fax: (612) 706-5555
Email: mjoyce@mail.actg.org

Listening Fitness*/Canada
Developed by Paul Madaule
Listening Technologies Inc.
599 Markham St.
Toronto, ON, Canada, M6G 2L7
Tel: (416) 531-8400
Fax: (416) 588-4459
Email: listen@idirect.com
Website: www.listeningfitness.com.

The Listening Program*/USA
Developed by Advanced Brain Technologies, LLC
P.O. Box 1088
Ogden, UT 84402
Tel: (888) 228-1798
Fax: (801) 627-4505
Email: info@advancedbrain.com.
Website: www.advancedbrain.com

Samonas Sound Therapy*/Germany
Developed by Ingo Steinbach
Klangstudio Lambdoma, Germany
Markgrafenufer 9
D-59071 Hamm, Germany
USt-ID-Nr: DE 125 299 034
Tel: (49) 2381-98-222-0
Fax: (49) 2381-98-222-88
Email: ist@sonas.com
Website: www.sonas.com

Sound Therapy for the Walkman/Canada
Developed by Patricia Joudry
Steele and Steele Sound Therapy
Box 616
Dalmeny, Saskatchewan
Canada S0K 1E0
Tel/Fax: (306) 931-2522
Email: soundtherapy@vsource.com
Website: www.intouchmag.com/soundtherapy.html

CLINICAL SOUNDWORK MODELS

The following clinics/organizations are examples of current soundwork practices used in a therapeutic or educational context.

Center for InnerChange

Ron Minson, M.D., and Kate O'Brien-Minson, Directors
55 Madison Street, Suite 400
Denver, CO 80206
Tel: (303) 320-4411
Fax: (303) 322-5550
Email: info@centerforinnerchange.com
Website: www.centerforinnerchange.com

Dr. Ron Minson, former Chief of Psychiatry at two of Denver's teaching hospitals, learned about the Tomatis Method in searching for help for his daughter. After studying with Dr. Alfred Tomatis in France, Dr. Minson and his wife, Kate, opened their center in Denver in 1990. Dr. Minson artfully combines traditional and alternative therapies. The Center for InnerChange specializes in a non-pharmacological approach by using sound as a natural way to improve brain function. With the Tomatis Listening Method at its core, other methods include cognitive behavioral therapy for both children and adults, family therapy, and allergy/nutrition consultations.

The Chalice of Repose Project

Therese Schroeder-Sheker, Director
St. Patrick Hospital
312 East Pine Street
Missoula, MT 59802
Tel: (406) 329-2810
Fax: (406) 329-5614
Email: info@saintpatrick.org
Website: www.saintpatrick.org/chalice

The Chalice of Repose Project is a unique end-of-life patient care program and graduate level school of music-thanatology. It includes a palliative-clinical practice and an educational program. The Project is a nonprofit, tax-exempt corporation housed within St. Patrick Hospital in Missoula, Montana, USA. The Project's mission is to lovingly serve the physical and spiritual needs of the dying with prescriptive music; to educate clinicians, healthcare providers, and the public about the possibility of a blessed death and the gift that conscious dying can bring to the fullness of life; and to integrate and model these contemplative and clinical values in daily practice.

Cymatics
Sir Peter Guy Manners, M.D., D.O., Ph.D.
Brentforton Scientific and Medical Trust
Brentforton Hall
Vale of Evesharm, Worcester
England WR11 5JH
Tel: (44) 1386-830537
Fax: (44) 1386-830918
Cymatic therapy is not applied through the auditory system, rather directly through the skin. A computerized instrument transmits resonant frequencies of sound into the body. Sound waves, within the audible range, pass through healthy tissues and reestablish healthy resonance in unhealthy tissues. Used by nurses, chiropractors, osteopaths, and acupuncturists, cymatic machines have been used in the USA since the late 1960s. Training is required.

The Davis Center for Hearing, Speech & Learning
Dorinne S. Davis, M.A. CCC-A, Director
98 Rt. 46
W. Budd Lake, NJ 07828
Tel: (973) 347-7662
Fax: (973) 691-0611
Email: info@thedaviscenter.com
Website: www.thedaviscenter.com
Providing multiple sound-based therapies in one location, The Davis Center is an example of the sound therapy centers of the future. Dorinne S. Davis is a licensed, certified audiologist. Her thirty years experience in Educational & Rehabilitative Audiology provide the foundation for the center's unique focus and evaluation protocol. The Davis Center assists people of all ages, particularly those with special needs, addressing symptoms related to Autism, PDD, ADD, ADHD, Dyslexia, and other Auditory Processing Disorders by offering a variety of specialized sound-based therapies for the enhancement of hearing, speech, and learning. Methods include Berard Auditory Integration Training (AIT), Tomatis, The Listening Program, and Lindamood Bell. Well-being issues are addressed through BioAcoustics.

Hearing and Learning Center/Beth Israel Medical Center
Jane R. Maydell, Ph.D., Director
Beth Israel Medical Center
10 Union Square East, Suite 2K
New York, NY 10003
Tel: (212) 844-8790
Fax: (212) 844-8791
Email: jmadell@bethisraelny.org
This full-service center provides diagnostic and treatment services to infants, children, and adults with a variety of hearing, speech, language, and learning disorders. Under the direction of Dr. Jane Madell, a certified and licensed audiologist, auditory verbal therapist, and

speech-language pathologist, the emphasis at the center includes hearing loss and disorders involving auditory processing, auditory attention, and auditory function. Therapies include speech-language therapy, auditory verbal therapy, auditory training, auditory integration training, The Listening Program, Fast ForWard, Earobics, and specific listening therapy. Reading services are also available using Lindamood Bell and Orton Gillingham methods. Extensive follow-up and support services include school visits, classroom evaluation, in-service training for school personnel, and evaluation and dispensing of assistive devices.

National Academy for Child Development (NACD)
Robert J. Doman Jr., Executive Director
National Headquarters:
The Weber Center
2380 Washington Blvd., 2nd Floor
Ogden, UT 84401

Mailing Address:
P.O. Box 380
Huntsville, UT 84317
Tel: (801) 621-8606
Fax: (801) 621-8389
Email: nacdinfo@nacd.org
Website: www.nacd.org

An international organization of parents and professionals dedicated to helping children and adults reach their full potential. Founded in 1979 by educator and lecturer Robert J. Doman Jr., NACD designs very specific home neurodevelopmental programs for infants, children, and adults. Client populations span comatose to highly gifted. Sound stimulation program of choice: The Listening Program.

New Visions
Suzanne Evans Morris, Ph.D., Director
1124 Roberts Mountain Road
Faber, VA 22938
Tel: (804) 361-2285
Email: mealtime@new-vis.com
Website: www.new-vis.com

New Visions provides continuing education and therapy services to professionals and parents working with infants and children with feeding, swallowing, oral-motor, and pre-speech problems. The New Visions Mealtimes catalog includes a wide variety of feeding and oral-motor materials and music recordings to support learning. New Visions was established in 1985 by Suzanne Evans Morris, Ph.D. Its programs are located in the Blue Ridge foothills of Nelson County, Virginia.

Pediatric Therapeutics
Sheila Smith Allen, M.A., O.T.R., B.C.P, Codirector
330 Main Street
Chatham, NJ 07928
Tel: (973) 635-0202
Fax: (973) 635-9609
Email: Ssmiallen@aol.com
Pediatric Therapeutics is a private therapy center, established in 1986, providing family-centered occupational, physical, and speech/language therapies to children from birth to twenty-one years. Soundwork is incorporated into a variety of clinical approaches by all disciplines in order to affect arousal, regulatory functions, attention, and adaptive behavior. It is an integral component of sensory integrative intervention. In both clinical treatment and home-programming, therapists and/or parents use an array of activities, music, and sound-based programs, ranging from basic breathing, movement, and soundmaking, to psychoacoustically engineered programs of listening to technologically advanced software. Specific sound-based tools include The Listening Program and its extensions, Sound Health Series, Metamusic, Music of Light, Ease, Sonas/Samonas, Interactive Metronome, Fast ForWord, and BrainBuilder.

Fred Schwartz, M.D.
314 Woodward Way NW
Atlanta, GA 30305
Tel: (404) 335-4242
Fax: (404) 355-0795
Email: drmusic@mindspring.com
Website: www.transitionsmusic.com
Dr. Schwartz is a board certified anesthesiologist, practicing at Piedmont Hospital in Atlanta, Georgia. He is a member of the International Society for Music in Medicine, the American Music Therapy Association, as well as APPPAH. He has used music in the operating room and delivery suite for over 20 years, and for the last 10 years has also produced music for pregnancy, childbirth, and babies. He is the author of an extraordinary research study entitled "Music, Stress Reduction and Medical Cost Savings in the Neonatal Intensive Care Unit," that details the history and current usages of music in neonatal ICUs. This study can be found at the Internet site listed above.

Strang-Cornell Cancer Prevention Center (affiliated with New York Hospital)
Mitch Gaynor, M.D., Director of Medical Oncology and Integrative Medicine
428 E. 72nd Street, Suite 100
New York, NY 10021
Tel: (212) 794-4900, ext. 161
Fax: (212) 794-0749
Email: mgaynor@strang.org

Since 1991, Dr. Gaynor has used sound as a complementary therapy in the form of chanting, music, and quartz crystal bowls with remarkable results.

Sound Listening and Learning Center
Billie Thompson, Ph.D., Director
301 E. Bethany Home Road, Suite A-107
Phoenix, AZ 85012
Tel: (602) 381-0086
Fax: (602) 957-6741

200 E. Del Mar, Suite 208
Pasadena, CA 91105
Tel: (626) 405-2386
Fax: (626) 405-2387
Email: info@soundlistening.com
Website: www.soundlistening.com

Billie M. Thompson, Ph.D., founded the Sound Listening and Learning Center in Phoenix, Arizona (1987) and in Pasadena, California (1994). The centers and their outreach programs across the U.S. provide experiences of accelerated learning and transformational change to children, adolescents, adults, families, schools, and corporations. She coedited the anthology, About the Tomatis Method, *edited and copublished Tomatis's English translations of his autobiography,* The Conscious Ear, *and his first book,* The Ear and Language. *Complementing the Tomatis Method, Dr. Thompson integrates Rubenfeld Synergy Method, Structure of Intellect, Neurolinguistic Programming, and unique humanistic psychology techniques in her work. She has new patents in the field of sound training.*

SOUNDWORKERS REFERRED TO IN *THE POWER OF SOUND*

Susan Alexjander
P.O. Box 428
Aptos, CA 95001
Tel: (831) 662-9450
Email: xjander@got.net

Vickie Dodd
Mind/Body Productions
P.O. Box 7312
Boulder, CO 80306
Tel: (303) 444-1766

Jonathan Goldman
Director/Sound Healers Association
P.O. Box 2240
Boulder, CO 80306
Tel: (303) 443-8181
Fax: (303) 443-6023
Email: jonathan@healingsounds.com
Website: www.healingsounds.com

Fabien Maman
Director/Academy of Sound, Color and Movement
4800 Baseline #E104-237
Boulder, CO 80303
Tel: (303) 926-0552 or (800) 615-3675
Email: tamado@earthnet.net
Website: www.tama-do.com

Suzanne Evans Morris, Ph.D.
Director/New Visions
See page 295

Ron Minson, M.D.
Director/Center for InnerChange
See page 293

Drew Pierson, Ph.D.
1835 Via El Capitan
San Jose, CA 95124
Tel: (800) 581-8178
Website: www.winterstale.net

Molly Scott, Ed.D., LMHC
Director/Creative Resonance Institute
327 Warner Hill Road
Charlemont, MA 01339
Tel: (413) 339-5501
Fax: (413) 339-0144
Email: Sumol@aol.com

Billie Thompson, Ph.D.
Director/Sound Listening and Learning Center
See page 297

Jeffrey Thompson, D.C.
Center for Neuroacoustic Research
California Institute for Human Science
701 Garden View Court

Encinitas, CA 92024
Tel: (760) 942-6749
Fax: (760) 942-6768
Email: drjeff@adnc.com
Website: www.jeffthompson.com and www.body-mind.com

SOUNDWORK SERVICES AND ORGANIZATIONS

Applied Music & Sound
Joshua Leeds, Creative Director
1001 Bridgeway PMB 716
Sausalito, CA 94965
Tel: (800) 788-0949
Fax: (888) 590-2678
Email: nusound@well.com or info@thepowerofsound.com
Website: www.appliedmusic.com
Specializing in application-specific audio programs, Applied Music & Sound recordings are designed to facilitate wellness, accelerate learning, and improve performance. Sophisticated sonic neurotechnologies (including filtration/gating or binaural frequencies) are often combined with psychoacoustically refined musical arrangements.

Bio-sonics
John Beaulieu, Director
BioSonic Enterprises, Ltd.
P.O. Box 487
High Falls, NY 12440
Tel: (914) 687-4767 or (800) 925-0159
Fax: (914) 687-0205
Email: JohnB310@aol.com
Website: www.biosonicenterprises.com
BioSonic Enterprises is dedicated to presenting creative classes and products on Music and Sound Healing, Energy Medicine, and Polarity Therapy.

Center for Bio-Medical Research
Michael H. Thaut, Director
The Center for Biomedical Research in Music at Colorado State University
Tel: (970) 491-7384
Fax: (970) 491-7541
Email: mthaut@lamar.colostate.edu
Website: www.colostate.edu/depts/cbrm
A university research center dedicated to auditory motor and cognitive neuroscience, neurologic rehabilitation, rhythmic perception, production, and synchronization, and the neuroscience of music and scientific foundation of music therapy.

The Georgiana Institute

Annabel Stehli, Director
Auditory Integration Training (AIT)—Digital Auditory Aerobics (DAA)
P.O. Box 10, 137 Davenport Road
Roxbury, CT 06783
Tel: (860) 355-1545
Fax: (860) 355-2443
Email: georgianainstitute@snet.net
Website: www.georgianainstitute.org

Annabel Stehli, author of The Sound of a Miracle: A Child's Triumph over Autism *and editor of* Dancing in the Rain, *introduced Auditory Integration Training to the United States two decades ago. In* The Sound of a Miracle, *Stehli recounts Georgiana's incredible journey through the horrid grip of autism to the wonderful miracle she received through Dr. Guy Berard's Auditory Integration Training (AIT).*

Healing HealthCare Systems, Inc.

100 W. Grove Street, Suite 175
Reno, NV 89509
Tel: (800) 348-0799
Fax: (775) 827-0304
Email: healhealth@aol.com
Website: www.healinghealth.com

HHS specializes in sound and music products and services facilitating hospital practices that serve both clinical and non-clinical needs of patients, families, and staff.

H.E.A.R. (Hearing Education and Awareness for Rockers)

Kathy Peck, Executive Director
PO Box 460847
San Francisco, CA 94146
Tel: (415) 409-EARS (3277)
Fax: (415) 409-LOUD (5683)
Email: hear@hearnet.com
Website: www.hearnet.com

H.E.A.R. is a non-profit organization dedicated to raising awareness of the real dangers of repeated exposure to excessive noise levels which can lead to permanent, and sometimes debilitating, hearing loss and tinnitus. Services available for musicians, music fans, and anyone needing help with their hearing.

House Ear Institute

2100 West 3rd Street
Los Angeles, CA 90057
Tel: (213) 483-4431
TDD: (213) 484-2642

HEI is a non-profit research and education center. It is also a clinic.

Metric Halo Laboratories
M/S 601 Building 8
Castle Point Campus
Castle Point, NY 12511-0601
Tel: (845) 831-8600
Fax: (603) 250-2451
Email: in-foo@mhlabs.com
Website: www.mhlabs.com
Applied Music & Sound uses a wonderful software called Spectrafoo, which portrays the frequency ranges of all sounds. This program was written by the wonderfully creative team known as Metric Halo.

The M.I.N.D. Institute
(Music Intelligence Neural Development Institute)
2070 Business Center Drive, Suite 210
Irvine, CA 92612
Tel: (949) 475-0492
Fax: (949) 475-0499
Email: matthew@MINDinst.org
Website: www.mindinst.org
The Music Intelligence Neural Development Institute is a community-based, non-profit, interdisciplinary basic scientific research institute, which was formed in 1997 by the team of scientists that did the dramatic and groundbreaking research that used music as a window into higher brain function. At the core of this research is the structured trion model of higher brain function that makes clear predictions about the relationship of music and the neural machinery of mammalian cortex. Results from behavioral studies confirming these predictions have received worldwide media and public attention. The goal of the MI is not only to understand the neural machinery of higher brain function and perform innovative behavioral studies, but to channel the results back into society to the benefit of education and medicine.

The Monroe Institute
62 Roberts Mountain Road
Faber, VA 22938-2317
Tel: (804) 361-1252
Fax: (804) 351-1237
Email: MonroeInst@aol.com
Website: www.monroeinstitute.org
The Monroe Institute, a nonprofit research, educational, membership-based organization, is devoted to the exploration of methods of accelerated learning through practical explorations and coordinated research efforts using an interdisciplinary approach.

Noise Pollution Clearinghouse
P.O. Box 1137
Montpelier, VT 05601
Tel: (888) 200-8332
Email: npc@nonoise.org
Website: www.nonoise.org
NPC is a national nonprofit organization with extensive online noise-related resources. NPC seeks to raise awareness about noise pollution; create, collect, and distribute information and resources regarding noise pollution; strengthen laws and governmental efforts to control noise pollution; establish networks among environmental, professional, medical, governmental, and activist groups working on noise pollution issues; assist activists working against noise pollution.

Open Ear Center
Pat Moffit Cook, Director
Bainbridge Island, WA 98110
Tel: (206) 842-5560
Fax: (206) 842-1968
Email: openear@nwlink.com or pat@openearjournal.com.
Website: www.openearjournal.com
The Open Ear Center offers training programs, workshops, and international intensives in the practical and professional use of crosscultural sound and music in healthcare and self-maintenance. Pat Moffitt Cook, the founder and director, is a pioneer in the use of crosscultural sound and music in healthcare. Her doctoral work in music paralleled extensive practical training and certification in methods of Auditory Stimulation and Sensory Integration (Tomatis Method, The Listening Program, LWP) and in Guided Imagery and Music (GIM). For over 22 years, Pat has traveled extensively throughout the world, recording and participating in musical rituals and the daily life of other cultures.

SHHH (Self Help for Hard of Hearing People, Inc.)
7910 Woodmont Ave., Suite 1200
Bethesda, MD 20814
Tel: (301) 657-2248
Fax: (301) 913-9413
TTY: (301) 657-2249
Email: National@shhh.org
Website: www.shhh.org
SHHH opens the world of communication to people with hearing loss by providing information, education, support, and advocacy.

Society for Auditory Intervention Techniques
P.O. Box 4538
Salem, OR 97302
Website: www.sait.com

The Society for Auditory Intervention Techniques (SAIT) is a non-profit organization which distributes information about auditory integration training (AIT) and other auditory-based interventions to professionals and parents.

Sound Remedies Catalog and Resource Guide
1001 Bridgeway PMB 716
Sausalito, CA 94965
Tel: (800) 788-0949
Fax: (888) 590-2678
Email: info@sound-remedies.com
Website: www.sound-remedies.com
The focus of the Sound Remedies Catalog and Resource Guide is the emerging field of soundwork. Sound Remedies contains categorized lists of music and sound programs, recommended reading, and resources.

Transitions Music
P.O. Box 8532
Atlanta, GA 30306
Tel: (404) 355-4242
Fax: (404) 355-9795
Email: wombsnd@mindspring.com
Website: www.transitions.com
Dr. Fred Schwartz is the founder of Transitions Music, a record company specializing in the use of womb sounds. His albums are widely used in both neonatal intensive care units and in the consumer sector.

SOUNDWORK PRODUCTS REFERRED TO IN *THE POWER OF SOUND*

The Listening Program
Developed by Advanced Brain Technologies, LLC
P.O. Box 1088
Ogden, UT 84402
Tel: (888) 228-1798
Fax: (801) 627-4505
Email: info@advancedbrain.com.
Website: www.advancedbrain.com
A sound-stimulation auditory retraining method consisting of eight specially developed CDs with a Guidebook and Listening Journal. The eight-week program can be used at home, school, or office—a CD player and headphones are the only equipment necessary. Designed primarily for children and adults with learning disabilities and other neurodevelopmental issues, The Listening Program is used thirty minutes per day, five days per week. It is available exclusively through therapists and health and educational professionals who have received specialized training in the administration of the program.

Sound Body, Sound Mind: Music for Healing with Andrew Weil, M.D.
Double CD with a 64-page book or double cassette (no book)
Upaya Records, 1998
Available in retail outlets or online at www.sound-remedies.com
A dynamic sonic tool for health, relaxation, and well-being, performed by The Arcangelos Chamber Ensemble. It facilitates deep, self-directed healing through pulse-entraining rhythms, timbres, and melodies combined with clinically tested soundwave technology. Using Sound Body *one is naturally coaxed into subconscious brainwave states conducive to self-directed healing with soothing music from Mozart, Mahler, Bach, and Brahms, rearranged to complement the frequency score. On the companion album* Sound Mind, *Dr. Andrew Weil speaks on music and sound in health, Anna Wise explains binaural frequencies, and Joshua Leeds elaborates on psychoacoustics.*

The Sound Health Series
Available from the Sound Remedies Catalog
1001 Bridgeway PMB 716
Sausalito, CA 94965
Tel: (800) 788-0949
Fax: (888) 590-2678
Email: info@sound-remedies.com
Website: www.sound-remedies.com
The Sound Health Series improves the function of the ear and brain by creating a sound capsule of natural full-spectrum sound. It uses psychoacoustically refined orchestrations of Mozart, Bach, Vivaldi, and others, performed by The Arcangelos Chamber Ensemble. Recordings from the Sound Health Series should be played throughout the day at a very gentle volume to improve auditory processing, to diminish the negative effects of noise pollution, and to enhance health, learning, and productivity. The Sound Health Series currently includes eight albums: Music for Concentration, Thinking, Learning, Productivity, Inspiration, and Motivation, as well as Music to Relax and De-Stress. The selections on the Music for The Power of Sound CD *all derive from the Sound Health Series.*

INTERNET RESEARCH RESOURCES

Cymatics—The Science of the Future?
Website: www.alphaomega.se/english/cymatics.html

Institute for Music Research/The University of Texas
Website: imr.utsa.edu

Music Department at the University of Queensland, Australia
Website: www.usq.edu.au/faculty/arts/music/Research.htm
Their archives are specific to the research of music in education.

MuSICA: The Music and Science Information Computer Archive located at the University of California at Irvine
Website: www.musica.uci.edu

Noise Pollution Clearinghouse
Website: www.nonoise.org

Sound Healers Association
Website: www.healingsounds.com/sha/shbib.html
Excellent bibliography of soundwork

Ultrasound Research Laboratory/Mayo Clinic
Website: www.mayo.edu/ultrasound/ultrasound.html

Notes

INTRODUCTION

1. National Institutes of Health, "Noise and Hearing Loss," consensus development conference statement, 22–24 January 1990.
2. Billie M. Thompson and Susan R. Andrews, "The Emerging Field of Sound Training," *Engineering in Medicine and Biology* 18, no. 2 (March–April 1999): 92.
3. Robert J. Doman Jr., "Sensory Stimulation," *Journal of the National Academy of Child Development* 1, no. 1 (1980).

CHAPTER 1: WHAT IS SOUND?

1. Paul G. Hewitt, *Conceptual Physics*, 7th ed. (New York: HarperCollins, 1993), 342.
2. Joachim-Ernst Berendt, *Nada Brahma: The World Is Sound* (Rochester, Vt.: Destiny Books, 1987), 18.
3. David Tame, *The Secret Power of Music* (Rochester, Vt.: Destiny Books, 1987), 206.
4. Ibid., 33.
5. Ibid., 33–68. Synchronistically, the loss of the five-thousand-year tradition of sound use to Western music took place within the period that also resulted in the modern makeover of China. Current concerts include *Sacred War Symphony* and *The Red Detachment of Women*.

CHAPTER 2: THE PHYSICS OF SOUND

1. Hermann Helmholtz, *On the Sensations of Tone: As a Physiological Basis for the Theory of Music*, trans. Alexander J. Ellis (1885; reprint, New York: Dover Publications, 1954), 1.
2. Hewitt, 322.
3. Ibid., 340.
4. Donald E. Hall, *Musical Acoustics* (Belmont, Calif.: Wadsworth Publishing, 1980), 6.
5. Helmholtz, 8.
6. Neil R. Carlson, *Physiology of Behavior* (Boston: Allyn and Bacon, 1994), 182.
7. Hewitt, 342.
8. Seth J. Putterman, "Sonoluminescence: Sound into Light," *Scientific American* 272, no. 2 (Feb. 1995): 46–51.

Chapter 3: The Mechanics of Hearing

1. Alfred Tomatis, *The Ear and Language* (Norval, Ont.: Moulin Publishing, 1996), 175. Dr. Alfred Tomatis has proposed an alternative concept about the pathway of sound and the role of the ossicles, however. He believes that sound is not transferred through the ossicles, as is the common belief—referred to as the Helmholtz-Bekesy concept. Tomatis states that "the peripheral bone that surrounds the tympanic membrane, especially in the lower area, conducts the sound toward the inner ear." Essentially it is the entire bony structure of the middle-ear chamber—not the ossicles—that transfers sound (vibrates) to the inner ear; the primary function of the ossicles is a muting device to protect the inner ear from dangerously loud sounds.
2. Bradford Weeks, "The Therapeutic Effects of High-Audition Music and Its Role in Sacred Music," in *About the Tomatis Method*, ed. T. Gilmor (Toronto: Listening Centre Press, 1989), 167.
3. Carlson, 183–90.
4. Weeks, 167.

Chapter 4: Resonance and Entrainment

1. Hewitt, 346.
2. Hall, 233.
3. Hewitt, 348.
4. Ibid.
5. K. C. Cole, *Sympathetic Vibrations* (New York: Bantam, 1985), 265.
6. Ibid., 265.
7. Randall McClellan, *The Healing Forces of Music: History, Theory, and Practice* (Rockport, Mass.: Element, 1991), 21.
8. Hewitt, 346.
9. Cole, 264.
10. M. H. Thaut, G. P. Kenyon, M. L. Schauer, and G. C. McIntosh, "The Connection between Rhythmicity and Brain Function," *Engineering in Medicine and Biology* 18, no. 2 (March–April 1999): 101.
11. Jonathan Goldman, "Sonic Entrainment," in *MusicMedicine*, ed. Ralph Spintge (St. Louis: MMB Music, 1992), 194–208; Goldman, "Sonic Entrainment," in *Music: Physician for Times to Come*, ed. Don Campbell (London: Quest Books, 1991), 217–33.
12. George Leonard, *The Silent Pulse* (New York: Dutton, 1978), 13.
13. Itzhak Bentov, *Stalking the Wild Pendulum: On the Mechanics of Consciousness* (Rochester, Vt.: Destiny Books, 1988), 31.
14. Ibid., 29.
15. F. Holmes Atwater, *The Monroe Institute's Hemi-Sync Process: A Theoretical Perspective* (Faber, Va.: The Monroe Institute, 1988).
16. Thaut, et al., 107.

Chapter 5: Frequency Medicine: The Work of Alfred Tomatis

1. Timothy Gilmor, Paul Madaule, and Billie Thompson, *About the Tomatis Method* (Ontario: Listening Centre Press, 1989), 7.
2. Ibid., 214.
3. Ibid., 7.
4. Alfred Tomatis, *The Conscious Ear* (New York: Station Hill Press, 1991), 12–35.
5. Ibid., 42.
6. Thompson and Andrews, 90.

7. Ibid., 91.

8. Billie M. Thompson, "Afterword," in *Ear and Language*, Alfred Tomatis, 200.

9. Thompson and Andrews, 93.

10. Tomatis, *The Conscious Ear*, 140–59.

CHAPTER 6: NEURODEVELOPMENTAL AUDITORY TRAINING: THE WORK OF ROBERT J. DOMAN JR.

1. Robert J. Doman, M.D., "Neurological Dysorganization and Antisocial Behavior," *Journal of the National Academy of Child Development* 6, no. 2 (1986).

2. Robert J. Doman Jr., "Sensory Stimulation."

3. *The Listening Program Guidebook*, ed. Joshua Leeds (Ogden, Utah: Advanced Brain Technologies, 1999), 77.

4. Ibid.

5. Ibid., 78–80.

6. Ibid., 53–54.

7. Ibid., 80–85.

CHAPTER 7: A NEW AWARENESS OF SOUND

1. Fred Schwartz, M.D., "Music as Anesthesia," in *Sonic Alchemy*, ed. Joshua Leeds (Sausalito, Calif.: InnerSong Press, 1997), 79–88.

2. T. Wigram, "The Physical Effects of Sound," *British Society for Musical Therapy Bulletin*, no. 7 (autumn 1989): 15.

3. Thompson and Andrews, 92.

4. *The Listening Program Guidebook*, 78.

5. Alfred Tomatis, *The Ear and Language* (Norval, Ont.: Moulin, 1996), 129.

6. *Merriam-Webster*, 1989.

7. Robert J. Doman Jr., "Dominance and Emotionality," *Journal of the National Academy for Child Development* 2, no. 2 (1982). A reprint of this article can be found on the Website of the National Association of Child Development (www.nacd.org).

8. Alfred Tomatis, interview in *About the Tomatis Method*, 210.

9. Reinhard Flatischler, "The Influence of Musical Rhythmicity in Internal Rhythmical Events," in *Music Medicine*, ed. Ralph Spintge (St. Louis: MMB Music, 1992), 241–48.

10. R. Murray Schafer, *The Soundscape* (Rochester, Vt.: Destiny Books, 1977), 227.

11. Reinhard Flatischler, *The Forgotten Power of Rhythm* (Mendocino, Calif.: LifeRhythm, 1992), 93.

12. Schafer, 226.

13. Flatischler, 242.

14. Schafer, 227.

15. Flatischler, 242.

16. Ibid., 248.

17. Ibid.

18. Anna Wise, *The High Performance Mind* (New York: Tarcher/Putnam, 1995), 3.

CHAPTER 8: SONIC SAFETY

1. Arenofsky, 22–24.

2. Claudia Kalb, "Our Embattled Ears: How to Protect Yourself," *Newsweek* 130, no. 8 (25 Aug. 1997): 75–77.

3. Mary Jo Burtka and Kathleen L. Yaremchuk, "Variations and Pitfalls of Noise-Induced Hearing Loss, *Hearing Loss* (May–June, 1997).

4. House Ear Institute Website (www.hei.org).

5. Burtka and Yaremchuk.
6. Stephen A. Falk and N. Woods, "Hospital Noise Levels and Potential Health Hazards," *New England Journal of Medicine* (Oct. 1973): 774–80.
7. U.S. Department of Labor, Occupational Safety and Health Administration, *Occupational Noise Exposure: Hearing Conservation Amendment, Part III. Federal Register* 46 (1981): 4078–179.
8. Kalb, 75.

CHAPTER 9: MUSIC AND SOUND IN YOUR LIFE

1. *Wall Street Journal,* 14 Jan. 1998.
2. Tomatis, *The Conscious Ear,* 144.
3. Nikki Landre, "Keys to Successful Music Lessons," *Discover* (Oct. 1996), 100.
4. *San Francisco Chronicle,* 9 Nov. 1998.
5. James Shreeve, "Music of the Hemispheres," *Discover* (Oct. 1996).
6. Felicity Hicks, "The Role of Music Therapy in the Care of the Newborn," *Nursing Times* 91, no. 38 (1995): 31–33.
7. N. M. Weinberger, "Elevator Music: More Than It Seems," *MuSica* 2, no. 2 (fall 1995): 1–5.
8. Peter Ostwald, "Music and Human Emotions," *Journal of Music Therapy* 3 (1966): 93–94.
9. J. H. Appleton, "Epilogue: Implications for Contemporary Music Practice," in *Psychology and Music: The Understanding of Melody and Rhythm* by T. J. Tighe and W. J. Dowling (Hillsdale, N.J.: Lawrence Erlebaum, 1993), 215–19.
10. Weinberger, 3.
11. Cathy H. McKinney, F. Tims, A. Kumar, and M. Kumar, "The Effect of Selected Classical Music and Spontaneous Imagery on Plasma B-Endorphin," *Journal of Behavioral Medicine* 20, no. 1 (1997): 85–99.
12. A highly practiced therapeutic approach that employs guided imagery is known as GIM, an acronym for Guided Imagery and Music. Created by Helen Bonny, GIM uses specially programmed classical music to generate a dynamic unfolding of inner experiences.
13. Elizabeth F. Brown and William R. Hendee, "Adolescents and Their Music: Insights into the Health of Adolescents," *Journal of the American Medical Association* 262, no. 12 (1989): 1659–63.
14. Hannelore Wass, J. Raup, K. Carullo, L. Martel, L. Mingione, and A. Sperring, "Adolescents' Interest in and Views of Destructive Themes in Rock Music," *Omega* 19, no. 3 (1988–89): 117–26.
15. Graham Martin, Michael Clark, and Colby Pearce, "Adolescent Suicide: Music Preference as an Indicator of Vulnerablility," *Journal of the American Academy of Child and Adolescent Psychiatry* 32, no. 3 (May 1993): 530–35.
16. James D. Johnson, M. Adams, L. Ashburn, and W. Reed, "Differential Gender Effects of Exposure to Rap Music on African Americans," *Sex Roles: A Journal of Research* 33, no. 7–8 (Oct. 1995): 597–605.
17. Christy Barongan and Gordon C. Nagayama Hall, "The Influence of Misogynous Rap Music on Sexual Aggression against Women," *Psychology of Women Quarterly* 19 (1995): 195–207.
18. Kevin J. Took and David S. Weiss, "The Relationship between Heavy Metal and Rap Music on Adolescent Turmoil: Real or Artifact?" *Adolescence* 29, no. 115 (fall 1994): 613–22.
19. Mary E. Ballard and Steven Coates, "The Immediate Effects of Homicidal, Suicidal, and Nonviolent Heavy Metal and Rap Songs on the Moods of College Students," *Youth and Society* 27, no. 2 (Dec. 1995): 148–68.
20. Ibid., 148.

21. Brown and Hendee, 1659.
22. Marty Munson and Therese Walsh, "Soothing Sounds: Even Raucous Tunes May Be Relaxing," *Health Front Journal: Prevention* 47, no. 10 (Oct. 1995): 42–44.
23. Suzanne B. Hanser and Larry W. Thompson, "Effects of Music Therapy Strategy on Depressed Older Adults," *Journal of Gerontology, Psychological Sciences* 49, no. 6 (1994): 265–69.
24. Rick Weiss, "Music Therapy: Doctors Explore the Healing Potential of Rhythm and Song," *Washington Post*, 15 July 1994: 10–12.
25. This research was conducted by neurologist Gottfried Schlaug of the Heinrich Heine University in Dusseldorf, Germany, and reported in *Discover* (Oct. 1996), 96.
26. Studies conducted by psychologist Frances Rauscher, currently of the University of Wisconsin at Oshkosh. Rauscher was a coresearcher at the University of California at Irvine with Gordon Shaw and Katherine Ky. Together they launched the Mozart effect studies in 1993. These seminal studies, reported in *Discover*, suggest that listening to music (specifically Mozart) temporarily enhances the brain's ability to perform abstract operations. The preschool study discussed here was published by the University of Calfornia, Irvine (*Omni*, winter 1995).
27. Research conducted by biophysicist Martin Gardiner of the Music School in Providence, Rhode Island, and reported in *Discover* (Oct. 1996).
28. Research conducted at the Chinese University of Hong Kong and reported 5 Nov. 1998 in *Nature*.
29. Study conducted by Dr. Frances Rauscher, K. D. Robinson, and J. J. Jens and reported 20 July 1998 in *Neurological Research*.
30. Research conducted by neuroscientist Anne Blood, McGill University, Montreal, Canada.
31. Research conducted by Lawrence Parsons, University of Texas, San Antonio.
32. Research conducted by Dr. Gottfried Schlaug, Beth Israel Deaconess Medical Center, Boston, Massachusetts.
33. Research conducted by Lawrence Parsons, University of Texas, San Antonio.
34. Studies conducted in 1993 by psychologist Frances Rauscher, Gordon Shaw, and Katherine Ky at the University of California, Irvine, and reported in *Discover*.
35. F. H. Rauscher, and G. L. Shaw, "Key Components of the Mozart Effect," *Perceptual and Motor Skills* 86, no. 3 (June 1998): 835–41.
36. Research conducted in 1994 by Esther Haskvitz at Springfield College, Springfield, Massachusetts, and reported in *Physical Therapy* (May 1994); and in 1991 by Gopi Tejwani, Ohio State University College of Medicine, and reported in the *Washington Post* (5 Feb. 1991).
37. *Washington Post*, 3 Oct, 1995.
38. Study conducted by Dr. Ira Grenadir, podiatrist and sports medicine specialist, Boston, Massachusetts, and reported in the *Washington Post* (5 Feb. 1991).
39. Research conducted by Dr. Bruce Becker, Eugene, Oregon, and reported in the *Washington Post* (5 Feb. 1991).
40. Research conducted by James Sundquist, Medical and Sports Music Institute of America, and reported in *Washington Post* (5 Feb. 1991).
41. Research conducted by Raymond Hull, Wichita State University, Kansas, and reported in the *New York Times* (21 June 1998).
42. Arenofsky, 22–24.
43. Medical and Sports Music Institute of America, the *Washington Post* (5 Feb. 1991).
44. Research conducted by Greg R. Oldham, organizational behaviorist and professor of business administration at the University of Illinois at Urbana-Champaign, and reported in the *Journal of Applied Psychology* (Oct. 1995).
45. Research conducted in 1996 by Joseph Ribak, Occupational Health and Rehabilitation

Institute at Loewenstein Hospital, and Tel-Aviv University.

46. Research conducted by Stephen A. Falk, M.D., and Nancy F. Woods, National Institute of Environmental Health Sciences, Research Triangle Park, North Carolina, and Duke University School of Nursing, Durham, North Carolina, and reported in the *New England Journal of Medicine* (11 Oct. 1973).

47. *New York Times* (22 Aug. 1993).

48. Donna Duvall and Alan Booth, "The Housing Environment and Women's Health," *Journal of Health and Social Behavior* (Dec. 1979): 410–17.

49. Susan L. Staples, "Human Response to Environmental Noise," *American Psychologist* 51, no. 2 (Feb. 1996): 143–50.

50. Research conducted by Karen Allen, State University of New York at Buffalo, and reported in the *Journal of the American Medical Association* (Nov. 1994).

51. Eileen Durham, "Relaxation Therapy Works," *RN* (Aug. 1991): 40–42.

52. Julie Anderson Schorr, "Music and Pattern Change in Chronic Pain," *Advances in Nursing Sciences* 15, no. 4 (June 1993): 27–36.

53. Hicks, 31.

54. Ibid., 33.

55. Ibid.

56. Falk and Woods.

57. Fred Schwartz, M.D., "Music as Anesthesia," in *Sonic Alchemy,* 97–100.

58. G. W. Grumet, "Pandemonium in the Modern Hospital," *New England Journal of Medicine* 328 (Feb. 1993).

59. McKinney, et al.

CHAPTER 10: A MATTER OF DISTINCTIONS

1. N. M. Weinberger, "Music Research at the Turn of the Millennium," *MuSica* 5, no. 3 (fall 1999): 9.

2. Ibid., 5.

3. McClellan, 181.

CHAPTER 11: THE BUILDING BLOCKS OF THERAPEUTIC SOUND

1. *Essential Dictionary of Music* (Los Angeles: Alfred Publishing, 1966), 92.

2. Kay Gardner, *Sounding the Inner Landscape: Music as Medicine* (Stonington, Maine: Caduceus Publications, 1990), 128.

3. Mitchell L. Gaynor, *Sounds of Healing* (New York: Broadway Books, 1999), 46.

4. Ibid., 25.

5. Goldman, *Healing Sounds,* 33.

6. Gardner, 218–19.

7. Goldman, *Healing Sounds,* 35.

8. Gardner, 220.

9. Goldman, *Healing Sounds,* 38.

CHAPTER 12: SONIC NEUROTECHNOLOGIES

1. Carlson, 2.

2. Alfred Tomatis, interview in *About the Tomatis Method,* 210.

3. *The Listening Program Guidebook,* ii.

4. *The Listening Program Guidebook,* 70.

5. Paul Madaule, the founder of the Tomatis Listening Centre in Toronto, has created at-home exercises to support auditory health that he calls Earobics. *When Listening Comes Alive* (Norval, Ont.: Moulin Press, 1993) 155.

6. Patricia Joudry, *Sound Therapy for the Walkman* (St. Denis, Sask.: Steele and Steele, 1984), 5.
7. Gilmore, et al., *About the Tomatis Method*, 2.
8. Thompson and Andrews, 94. As of this writing, SAIT has reorganized under the name Society for Auditory Intervention Techniques, acknowledging and embracing other valid approaches to auditory-based interventions (www.sait.org).
9. Further information about The Listening Program can be found through Advanced Brain Technologies.
10. In the Tomatis Method, filtration goes as high as 8000 Hz. In the at-home version of The Listening Program, maximum filtration is 3500 Hz.
11. *The Listening Program Guidebook,* 74.
12. Sheila Ostrander and Lynn Schroeder, *Superlearning 2000* (New York: Delacorte Press, 1994), 103.
13. Thompson and Andrews, 95–96.
14. Ibid., 90.
15. Ibid., 95.
16. The author serves as a producer, writer, and instructor in the use of The Listening Program.
17. Advanced Brain Technologies. P.O. Box 1088, Ogden, UT 84402. (888) 228-1798. Fax (801) 627-4505. Email: info@advancedbrain.com. Website: www.advancedbrain.com.
18. Madaule, *When Listening Comes Alive.*
19. Listening Technologies Inc. 599 Markham St.,Toronto, ON, Canada, M6G 2L7. (416) 531-8400. Fax (416) 588-4459. Email: listen@idirect.com. Website: www.listeningfitness.com.
20. Gerald Oster, "Auditory Beats in the Brain," *Scientific American* (1973): 96.
21. F. Holmes Atwater, *The Hemi-Sync Process* (Faber, Va.: Research Division, The Monroe Institute, 1999), 2–3.
22. Oster, 95.
23. 440 Hz corresponds to the A above middle C on the piano and is the note that orchestras tune to.
24. Suzanne Evans Morris, Ph.D., is a speech-language pathologist in private practice near Charlottesville, Virginia. With more than thirty-five years of clinical experience, she is internationally known for her work in identifying and treating young children with pre-speech and feeding disorders. She has studied neurodevelopmental treatment approaches extensively and is a speech instructor for the Neurodevelopment Treatment Association. An advocate of therapeutic auditory programs, she is an active member of the professional division of The Monroe Institute.
25. The Monroe Institute has worked with some 3,000 test subjects in a controlled laboratory setting. Each of these test subjects had a minimum of twenty individual tests. This gives The Monroe Institute a test base of over 60,000.
26. Morris points out that frontal lobe synchronization is not the only effect of Hemi-Sync. "TMI's lab work has focused a lot on synchronization in these areas because of their interest in more expanded states of consciousness. However, their brain mapping studies also have shown synchronization in many other areas. In addition, I see a very clear influence of Hemi-Sync with infants and young kids whose frontal lobes aren't even functional yet from a neuroanatomical/neurophysiological perspective."
27. Michael Hutchison, *Mega Brain Power* (New York: Hyperion, 1994), 62–63.
28. Wise, 3.
29. Oster, 94–102.
30. R. Swann, S. Bosanko, R. Cohen, R. Midgely, and K. M. Seed, *The Brain—A User's Manual* (New York: G. P. Putnam's Sons, 1982), 92.

31. Oster, 94–102.
32. Leslie France, "What Is Hemi-Sync?" *Focus* (fall 1990): 9.
33. The four major brainwave states are as follows: Beta waves (13–22 Hz) are found in our normal, waking state of consciousness. One is alert with a focus on the everyday activities of the world. Alpha waves (8–12 Hz) accompany states of relaxed wakefulness, such as day-dreaming and meditation. Alpha waves are blocked by sensory awareness, conceptual thinking and strong emotions. Theta waves (4–7 Hz) are found in states of high creativity, very deep meditation and as one drifts to sleep. Delta waves (.5–3.5 Hz) are found in the deepest part of the sleep cycle and in unconsciousness.
34. France, 8.
35. Robert Monroe lived from 1915 to 1995.
36. Unpredictably and without his willing it, Monroe found himself leaving his physical body to travel via a "second body" to locales far removed from the physical realities of his life. These have been described as out-of-body experiences.
37. The Monroe Institute, a nonprofit research, educational, membership-based organization, is devoted to the exploration of methods of accelerated learning through practical explo-rations and coordinated research efforts using an interdisciplinary approach.
38. Some of the current explorations of this technology are written about in the *Hemi-Sync Journal,* a publication of The Monroe Institute's professional division. They show the wide range of applicability currently taking place: "Accelerating Corporate Change," "Teen Tapes: A Pilot Study," "Studying Hemi-Sync on Animals," "Hemi-Sync and AIDS," "Hemi-Sync and Archetype Emergence in Jungian Psychotherapy," "Hemi-Sync Uses in the Military," and "Recapturing the Intuitive in Therapy and Education."
39. Atwater, *The Hemi-Sync Process,* 2.
40. P. Kliempt, D. Ruta, S. Ogston, A. Landeck, and K. Martay, "Hemispheric-Synchroniza-tion during Anaesthesia," *Anaesthesia* 54, no. 8 (1999): 760–73.
41. J. D. Lane, S. J. Kasian, J. E. Owens, and G. R. Marsh, "Binaural Auditory Beats Affect Vigilance, Performance, and Mood," *Physiology and Behavior* 63, no. 2 (1998): 249–52.
42. Ibid., 251.
43. Ibid., 252. In her peer review of this material, Suzanne Evans Morris makes an excellent point regarding the "type-casting" of specific brainwave states and their applications. Beta is generally associated with mental alertness. Theta and delta brainwaves are generally associ-ated with sleep. However, Morris points out that theta BBF frequencies are also quite effec-tive for states of high receptivity for learning and an open focus type of concentration (imagining, conceptualizing, stimulating creativity, etc.). She finds beta BBF frequencies are conducive to a narrow focus of concentration (writing reports, memorization, doing taxes, etc.) Morris believes there are a "Multiplicity of ways in which different sound frequency combinations for BBFs can support the intention of the individual using the recordings."
44. Gilbert O. Sanders and Raymond O. Waldkoetter, "A Study of Cognitive Substance Abuse Treatment with and without Auditory Guidance" (paper presented at The Monroe Insti-tute Professional Seminar, 1996).
45. Suzanne Evans Morris, "Music and Hemi-Sync in the Treatment of Children with Devel-opmental Disabilities," *Open Ear* 2 (1996): 14–17.
46. Ibid., 15.
47. Ibid., 17.
48. Lane et al., 249–52.

CHAPTER 13: APPLIED PSYCHOACOUSTICS FOR HEALTHCARE PRACTITIONERS

1. Kliempt et al., 760–73.
2. Vickie Dodd, *Turning the Blues to Gold: Soundprints* (Boulder, Colo.: Wovenword Press, 1999), back cover.
3. Hutchison, 111.
4. George Patrick, "The Effects of Vibroacoustic Music on Symptom Reduction," *Engineering in Medicine and Biology* 18, no. 2 (March–April 1999): 97–100.
5. Hutchison, 110.
6. John Beaulieu, www.biosonicenterprises.com.
7. Hewitt, 344.
8. Physical Acoustics Laboratory at Boston University website (http://paclab.bu.edu/index.html).
9. R. H. Lee, ed., *Scientific Investigations into Chinese Oui-gong* (San Clemente, Calif.: China Healthways Institute, 1992), 18.
10. P. G. Manners, *Techniques and Theories for the Emerging Pattern of Current Research* (Bretforton, Vale of Worcestershire, U.K.: Bretforton Hall Clinic, nd.).
11. McKinney et al.
12. K. M. Stevens, "My Room—Not Theirs! A Case Study of Music during Childbirth," *Journal of the Australian College of Midwives* 5, no. 3. (Sept. 1993): 27–30.
13. Go to www.thepowerofsound.com for excerpts from *The Luminous Wound* by Therese Schroeder-Sheker, founder of the Chalice of Repose Project.
14. W. J. Gardner, "Suppression of Pain by Sound," *Science* 132 (July 1960): 32–33.
15. R. Spintge and R. Droh, "Towards Research Standards in MusicMedicine/Music Therapy: A Proposal for a Multimodel Approach," in *MusicMedicine*, 345–49.
16. E. Podolsky, ed., *Music Therapy* (New York: Philosophical Library, 1954).
17. Burton Goldberg Group, *Alternative Medicine* (Fife, Wash.: Future Medicine Publishing, 1993), 444–45.
18. Ibid.
19. Spintge and Droh; Rosalie Rebollo Pratt and Ralph Spintge, M.D., eds., *MusicMedicine*, Vol. 2 (St. Louis: MMB Music, 1996).
20. Daniel J. Schneck and Judith K. Schneck, eds., *Music in Human Adaptation*. (St. Louis: MMB Music, 1997).
21. Gordon L. Shaw, *Keeping Mozart in Mind* (New York: Academic Press, 2000).
22. A valuable addition to *Applied Psychoacoustics for Healthcare Practitioners* has been provided by Sheila Smith Allan, codirector of Pediatric Therapeutics in Chatham, NJ. Her article, entitled "The Clinical Use of Sound to Facilitate Performance and Learning (From an OT/SLP/PT Perspective)," can be found online at www.thepowerofsound.com.

EPILOGUE

1. Information regarding the Noise Pollution Clearing House can be found in "Soundwork Resources."

APPENDIX A: THE ANATOMY OF PSYCHOACOUSTIC MUSIC CREATION: THE POWER OF SOUND CD

1. The album was titled *Safe Passage: Affirming Songs of Hope and Healing* (Sausalito, Calif: InnerSong Press, 1991).

2. *San Francisco Chronicle* (9 Nov. 1998), "Human Brain Resonates to Music."
3. This example from The Listening Program does not include the filtration and gating processing that is actually found on the program. It was included on the enclosed CD for dynamic panning, nature, and rhythmic contour examples only. An edited version of this piece is found on the Sound Health Series album *Motivation.*

APPENDIX D: TOMATIS: REVISING THE MAP OF THE MUSICIAN'S ODYSSEY

1. Tomatis, *The Conscious Ear,* 40.
2. Paul Madaule, "The Tomatis Method for Singers and Musicians," in *About the Tomatis Method,* 77.
3. Madaule, "The Tomatis Method for Singers and Musicians," 79.
4. Timothy Gilmor, "Overview of the Tomatis Method," in *About the Tomatis Method,* 27.
5. Ibid.
6. Madaule, "The Tomatis Method for Singers and Musicians," 84.
7. Alfred Tomatis, interview in *About the Tomatis Method,* 225.

Bibliography

Beaulieu, John. *Music and Sound in the Healing Arts.* New York: Station Hill Press, 1987.

Bentov, Itzhak. *Stalking the Wild Pendulum: On the Mechanics of Consciousness.* Rochester, VT: Destiny Books, 1988.

Berendt, Joachim-Ernst. *Nada Brahma: The World is Sound.* Rochester, VT: Destiny Books, 1987.

Brewer, Chris and Don Campbell. *Rhythms of Learning.* Tucson, AZ: Zephyr Press, 1991.

Campbell, Don. *Music Physician for Times to Come.* Wheaton, IL: Quest Books, 1991.

———. *The Mozart Effect.* NY: Avon Books, 1997.

———. *The Mozart Effect for Children.* New York: Morrow, 2000.

Carlson, Neil R. *Physiology of Behavior.* MA: Allyn and Bacon, 1994.

Cole, K. C. *Sympathetic Vibrations: Reflections on Physics as a Way of Life.* NY: Bantom. 1984.

Clynes, Manfred. *Music, Mind, and Brain: The Neuropsychology of Music.* NY: Plenum Press, 1982.

Dewhurst-Maddock, Olivea. *The Book of Sound Therapy; Heal Yourself with Music and Voice.* NY: Fireside/Simon & Schuster, 1993.

Dodd, Vickie. *Turning the Blues to Gold; Soundprints.* Boulder, CO: Wovenword Press, 1999.

Flatischler, Reinhard. *The Forgotten Power of Rhythm.* Mendocino, CA: LifeRhythm, 1992.

———. "The Influence of Musical Rhythmicity in Internal Rhythmical Events." *MusicMedicine.* Ed. Ralph Spintge. MO: MMB Music, 1992.

Gardner, Kay. *Sounding the Inner Landscape; Music as Medicine.* Stonington, ME: Caduceus Publications, 1990.

Gass, Robert. *Chanting: Discovering Spirit in Song.* NY: Broadway Books, 1999.

Gaynor, Mitchell. *Sounds of Healing.* NY: Broadway Books. 1999.

Goldman, Jonathan. "Sonic Entrainment." *MusicMedicine.* Ed. Ralph Spintge. MO: MMB Music, 1992. 194-208.

———. "Sonic Entrainment." *Music: Physician For Times To Come.* Ed. Don Campbell. London: Quest Books, 1991. 217-233.

Hall, Donald E. *Musical Acoustics.* Belmont, CA: Wadsworth, 1980.

Hay, Louise L. *You Can Heal Your Life.* Santa Monica, CA: Hay House, 1984.

Helmholtz, Hermann. *On the Sensations of Tone.* New York: Dover, 1885.

Hewitt, Paul G. *Conceptual Physics.* (7th Edition). NY: HarperCollins. 1993.

Hoffman, Janalea. *Rhythmic Medicine; Music with a Purpose.* Leawood, KS: Jamillan Press, 1995.

Hutchinson, Michael. *Mega Brain: New Tools and Techniques for Brain Growth and Mind Expansion.* NY: Ballantine Books, 1987.

———. *Mega Brain Power: Transform Your Life with Mind Machines and Brain Nutrients.* NY: Hyperion, 1994.

Joudry, Patricia. *Sound Therapy for the Walkman.* St. Denis, Sask. Steele and Steele, 1984.

Jourdain, Robert. *Music, The Brain, and Ecstacy.* NY: Avon Books, 1997.

Kahn, Hazrat Inayat. *The Music of Life.* New Lebanon, NY: Omega Publications, 1983.

Kenyon, Tom. *Brain States.* FL: United States Publishing, 1994.

Leeds, Joshua. *Sonic Alchemy: Conversations with Leading Sound Practitioners.* Sausalito, CA: InnerSong Press, 1997.

Le Mee, Katherine. *Chant: The Origins, Form, Practice, and Healing Power of Gregorian Chant.* NY: Bell Tower, 1994.

Leonard, George. *The Silent Pulse: A Search for the Perfect Rhythm that Exists in Each of Us.* NY: Dutton, 1978.

Lozanov, Georgi. *Suggestology and Outlines of Suggestopedy.* Gordon and Breach Science Publishers. NY, NY. 1978.

Madaule, Paul. *When Listening Comes Alive.* Norval, Ontario: Moulin Publishing. 1993.

Maxfield, Melinda C. "The Journey of the Drum." *Music and Miracles.* Ed. Don Campbell. Wheaton, IL: Quest Books, 1992. 137-155.

McClellan, Randall. *The Healing Forces of Music.* MA: Element, 1991.

Newham, Paul. *The Singing Cure: An Introduction to Voice Movement Therapy.* MA: Shambhala, 1994.

Oster, G. "Auditory Beats in the Brain." *Scientific American* 1973, Vol. 229, 94-102.

Ostrander, Sheila, and E. Schroeder. *Superlearning 2000.* NY: Delacorte Press, 1994.

Redmond, Layne. *When the Drummers were Women.* NY: Harmony, 1997.

Schafer, R. Murray. *The Soundscape.* VT: Destiny Books, 1977.

Schneck, Dr. Daniel and Judith K. Schneck (editors). *Music in Human Adaption.* St. Louis: MMB, 1997.

Shaw, Gordon L. *Keeping Mozart in Mind.* San Diego: Academic Press. 2000.

Spintge, Ralph. *Music Medicine.* MO: MMB, 1992.

———. *Music Medicine,* Vol. 2. MO: MMB, 1996.

Stockhausen, Karlheinz. *Towards a Cosmic Music.* Dorset, England: Element, 1989.

Tame, David. *The Secret Power of Music.* Rochester, VT: Destiny Books, 1984.

Tomatis, Dr. Alfred. Interview. *About the Tomatis Method.* Ed. Billie Thompson. Toronto: The Listening Centre Press, 1989. 209-225.

———. *The Conscious Ear.* New York: Station Hill Press, 1991.

———. *The Ear and Language.* Ontario, Canada: Moulin Publishing, 1996.

Wise, Anna. *The High Performance Mind: Mastering Brainwaves for Insight, Healing, and Creativity.* NY: Tarcher/Putnam, 1995.

thepowerofsound.com

The field of soundwork continues to expand as new discoveries about the effects of music and sound become known. To stay abreast of developments in the field and encourage collaborative sound applications, a new website has been created by Joshua Leeds: thepowerofsound.com. Information at the site includes:

- Frontiers of Soundwork: A series of exceptional interviews with and excerpts from the work of leading soundwork practitioners

- The Sonic Activist: A networking source for those interested in sonic activism

- Soundwork Resources: A comprehensive reference list of people and organizations involved in soundwork

- Sound Remedies: Psychoacoustically designed music and sound products available online

- Information about Joshua Leeds's schedules of seminars and appearances

Index

About the Author

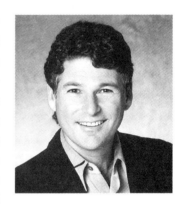

Joshua Leeds is a composer, producer, and sound researcher. He is one of few published authorities in the exciting new field of psychoacoustics—the study of the effects of music and sound on the human nervous system. Since 1986 he has produced more than twenty-five recordings, collaborating with leaders in health, psychology, and neurodevelopment. Cocreators include Louise L. Hay, Andrew Weil, M.D., Bernie Siegel, M.D., Anna Wise, Advanced Brain Technologies, and The Arcangelos Chamber Ensemble.

Since 1991 Joshua has published numerous magazine articles focusing on the therapeutic applications of music and sound. American and European publications include the peer-reviewed *American Journal of Acupuncture, Open Ear Journal, New Age Retailer,* and *Caduceus.* He is the author of *Sonic Alchemy: Conversations with Leading Sound Practitioners* (InnerSong Press), and editor of *The Listening Program.*

Joshua is the cofounder and director of Applied Music & Sound. Specializing in the creation of audio programs for health, learning, and productivity, AMS soundtracks are widely distributed in consumer, education, and therapeutic sectors. Joshua resides in the San Francisco Bay Area.